Surgery of Pediatric
Anorectal Malformations

Surgery of Pediatric Anorectal Malformations

Subir K. Chatterjee

MBBS Calcutta, FRCS England, PhD Calcutta, FAMS India

Professor of Surgery, Vivekananda Institute of Medical Sciences, Kolkata,
Head, Department of Surgery, Park Children's Center for Treatment and Research, Kolkata
Medical Director, Park Medical Research Society, Kolkata

Viva Books Private Limited

New Delhi • Mumbai • Chennai • Kolkata • Hyderabad • Bangalore

First Published, 2005

VIVA BOOKS PRIVATE LIMITED

- 4262/3, Ansari Road, Daryaganj, New Delhi 110 002
  E-mail: viva@vivagroupindia.net

- 215-216 New Apollo Estate, 2nd Floor, Mogra Lane, Andheri (E), Mumbai 400 069
  E-mail: vivamumbai@vivagroupindia.net

- Jamals Fazal Chambers, 26 Greams Road, Chennai 600 006
  E-mail: vivachennai@vivagroupindia.net

- B-103, Jindal Towers, 21/1A/3 Darga Road, Kolkata 700 017
  E-mail: vivakolkata@vivagroupindia.net

- 7, GF, Sovereign Park Aptts., 56-58, K. R. Road, Basavanagudi, Bangalore 560004
  E-mail: vivabangalore@vivagroupindia.net

- 101-102, Moghal Marc Apartments, 3-4-637 to 641, Narayanguda, Hyderabad 500029
  E-mail: vivahyderabad@vivagroupindia.net

ISBN 81-309-0168-4

Published by Vinod Vasishtha for Viva Books Private Limited,
4262/3 Ansari Road, Daryaganj, New Delhi 110 002.

Printed and bound at Sanat Printers, Kundli.

CONTENTS

FOREWORD

Professor Subir K Chatterjee is a scholarly member of *Chatterjees of India*. He has proved himself to be a highly regarded leader living up to the very high standards set by his forbears. Not only has he developed a centre which spans a very exciting era of rapid advances, but in spite of a huge clinical workload, he has been able to publish over 130 articles on his experiences embodying original concepts in the embryogenesis and surgical correction of a multiplicity of unique anomalies presenting as neonates and older children.

He is recognised nationally and internationally with a handsome array of accolades including the RK Gandhi Medal 2004. His book entitled "Anorectal Malformations" (Oxford University Press 1993) was indeed the culmination of his experience and studies of this complex of anomalies involving often all three systems associated with the development of the cloaca — the urinary, genital and alimentary tracts. He gave a masterly review of all significant contributions to date, including old and new classifications of the anomalies, diagnostic methodology and corrective surgical techniques. In this book he adds his own views based on a wealth of personal experience. A book of this nature written by a single author is a rarity, and a valuable factual presentation of a lifetime of surgery of crippled children together with the results of his treatment.

This new book, contains much of the content of the previous book and is now repeated not because it needs correction but it is now out of print, and many advances have occurred in the last ten years. The author himself has additional thoughts based on a variety of anomalies presenting to him in this very highly populated part of the world. The material has been arranged differently — he has switched to a more practical approach has been followed in which the chapter title leads the reader directly to the diagnostic signs of each anomaly and the paths of investigations that are necessary to portray the abnormal visceral and muscular anatomy prior to surgery.

Teaching has always been at the forefront of his surgical philosophy. He regards surgical teaching as a duty to his juniors whether at the bedside, in the operating room or in the laboratory. He is the Founder–Editor-in-Chief of the Journal of the Indian Association of Pediatric Surgeons; this journal first appeared in 1995. Many Professors of Pediatric Surgery and Pediatric Surgeons in India have received training in the departments of surgery headed by Professor Chatterjee.

Professor Chatterjee has retired from active surgery in his major teaching hospital appointments in Calcutta. He now heads the Park Medical Research Society and is Chief of Surgery of the Park Children's Centre.

We as pediatric surgeons welcome his new book and request him to remain vigilant in the years to come with a view to a further update.

F Douglas Stephens
Department of Surgery
Royal Children's Hospital
Melbourne, Australia

INTRODUCTION — WHY AN UPDATE?

Thirteen years ago I wrote a book entitled 'Anorectal Malformations'. It incorporated the available data on this subject, an analysis of the vast material that it was my good fortune to encounter in 4 institutions in what was then the city of Calcutta, and my personal views regarding classification and management.

Over the years, the scenario has changed radically. Advances in information technology have penetrated into every sphere of our life. The fabric of medicine as a whole is no longer what it was and hence every segment of this vast subject needs reappraisal. An update of our knowledge about anorectal malformations (ARM) and about the management of patients born with this has therefore become essential

The earlier book had ended with a question "**What of the future?**" Three points were brought up.

Prevention

A great deal is now known about embryogenesis. Fetuses and embryos can now be studied by a host of powerful instruments. ARMs can be reproduced in the laboratory by administering teratogenic agents; they can also be reproduced genetically by crossbreeding of animals with a hereditary trait. However a method to prevent the anomaly from occurring in humans has not yet been discovered. Hopefully the secret will be revealed fairly soon. It is likely that the gene responsible for the development of the anorectal region is closely positioned to other genes that might be responsible for the development of the esophagus, heart, urogenital organs, spine and lower limbs. ARMs and various anomalies associated with it, namely, esophageal, cardiac, urogenital and skeletal occur when the character of the genes are altered either by heredity or by a teratogenic agent.

The incidence of the malformation as a whole has certainly come down over the years, more in certain groups and less in others. A study of the changing distribution in different communities will no doubt provide clues to etiology and hence to prevention.

Antenatal Diagnosis

With prenatal ultrasonography many of the anomalies associated with ARM can be diagnosed and the presence of intestinal obstrucation can be detected. However, the precise nature and site of the ARM still eludes prenatal discovery by ultrasonography. ARM has recently been diagnosed prenatally by a new refinement of MRI (Kuwashima *et al*, 2001) and hopefully the technique will soon be in general use.

Management

There is no doubt that in our area better antenatal services are now available and healthier babies are born than in an earlier era. There is a much greater awareness about this condition in the minds of health providers and the general public. Hence detection now takes place earlier than before. Organization of neonatal services and of transport services has improved in certain parts but not to the desired extent in other parts of the developing world. Newer safer methods of emergency care and of both primary and secondary reconstruction have certainly developed. Three problems still remain to be solved, namely multiple malformations, very high lesions and sacral truncation. However, newer methods of supportive therapy have made the lives of the patients born with these conditions a lot easier. At the same time newer methods of assessment of results have been devised, and these enable better objective comparison of the results of different methods of management.

THE PRESENT SCENARIO

A lecture given in 1987 by a close friend of mine, Durham Smith, was entitled "The bath water needs changing but don't throw out the baby". It is indeed essential that the basic tenets that have been established over many decades are not discarded, but modified and added upon. This is what this book proposes to do.

The bulk of the new material I have studied has come from our private Clinic the Park Children's Center for Treatment and Research (PCC). My colleagues in this Clinic, namely Professor Amal Kumar Chakravarti, Professor Dhananjay Basak, Professor Jahurul Haque, Dr Ashoke Kumar Basu, Dr Sugato Banerjee, Dr Uday Sankar Chatterjee, Dr Debashish Mitra and Dr Kuntal Bhowmick have very kindly allowed me to use their material. A small portion has come from the Vivekananda Institute of Medical Sciences. Professor Sachhidananda Das who was the Head of the teaching Department of Pediatric Surgery, Nilratan Sarkar Medical College (NRS) from 1994 to 2002 has very kindly placed much of his material at my disposal and has collaborated in the writing of several chapters. His successor, Professor Nripen Samanta has very kindly allowed me to use some data collected by him up to the present time.

The above mentioned 3 institutions are located in the metropolitan city of Kolkata, formerly Calcutta, the capital of the State of West Bengal and the hub of Pediatric Surgical activity in Eastern India. Over 80 million people stay in the State of West Bengal. In this State the crude birth rate is 20 per 1000 and the infant mortality rate is 50 per 1000 live births. This compares favorably with the all-India figures. India's population is of over 1 billion, its crude birth rate is 26 per 1000 and its infant mortality rate 70 per 1000 live births. In West Bengal a significant difference exists between the figures for the rural and the urban areas. About 2/3 of the population live in the rural areas. Although there has been a progressive increase in total per capita income there is still considerable economic disparity between the urban and rural areas and between the rich and the poor. An estimated 36% still live below the poverty line. The majority of the population reaches a center capable of dealing with ARM by travelling in crowded trains and buses or in slow moving surface vehicles or in country boats. On the other hand the urban elite can afford almost anything that their counterparts in the developed world can.

In an earlier era the bulk of pediatric surgical work in Eastern India was carried out in Calcutta. Today there are pediatric surgeons living in many of the smaller towns of West Bengal and there are some who live in the metropolis but travel to peripheral centers. While NRS still remains the largest center for pediatric surgery in the public sector and the only center entrusted with postdoctoral teaching, there are now six new pediatric surgery units in this sector. Similarly in the private sector, while the PCC still remains the center with the largest intake of surgical neonates, six new units have come up in the private sector also and more are in the pipeline. Pari passu, the hinterland of Kolkata has shrunk over the last two decades. Surgeons with training in pediatric surgery are found in most of the States of Eastern India; some of them work in organized Pediatric Surgery units in Medical Colleges; others practice both adult and pediatric surgery in hospitals and private clinics (Fig). Pediatric Surgery units have also been set up in a number of Medical Colleges in two of our neighboring countries, Bangladesh and Nepal.

In spite of all this, NRS has seen 465 patients with ARM in the last 2 years; of these 270, namely about 60% were neonates. In the same period, PCC has seen 68 cases; only 30% of these were neonates; the others arrive after initial management elsewhere. Of the NRS patients, 33% were girls; In PCC 42% were girls. While almost 90% of the NRS cases come from the rural areas around the metropolis, PCC patients come mainly from the metropolitan area and from the smaller cities and towns of West Bengal as well as from those of our neighboring States and neighboring countries.

Compared to other neonatal surgical emergencies ARM is relatively easily diagnosed. Hence in NRS ARMs constitute about 30% of all neonatal surgical admissions; also there are 3 times as many neonates with ARM than with Esophageal atresia (EA). On the other hand, in PCC only 10% of neonatal surgical admissions have ARM and there are many more babies with EA than with ARM.

It is apparent that the incidence of ARM is much higher in the lower socioeconomic groups of our region. A detailed study of epidemiology will probably show in the future that either a nutritional deficiency or an environmental toxin is responsible for the distribution of the malformation, with or without an underlying genetic factor.

It is also apparent that the condition is being picked up much earlier than before and patients are reaching centers able to deal with the condition much earlier than before. It follows that in the absence of universal health insurance, the management of the condition has to be tailored to the socioeconomic status of the family.

Many years ago, Willis Potts, one of the father figures of Pediatric Surgery in the United

States of America had written, “A properly functioning rectum is an unappreciated gift of greatest price. The child who is so unfortunate as to be born with an imperforate anus may be saved a lifetime of misery and social seclusion by the surgeon who with skill, diligence and judgment performs the first operation on the malformed rectum”.

While participating in a number of conferences and workshops in the last 2 years, very many young surgeons working in SAARC countries have confronted me. They have asked me about my earlier book, which is out of print in India, about my views on recent advances and about how problems should be managed in situations with limited resources. These young surgeons need to be helped, hence this update. The earlier book was based on a study of 1250 patients; in the intervening years, 858 patients have been studied, these include the patients attending Park Children’s Center and also the patients admitted under the care of Professor S Das at the NRS Medical College between 1994 and 2002.

This book would not have been completed without the help of a large number of persons, to all of whom I remain greatly indebted, namely my surgical colleagues who have already been named, my office staff Mr. Kamalesh Chakraborty and Mr. Niranjan Sarkar, my artist Mr. Susanta Sinha, Mr. Indranil Roy of Laserworld and Phototype setter Mr. Tarun Goswami. I am very grateful to Professor Douglas Stephens whom I have known for over 3 decades for writing a foreword, to numerous Pediatric Surgeons from all over the globe and to my family for their constant encouragement and support.

CHAPTER 1

EVOLUTION

Ancient Indian literature, replete with information about so many other conditions, has nothing to say about anorectal anomalies. Paul of Aegina (AD 625-690) has been credited by Western authors to have been the first to have maintained by dilatation with bougies the opening in the rectum made by a blind plunge with a bistoury. From then until the end of the eighteenth century there was little progress in the management of this condition.

The Early Days

The anatomy of the area was recorded in detail by Vesalius in his famous book "De Humani Corpori Fabrica" as early as 1543. He described the dual function of the levator 'to support the bottom of the pelvis and to elevate the anus and the rectum', and found that the external sphincter was 'wonderfully joined to the insertion of the muscle raising the seat'. Subsequently, Santorini described more accurately the origin of the levator ani and the three parts of the external sphincter in greater detail in his book "Observations Anatomicae" in 1724.

Progress in management occurred in two directions. Firstly, puncture or blind groping of the perineum with trocar or bistoury was superceded by a midline incision and visual search for the imperforate rectal culdesac, and successful results were claimed by Bell (1787), Mantell (1789) and Kennedy (1800) in England. Secondly, relief of intestinal obstruction by iliac colostomy suggested by Littre as early as 1710, was in fact obtained by Duret (1793) and Desault (1794) in France.

1801 – 1850

This half century witnessed important steps in the evolution of the perineal operation. Dieffenbach, in 1826, performed the first transplant backwards of a rectovaginal fistula and resutured the divided sphincters in front of the new anus. Roux de Brignolles, in 1833, reached the blind rectum after a perineal dissection strictly in the midline. In 1835, Amussat reported his operation on a female infant with a rectovaginal fistula (actually, the baby had rectal atresia and a blind vaginal fistula). Having found the blind termination of the rectum by dissection upward from the perineum limited strictly to the midline, in the interest of the sphincters, he drew the gut down and sutured the mucosa accurately to the skin margins without undue tension. Thus was established the principle that epithelial continuity between the bowel mucosa and the perineal skin was essential for a successful result. Amussat is also credited to have been the first to identify five separate varieties of this malformation.

1851 – 1900

Events in the second half of the nineteenth century can be grouped under three headings.

Firstly, the first treatise devoted exclusively to the 'etiology, pathology and treatment of congenital malformations of the anus and rectum' was published from New York in 1860. Its author, Bodenhammer, devised the first systematic classification based on a study of 287 cases, largely autopsy specimens.

Secondly, extensions of the operative field were suggested in three directions. One, rectovaginal fistula was treated by dividing the posterior vaginal wall, fourchette and perineum in the midline and by resuturing these in front of the new anus. Two, a midline division of the coccyx and lower sacrum, a partial or total excision of the coccyx or partial excision of the sacrum or a parasacral exposure was used by a number of authors following the lead of Amussat. Three, a deliberate incision into the pelvic peritoneum to bring down the gut was suggested and carried out. Matas (1897) supported this approach stating that "the intraperitoneal exploration of the pelvis is not only a legitimate procedure but is one of the marked advances in the treatment of this class of cases".

Thirdly, abdominoperineal procedures began to be evolved. Three types of operation were carried out. One, a probe was passed through an iliac colostomy to push down the terminal gut and the perineum incised against the impinging tip. Two, after failure to locate the accessible bowel by perineal dissection, the abdomen was opened in the midline, and the position of the gut determined. Then with the finger in the abdomen as a guide, the perineal incision was deepened until the peritoneal cavity was opened and the rectum was pulled down into the perineum. Three, the reverse procedure, of opening the abdomen first and then incising the perineum through the peritoneal cavity was also done.

In 1892, Harrison Cripps reported on 5 cases, three boys without a visible opening of the bowel and two girls with the bowel opening in the vagina. They were operated in the lithotomy position with an incision 'made in the midline over the site of the anus to the tip of the coccyx'. Four were treated in the neonatal period. The bowel could be brought down after splitting the sphincters in the posterior midline and could be stitched to the skin but the opening tended to contract. The followup is very short, but this appears to be the first recorded sagittal anorectoplasty.

1901 – 1950

In this half century our understanding of the malformations advanced considerably but the techniques advocated earlier in dealing with them were largely forgotten. The choice of treatment lay between colostomy and perineal exploration. The choice was based until 1930 on a clinical examination of the perineum and sometimes upon needling. In 1930, Wangensteen and Rice published an epochmaking paper entitled 'Imperforate anus - a method of determining the surgical approach'. They carried out a radiological examination of the neonate held in the inverted position. The gas in the intestines was shown to rise and delineate the blind rectal pouch. The distance between the fundus of this gas shadow and a marker placed on the surface at the site normally occupied by the anus was a measure of the ease or difficulty of the perineal exploration. If the distance was 1.5 cm. or less the lesion was labelled 'low' and a successful perineal operation was predicted.

Another milestone was reached in 1934, when Ladd and Gross of Boston announced their classification of these malformations. They grouped the lesions into four types as follows:

Type 1 : patent anus and rectum, but a stenosis either at the anus or in the rectum.

Type 2 : imperforate anus, the obstruction being membranous in character.

Type 3 : imperforate anus, the rectal pouch ending blindly some distance above it.

Type 4 : anus and lower rectum normal, upper rectum ending blindly and separated by a variable distance from the lower pouch.

They noted associated fistulas in a very large percentage of their cases, mostly in those belonging to Type 3. The fistulas were classified as follows:

In males : Rectovesical
Rectourethral
Rectoperineal

In females : Rectovaginal
Recto-fossa navicularis
Rectoperineal

During this period, the embryological background of the malformations was expounded in different ways by Keith (1908, 1948), Keibel and Mall (1912) and others and new classifications based on these considerations were proposed from time to time.

Finally towards the end of this period, the primary abdominoperineal procedure for high lesions was revived. Norris first successfully performed it in 1943 and Rhoads did it in 1944. However, Rhoads, Pipes and Randall reported their results in 1948, in a paper entitled "A simultaneous abdominal and perineal approach in operations for imperforate anus with atresia of the rectum and recto sigmoid", and Norris, Brophy and Brayton followed in 1949 with their paper entitled 'Imperforate anus: a case series and preliminary report of the one stage abdominoperineal operation'.

At the end of this half century, the management of ARM passed into the hands of a select group of surgeons dedicated to serve infants and children, interested not only in saving lives but in restoring normalcy.

1951 – 1970

In 1951 was published a lecture that Denis Browne had delivered in the Royal College of Surgeons of England a year earlier. It was entitled "Some congenital deformities of the rectum, anus, vagina and urethra". Browne explained the necessity of classifying the Ladd three type of ARM into high and low depending upon whether the gut terminated above or below the pelvic floor. He emphasized the importance of preserving the levator ani intact and the advantages of using the presacral route in correcting high anomalies. He also introduced the term 'covered anus' for a group of low anomalies where a normally formed anus was 'covered over' resulting in narrowing or total obliteration of the orifice or its anterior extension just under the surface. The embryological explanation offered was excessive posterior fusion of the genital folds (1955).

It was left to Douglas Stephens of Melbourne to work out the detailed anatomy of anorectal malformations and their relation to the levator ani. Stephens described this work in detail in a series of papers between 1953 and 1959 and published a book in 1963. He classified the malformations into two groups (a) those of the anus and (b) those of the rectum; and described their anatomy in males and in females.

Stephens with Kelly (1969) modified the Wangensteen-Rice Xray technique to correlate the level of the blind end of the gut to the skeleton of the pelvis (Fig. 1.1). Three lines were described.

1. The Pubo-Coccygeal line or P-C line, stretching from the upper border of the symphysis to the sacrococcygeal junction. The anterior end is the center of the boomerang shape of the pubic bone and the posterior end is just caudal to the fifth ossific center of the sacrum. It cuts through the ischial shadow at the junction of its upper fourth and lower three-fourths, and this fact can be utilized in drawing the line when the lower sacral segments are deficient. This line corresponds to the origin of the levator ani.
2. The Ischial line is drawn parallel to the P-C line through the I point, which is the lowest part of the ossified ischial bone. It corresponds to the upper surface of the bulb of the male urethra and the upper limit of the perineal body and the triangular ligament; it also indicates the lowest point of the levator ani.
3. The anal pit line is drawn parallel to the two previous lines through the A point; this is the site of the normal anus, and is reached by continuing the P-I line caudally for an equal distance.

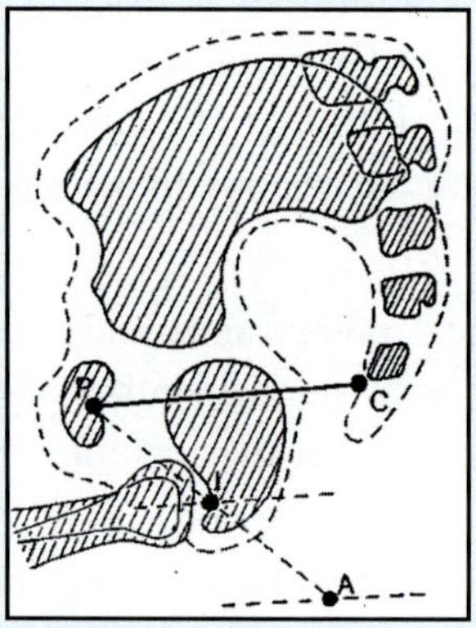

Fig. 1.1 Diagram of neonatal pelvic skeleton showing P, C and I points and pubococcygeal, ischial and anal pit lines.

When the gas shadow was at or above the P-C line, the lesion was considered high or supralevator; when it was below the I line it was considered low or translevator, and when it fell between the two lines it was named intermediate

It was emphasized that the Xray was of value only if this was correctly centered over the greater trochanter of the baby after he was held inverted for three minutes with the hips slightly extended (Figs. 1.2-4).

Stephens' most significant contribution to surgical practice was his elucidation in 1953 of the technique of preserving the puborectalis sling by dissecting the presacral space through the sacrococcygeal joint. The joint was reached by a midline vertical incision with the patient prone. The joint was opened up and the incision extended trans-

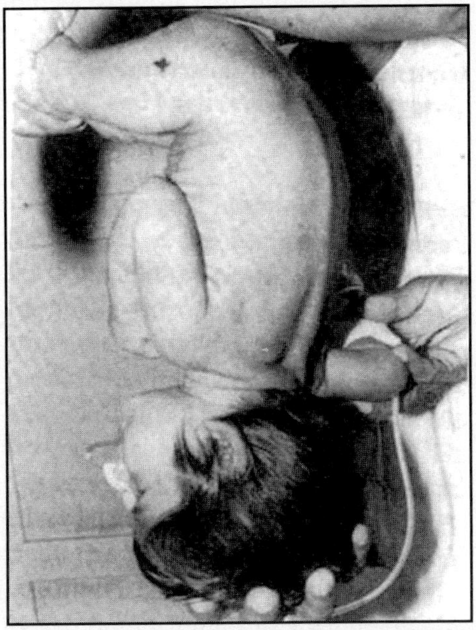

Fig. 1.2 Position of the baby for invertogram; the Xray tube is centered on the greater trochanter marked +.

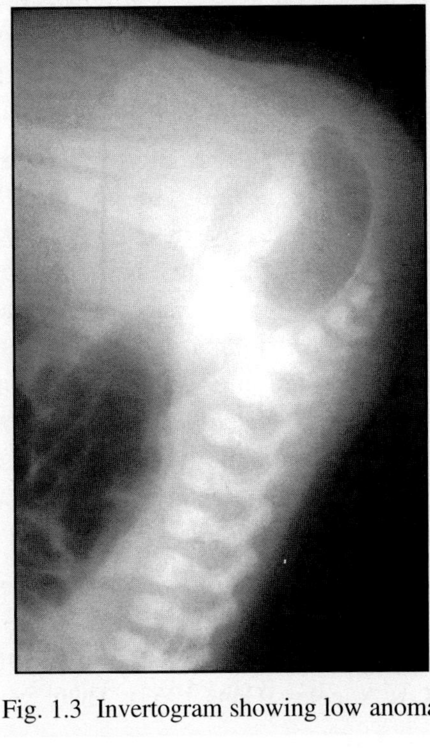

Fig. 1.3 Invertogram showing low anomaly.

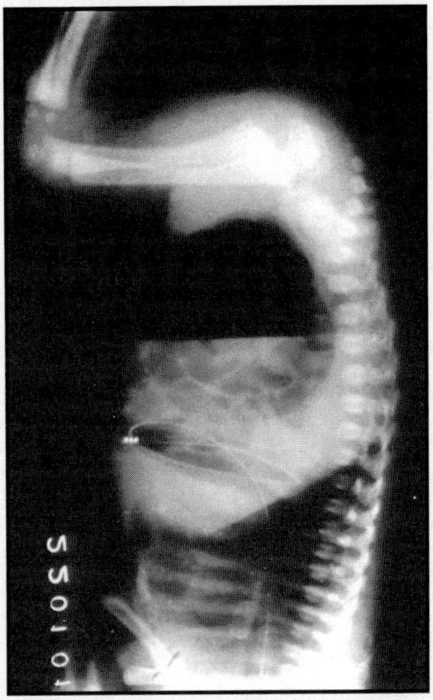

Fig. 1.4 Invertogram showing high anomaly.

versely over both the gluteus maximus muscles to allow the introduction of a pair of retractors 5 cm. wide. If the bowel ended below the 4th sacral vertebra, it could be dissected free and anterior fistulas closed and divided. The bowel was closed temporarily and a second incision was made at the normal anal site. The levator sling was identified behind the urethra or vagina and a tunnel created working both from above and from below. The tunnel was dilated and the bowel was then pulled through it to reach the surface. It was then sutured in place and the wounds closed. The operation was named Sacro Perineal Reconstruction or SPR. If the bowel ended above the 4th sacral vertebra, the levator sling was defined from above and below and a Penrose drain left in. The patient was then turned over for a laparotomy and the terminal bowel mobilized from above could be pulled through the sling in the line of the Penrose drain to reach the surface. The operation then became Sacro Abdomino Perineal Reconstruction or SAPR.

Stephens felt that in malformations of the rectum, the levator ani musculature was well developed and provided the main sphinctericmechanism available for reconstruction, while the internal and external sphincters were of negligible value.

Throughout the 1950s a vast amount of literature on ARM emanated from the rapidly developing North American centers of Pediatric Surgery, notably Boston, New York and Chicago. In most of this the emphasis was on Ladd's classification, on assessing the distance between the blind end of the gut and the surface by Wangensteen-Rice technique, and on accurate placement of the gut through the external sphincter by both perineal and abdominoperineal procedures.

The Rhoads procedure was the operation of choice for high lesions. In his 1953 textbook, 'The surgery of infancy and childhood', Gross described the technical details of the operation and commented that 'while the procedure has some drawbacks, particularly because of neuromuscular weakness which sometimes accompany it, it offers the tremendous advantage of being able to remedy the most extensive rectal malformation and any coexisting fistula in one sitting, even for a newborn baby. While the operation has great merit it should not be performed if it is possible to treat a particular anomaly by the perineal operation alone'.

In 1954, Potts and his colleagues described details of a perineal procedure to deal with vestibular fistula in girls, without any mention of the levator ani muscle; extensive freeing of the rectum from the perineal body was advised.

However, in 1960, Scott, Swenson and Fisher wrote as follows: 'The most important factor in the diagnosis, treatment and prognosis of imperforate anus is the relationship between the bowel and the levator ani. Cases may be divided into those in which the bowel ends above and those in which the bowel passes through this muscle to open in the vulva or perineum;' They studied 63 cases, 33 being high and 30 low; the marked difference in results of treatment in the two groups were emphasized and it was hinted that in the high anomalies the results were better in those in whom a puborectalis sling could be palpated behind the pulled through rectum.

In the years that followed, there was intense activity all over the world in devising new classifications, new operations and new procedures to diagnose the different types and to assess the result of treatment.

On the basis of Denis Browne's classification, Partridge and Gough in 1961 analyzed 323 cases seen over a 10-year period in London. The treatment advocated included an operation described as 'cutback' by Browne, as a simpler alternative to anal transplant for certain types of low anomalies. Abdominoperineal pullthrough was advised for high anomalies with every effort to carry this out through the levator sling.

New classifications based on large series of cases were suggested from Capetown (Louw 1965), New York (Santulli 1965) and Los Angeles (Gans 1963). There was a considerable difference of opinion on the meaning of simple words, and exchange of ideas became progressively more difficult (Bill 1964).

As far as new operative techniques are concerned, the most striking one was to pull through the proximal bowel in the endorectal plane after dissecting in the submucous space and excising the mucosa of the terminal bowel. Rehbein (1959) and Romualdi (1960) first suggested this modification of the abdominoperineal operation without respecting the pubo-rectalis sling; it was later modified so that the gut traversed the endorectal plane as well as the space between the puborectalis sling. The endorectal pullthrough had the advantages of preserving with certainty the pelvis nerves and the afferent impulses from the muscular shell of the rectum. When Rehbein failed to identify the sling during laparotomy, he turned the patient over to expose the sling by the presacral route and then completed the pullthrough face up (1967). Kiesewetter (1967) on the other hand, began his reconstruction by delineating the sling from the back and then turned the patient over to complete the pullthrough like a Rehbein procedure. The Kiesewetter-Rehbein operation can be named Sacro Abdomino Endorectal Perineal Reconstruction or SAEPR.

The abdominoperineal operations described by Santulli (1962) and Swenson and Donnellan (1967) had more advocates. These were modifications of the original Rhoads operations but the pullthrough was done through the levator sling. Santulli defined the sling from above and Swenson and Donnellan defined it from below. The landmark of the sling was the posterior wall of the urethra or vagina; its identification was equally difficult from both routes

A significant suggestion was made by Hiatt and Santulli (1963) that sensation could be improved if long skin flaps are cut and turned into the new anal canal. Nixon (1968) called this principle 'inversion proctoplasty' and wrote that 'it was based on the unorthodox opinion that 'the proctodeum is not agenetic, but everted'.

On the diagnostic side, the value, limitations and technique of inversion radiography were studied by many. Simultaneously, contrast radiography developed by leaps and bounds, with the introduction of image intensifiers and new contrast fluids.

In 1969, Kelly working with Stephens came out with a method of assessing results on the basis of clinical and radiological findings using a scoring system; this has become known as the Kelly Code (Table 1.1).

Our first publication on the subject also appeared in 1969; we reported a series of girls who had a double termination of the alimentary tract.

In March 1970, a Pediatric Surgery Congress was held in Melbourne to celebrate the Centenary of the Royal Children's Hospital. All intending participants received a brochure entitled 'A Proposed International Classification of Anorectal Anomalies', with a covering letter which said 'The opportunity afforded by the meeting of so many pediatric surgeons interested in this complex subject of anorectal malformations should not pass without a determined effort to resolve some of the differences of opinion on a number of important problems'. The letter invited opinion from those who felt strongly enough about the topic in question.

TABLE 1.1: The Kelly Code (Stephens & Smith)

A. Clinical		
Continence	: 2	normal under all circumstances, no soiling
	1	occasional escape of faeces and flatus, occasional accidents
	0	no control, frequent accidents
Staining	: 2	always clean
	1	occasional staining
	0	always stained
Sphincter Squeeze	: 2	strong & effective
	1	weak & partial
	0	none
B. Radiological		
Leak Round Rectal catheter	: 2	none with size 13-14
	1	leak with 13-14, but none with 26
	0	leak with 26
Rectal Sensation	: 2	appreciates filling 100-400ml. and defaecates on command
	1	appreciates filling over 400 ml. and delayed defaecation
	0	no sensation, leakage
Appearance of Bowel	: 2	normal angulation, diminishes on defaecation, restores on command to stop.
	1	diminished angulation and movement
	0	no angulation or movement

An International Classification was in fact put up by a panel consisting of AH Bill, S Cywes, SL Gans, WB Kiesewetter, JH Louw, RV Magnus, HH Nixon, F Rehbein, TV Santuli, ED Smith and FD Stephens. The panel 'recognized that no single classification of these anomalies is ideal. Each falls short as a pure anatomic, embryologic, therapeutic or prognostic classification. We believe that the classification will best serve all of these interests and form a basis of common language for these anomalies'. The classification published in 1970 reads as follows (Table 1.2).

TABLE 1.2: The Melbourne Classification (Santulli *et al*, 1970)

Male	Female
A. Low (Translevator)	
1. At Normal Anal site	1. Same
a) Anal stenosis	a) Same
b) Covered anus-complete	b) Same
2. At perineal site	2. Same
a) Anocutaneous fistula (Covered anus-incomplete)	a) Same
b) Anterior perineal anus	b) Same
	3. At Vulvar Site
	a) Anovulvar fistula
	b) Anovestibular fistula
	c) Vestibular anus
B. Intermediate	
1. Anal Agenesis	1. Same
a) Without fistula	a) Without fistula
b) With fistula Rectobulbar	b) With fistula
	i) Rectovestibular
	ii) Rectovaginal-low
2. Anorectal Stenosis	2. Same
C. High Supralevator	
1. Anorectal Agenesis	1. Same
a) Without fistula	a) Without fistula
b) With fistula	b) With fistula
i) Rectourethral	i) Rectovaginal-high
ii) Rectovesical	ii) Rectocloacal
iii) Rectovesical	
2. Rectal Atresia	2. Same
D. Miscellaneous	
E. Imperforate Anal Membrane Cloacal Exstrophy, Others	

Before the year was over, it became obvious that the proposed classification would not meet with universal acceptance. Gans who was one of the panellists immediately published a critical analysis and revived a modified form of his own earlier classification (1970). He dispensed with all reference to high and low, supralevator and translevator, and simply suggested four groups. These were:

1. Ectopic anus
2. Imperforate anus with two subtypes-anal atresia and anorectal atresia
3. Rectal atresia
4. Anal and rectal stenosis

1971 – 1980

The decade began with the publication in 1971 of a book by Stephens and Smith entitled "Anorectal malformations in Children". This book became a bible for all workers in this field; in it was set forth all the important published information on the subject and more particularly the contributions of the Melbourne group. The anatomical findings of each malformation as disclosed by clinical examinations, Xrays, surgical operations and autopsies were described. The developmental defect responsible for each was discussed, the management policy enunciated and the steps of the operative procedures delineated. Finally methods of assessing results were devised and the actual results analyzed. Apart from the malformations that entered the official classification, a very large number of miscellaneous rare anomalies were separately listed by the authors; some of these were described.

Soon after, members of the Surgical Section of the American Academy of Pediatrics received a questionnaire prepared on the basis of the 1970 classification. Information obtained in reply to this regarding incidence, management and results of treatment was published by Santulli and his colleagues on the basis of 1166 cases (1971).

In 1972 Wilkinson classified his material into four groups but these were different.

1. Anorectal stenosis
2. Covered anus
3. Anorectal atresia with several sub groups - perineal fistula, low vaginal fistula, high vaginal fistula, urethral fistula and no fistula.
4. Rectal atresia

Cremin *et al* in 1973 introduced a new dimension into invertograms, namely the M point. This was the junction of the upper two-thirds and the lower third of the ischial body and was thought to correspond to the level of the puborectalis sling. Our own opinion about the false positive and false negative results of invertography was published in 1976.

Ultrasonography was harnessed to delineate ARMs by Willital in 1971. This was initially performed by placing the baby in the lithotomy position, and obtaining sector scans of the pelvis by moving the transducer parallel to the table over the perineal skin at the level where the anus would normally be located. Subsequently, in 1979 Schuster showed that a more pictorial representation would be obtained by keeping the baby supine and scanning in the sagittal plane over the full bladder (Figs. 1.5-6).

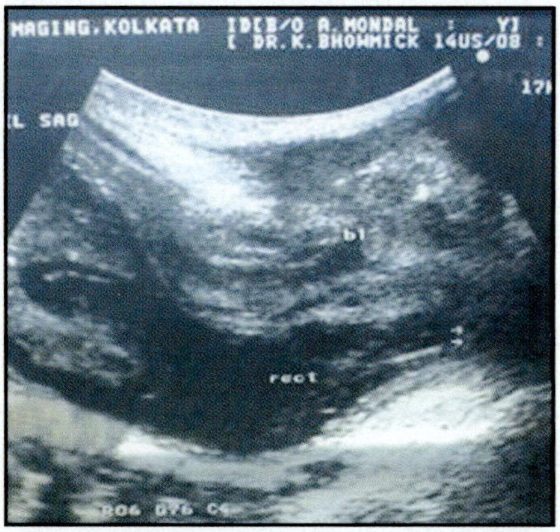

Fig. 1.5 Ultrasonogram of neonate with low anomaly.

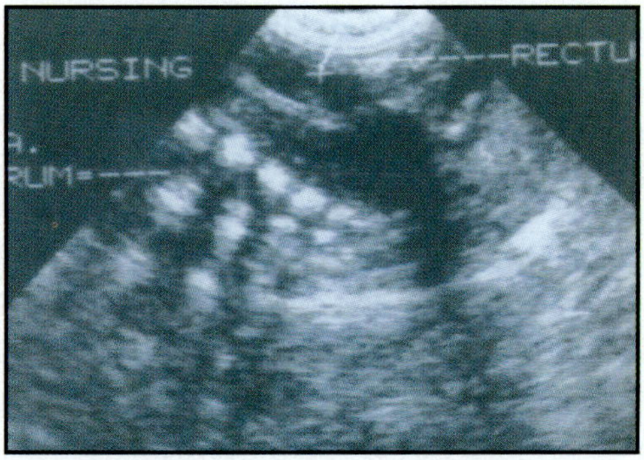

Fig. 1.6 Ultrasonogram of neonate with intermediate anomaly.

The CT scanner was introduced in this decade but it was not utilized to study ARM.

In the 1970s fibreoptic endoscopes began to be miniaturized and with their aid the human eye could penetrate the lower urogenital tract and fistulas connected with it on progressively smaller patients and with progressively greater accuracy (Gans 1971).

Two significant technical successes were reported in the second half of the decade.

First, a new abdominoperineal operation was proposed from Lyons by Mollard *et al* in 1978. The levator sling was identified through a curved perineal incision made behind the scrotum with its two posterior ends 1 cm. lateral and anterior to the new anal site. A tunnel was created behind the posterior urethra by gently retracting the muscle fibers posteriorly and laterally and enlarging the space with dilators. The abdominal part of the procedure resembled a Rehbein procedure. The proximal bowel was pulled through the endorectal pouch and then through the levator sling. It was finally brought out to the normal anal site through a separate stellate incision. Mollard pointed out the advantages of his incision over the original Swenson-Donnellan method wherein the sling was approached through an incision at the normal anal site, and also over methods that approached the sling solely from the abdomen or from the back.

Second, considerable information on the problem of cloacal anomalies emanated from Boston; Hendren (1977) described the structural and functional malformations that were present in his patients and advocated a one stage complete correction of all defects some time after a preliminary neonatal colostomy.

1981 – 1990

The events of this decade are Posterior Sagittal AnoRectoPlasty (PSARP), Wingspread, Advances in medical imaging and Animal models.

Posterior Sagittal Anorectoplasty (PSARP)

The technique of this operation was first published by deVries and Pena in 1982, but it had been presented earlier by Alberto

Pena in Acapulco, Mexico in October 1980. Innumerable publications have appeared since then. The reaction of pediatric surgeons of this procedure, in Pena's own words "varied from very enthusiastic, unconditional acceptance to almost violent rejection". No pediatric surgeon interested in ARM could afford to remain unmoved.

The operation was not really new. It had been advocated by the pioneers of the preceding century but for obvious reasons they did not succeed, and much safer methods were devised. The exposure that was most favored in the 1970s was the sacroperineal (Stephens), but 'our inability to see what we were doing' in the course of this exposure, wrote Pena, 'prompted us to expose more of the surgical area and design a new operation'.

The principles of the operation were as follows:

1. perform a prereconstruction colostomy;
2. place the patient prone with a catheter in the urethra;
3. incise the perineum sagittally over a variable length;
4. divide all tissues strictly in the midline till bowel, urethra and/or vagina are reached;
5. identify all striated muscles with an electric stimulator;
6. ensure strict hemostasis;
7. disconnect and close fistulas under direct vision;
8. taper the bowel so that it lies within the muscle complex;
9. repair meticulously all divided muscles;
10. suture the bowel to the skin at the normal site and close the wound; over and do an abdominoperineal pullthrough;
12. if the bowel is very low, repair without colostomy and without tapering; and
13. carry out a program of dilatations even after colostomy closure.

The greatest theoretical value of the exposure was that it allowed surgeons to see and show the structure and function of the region in a manner that was not possible earlier on a living subject.

Wingspread 1985

In May 1984, Douglas Stephens convened a workshop at Wingspread, Wisconsin, USA; the Department of Surgery, Children's Memorial Hospital, Chicago and the Johnson Foundation were the sponsors; India was represented by T Dorairajan and myself. The proceedings were reported by Stephens and Smith in 1986.

The prime object of the workshop was to **review classifications and propose a simple, practical 1984 classification**. This was thought necessary because the 1970 classification was considered 'too detailed, too complex and too unwieldy for common use and teaching'.

At Wingspread, an attempt was made to distinguish lesions on the basis of three criteria.

1. **Incidence;** namely whether the lesions were common or rare; lesions thought rare were left out.
2. **Level;** namely whether high, intermediate or low.

   High lesions were supralevator, in which 'bowel of normal or greater caliber terminated above the levator ani and may lie on or above its elevated hammock', above the P-C line.

Intermediate lesions were supralevator in which 'bowel of normal or greater caliber terminates above the levator ani but lies within the walls of a deepened hammock', between the P-C line and the I line.

Low lesions were translevator in which 'bowel of normal or greater caliber penetrates and is surrounded by levator ani, below the I line. (deVries & Cox,1985).

3. **The presence and site of a Fistula**
   The classification that emerged read as follows (Table 1.3).

TABLE 1.3: The Wingspread Classification, 1984

Male	Female
High	High
1. Anorectal Agenesis	1. Anorectal Agenesis
a) with rectoprostaticure-thral fistula	a) with rectovaginal fistula
b) without fistula	b) without fistula
2. Rectal atresia	2. Rectal atresia
Intermediate	Intermediate
1. Rectobulbar urethral fistula	1. Rectovestibular fistula
2. Anal agenesis without fistula	2. Rectovaginal fistula
	3. Anal agenesis without fistula
Low	Low
1. Anocutaneous fistula	1. Anovestibular fistula
2. Anal stenosis	2. Anocutaneous fistula
	3. Anal stenosis
3.Rare Malformations	Cloaca
	Rare Malformations.

Our comments at the time were as follows:

1. It is difficult to distinguish between common and rare for two reasons.

   Firstly, while many lesions are universally common, some lesions that practically never occur in one part of the world may not be at all infrequent in another part. We shall discuss 2 such lesions at length in later chapters. Secondly, lesions common at one period of time become rare at another period. For example, rectovesical fistula was very commonin the USA both in the Ladd and Gross classification of 1934 and also in the material studied by me in the Children's Hospital Chicago between 1957 and 1966; however it was deleted from the Wingspread list in 1984 because it was rare.
2. It is difficult to draw hard and fast lines between the 3 levels. While many lesions are undoubtedly high or intermediate or low, some fall in the gray zones between high and intermediate and between intermediate and low.
3. All fistulas are not static; some change after birth. A fistula clearly defined at birth may disappear by the time definitive surgery is carried out. A fistula high at birth may descend with growth; thus high rectovaginal fistulas may become low, and rectocloacal fistulas may become rectovaginal.

   Pena's own comments were that we should consider a spectrum of anomalies rather than a number of distinct anomalies in watertight compartments, and that a classification should have therapeutic implications.

The second object of Wingspread was to **determine criteria for assessment of results of treatment** 'in view of the many surgical techniques to reconstruct the anorectogenital passages', more correctly anorectourogenital passages. A nonscoring type of clinical assessment was devised. This is shown in Table 1.4.

TABLE 1.4: The Wingspread chart for Assessment, 1984

1. Clean
1.1 No accumulated feces
  1.11 No therapy
  1.12 Occasional therapy
  1.13 Therapy dependent
1.2 Accumulated feces
  1.21 No therapy
  1.22 Occasional therapy
  1.23 Therapy dependent
2. Staining
2.1 No accumulated feces
  2.11 No therapy
  2.12 Occasional therapy
  2.13 Therapy dependent
2.2 Accumulated feces
  2.21 No therapy
  2.22 Occasional therapy
  2.23 Therapy dependent
3. Intermittent fecal soiling
3.1 No accumulated feces
  3.11 No therapy
  3.12 Occasional therapy
  3.13 Therapy dependent
3.2 Accumulated feces
  3.21 No therapy
  3.22 Occasional therapy
  3.23 Therapy dependent
4. Constant fecal soiling
  4.1 No accumulated feces
  4.11 No therapy
  4.12 Occasional therapy
  4.13 Therapy dependent
  4.2 Accumulated feces
  4.21 No therapy
  4.22 Occasional therapy
  4.23 Therapy dependent

Related Complications
1. Anorectal
  a) abnormal position
  b) stenosis
  c) prolapse
  d) fistula
  e) lack of contractility
  f) abnormal length
2. Urinary
3. Genital
4. Other

In this chart, 4 basic levels of fecal continence were defined, namely clean, staining, intermittent fecal soiling and constant fecal soiling. Each level was subdivided to take into account accumulation of feces in the distal bowel and response to therapy. In addition there was provision to record information about the structure of the anus and about urinary and genital function.

Patients who did well improved on the chart with passage of time, and became less therapy dependent. Those who did not regressed or remained static. The position of a patient not receiving treatment could be improved by offering occasional treatment and the position of one receiving occasional treatment could be improved by offering continuous treatment. On the other hand discontinuance of treatment could lead to deterioration of status.

We found the charts very useful for assessing progress and for suggesting therapy and also for comparing the results of different methods of management.

The third object of Wingspread was **to adopt a scheme for identification of ARM, recording of surgical procedures and chronological events** 'for the comparison of one technique against another'. The Registration forms proposed by the Japan Study Group was accepted with minor modifications. They are tabulated below:

TABLE 1.5: Registration Form (Male)

Name______________Registration No.____________Date of Birth______________

19________Date of Description ______________________ Age ____________
Institute ______________________

1. Birth Weight _____gms. Gestational Age ____ wks. 2. Initial Symptom _______

3.Perineum - Description ____

____

____

Photo or drawing of perineum :

Abdominal skin fold-Describe :

Anal mark, yes/no - if yes : pit flat

Pigmentation, yes/no

Hypospadias, yes/no Bifid scrotum, yes/no Dentate line, yes/no

Other features :

4. External Fistula: Size (Fr…..) Direction: upwards backwards both Length… mm bouginage before investigation, yes/ no
5. Meconium in Urine, yes/no
6. Digital examination, Endoscopic Examination findings

7. Invertogram (…………hrs. after birth)

8. Radiopaque Dye Studies (age………..…)

9. Sacral vertebrae Sketch A-Pview

Classification			
diagnosed	clinically	surgically	by autopsy
Associated Anomalies ;	Urogenital:		Others :

TABLE 1.6: Registration Form (Female)

Name ________________Registration No.____________ Date of Birth__________

19_________Date of Description ______________________ Age ____________

Institute _______________________

1. Birth Weight _____gms. Gestational Age ____ wks. 2. Initial Symptom ______

3. Perineum - Description ____

____

____

Photo or drawing of perineum :

Abdominal skin fold-Describe :

Anal mark, yes/no - if yes : pit flat

Pigmentation, yes/no Hymen, yes/no Double Vagina, yes/no Labial fusion, yes/no

Perineal canal, yes/no

Perineal groove, yes/no

Dentate line, yes/no

Other features :

4. External Fistula: Size (Fr.....) Direction: upwards backwards both Length..... mm bouginage before investigation, yes/no

5. Meconium in Urine, yes/no

6. Digital examination, Endoscopic Examination findings

7. Invertogram (............hrs. after birth)

8. Radiopaque Dye Studies (age.............)

9. Sacral vertebrae Sketch A-Pview

Classification			
diagnosed	clinically	surgically	by autopsy
Associated Anomalies ;	Urogenital:		Others

We have not found the forms very useful for the following reasons:

1. many of our patients reach us after neonatal management elsewhere;
2. the surface appearance of the perineum should undoubtedly be studied carefully but the only features we have found useful are an obvious bulge and an actual or potential opening of the bowel;
3. visible external genital anomalies are also relatively less important than many invisible anomalies;
4. invertograms have become relatively less important than other imaging parameters.

For those who attended, Wingspread was indeed a memorable occasion. Lasting friendships were established, and these have endured longer than the classification, the assessment methods and the registration forms.

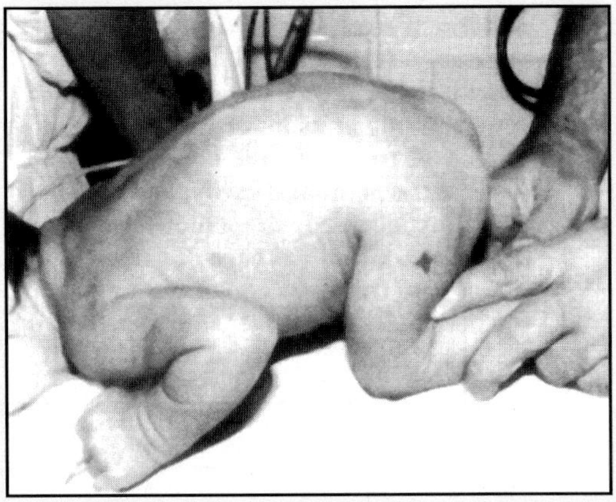

Fig. 1.7 Position of the baby for prone crosslateral Xray.

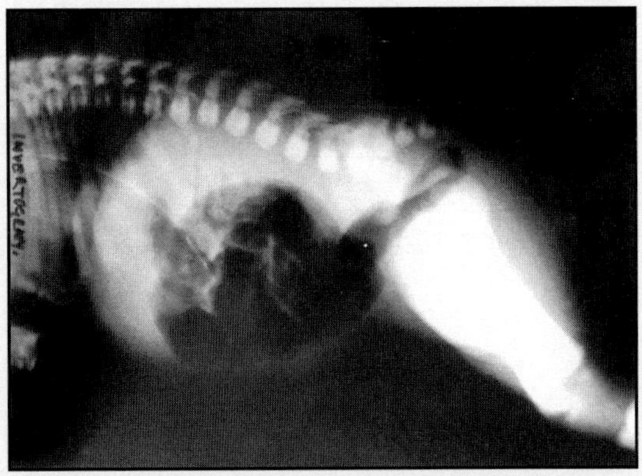

Fig. 1.8 Prone crosslateral Xray of low anomaly.

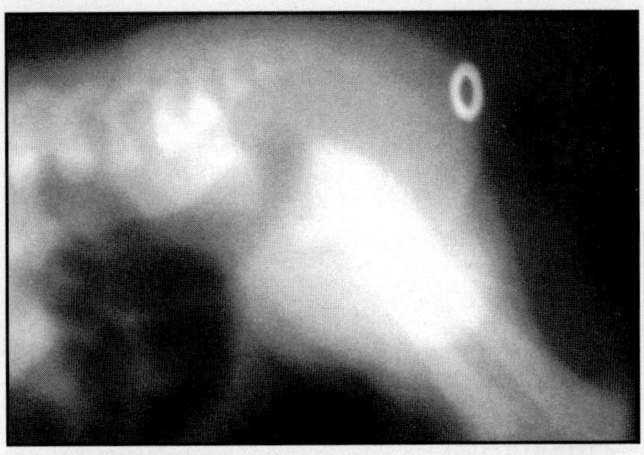

Fig. 1.9 Prone crosslateral Xray of high anomaly.

Advances in Imaging

In 1983 Narasimharao and his colleagues in Chandigarh developed a refinement of invertography named prone crosslateral Xray. The baby is placed in the knee chest position with the thighs at right angles to the trunk. The Xray tube is placed on one side centered on the greater trochanter and the film is placed on the other side (Figs. 1.7-9).

Ikawa first reported the value of the CT scan for patients with ARM in 1985. With axial sections he showed the disposition of the striated muscles in patients not submitted to reconstructive surgery (Figs. 1.10-12) and also in those submitted to these procedures. A CT scan could show whether a poor result was due to failure to pull the

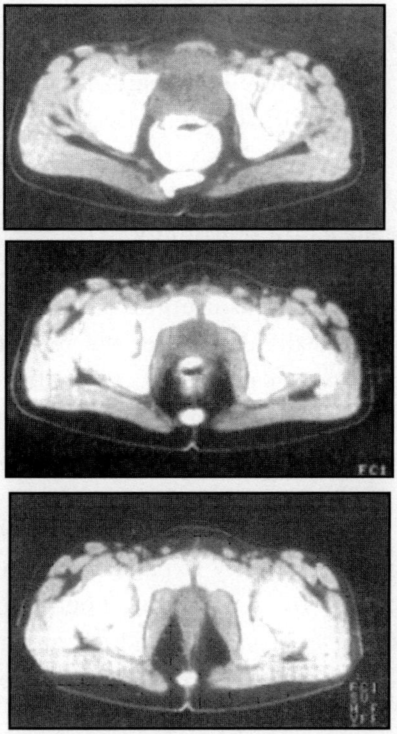

Fig. 1.10-12 CT scans, horizontal, of pelvis of 6 year old with ARM left with colostomy; cut at 3rd, 4th and 5th sacral vertebras.

bowel through the sphincter complex or to intrinsically hypoplastic striated muscles. It was therefore of great value in selecting patients for revisional surgery.

In 1987, Tam *et al* pointed out the advantages of performing a direct longitudinal scan on a neonate. They placed the neonate in the plane of the CT scanner and recorded a sagittal and two parasagittal scans. This enabled an accurate assessment of the level of the lesion, of fistulas and of associated anomalies if any. Resolution for tissue, meconium and gas was excellent (Fig. 1.13).

Also in 1987, Pringle *et al* reported on the use of MRI in delineating the anatomy

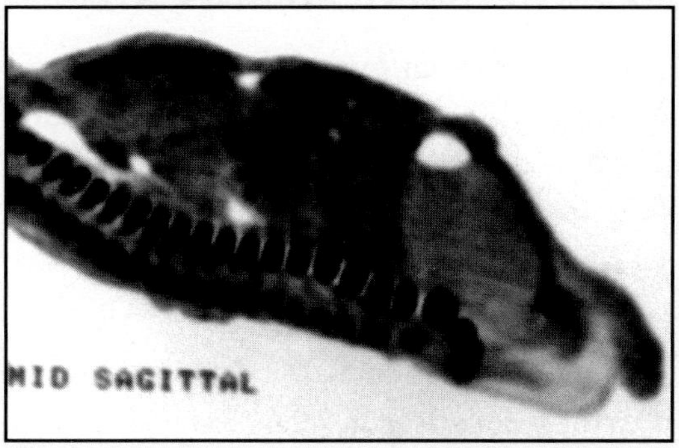

Fig. 1.13 CT scan longitudinal of neonate with high anomaly.

of ARM before and after reconstructive surgery. The anatomy was seen more clearly than in CT, specially associated anomalies of the spinal column and spinal cord and of the urogenital organs.

Animal Models

Although it had been known for some time that ARMs occur in farm animals, this information only began to be utilized in the 1980s. vander Putte and his colleagues in the Netherlands found that the anomalies in piglets closely resembled human ARMs and that in a particular herd, they occurred in response to a hereditary trait. Sufficient numbers became available for study as a result of inbreeding. In 1987 Lambrecht and Lierse found a species of mice with similar traits in Germany.

Animal models have helped in studying the normal and abnormal embryological events of the region and also the precise anatomical arrangements of the striated muscle complex, the internal sphincter and the associated fistulas. They have also provided an opportunity to perform reconstructive operations.

THE 1990s AND BEYOND

This has been an eventful period in many spheres of human endeavor, and many different modalities have been harnessed to solve problems posed by ARM.

Imaging

MRI, the imaging modality developed in the previous decade has been extensively on newborns as well as on older patients, either before reconstruction or after. In many centers it has become the investigation of choice.

Anal Endosonography has been used on adults since 1990 to show the state of the sphincters around the lower bowel. This is done by introducing an ultrasound probe into the rectum and gradually withdrawing it down the length of the anal canal. The pubiorectalis, the external sphincter and the internal sphincter could all be delineated, and the results of surgery could be assessed. Its use on children was first reported in 1994 by Emblem *et al*; its efficacy was compared with manometry and subsequently with MRI.

Embryology

The work done in the 1980s has been consolidated and a great deal of information obtained by using new methods of magnification. New animal models have been studied both to obtain data about normal development and also abnormal development. Malformations resembling those in humans have been produced in animals by experimental mating and by administering teratogenic drugs to pregnant animals. Details will be discussed in Chapter 4.

Laparoscopy

In 2000, Georgeson and his colleagues first described the role of Laparoscopy in assisting the pullthrough in high anorectal malformations. They treated 4 neonates without a colostomy and 7 older children who had had a colostomy. The dissection of the rectum was done laparoscopically and the fistula to the urethra or vagina was clipped and divided. After the rectum was retracted out of the pelvis, the pelvic floor could be visualized and the space between the two bellies of the pubococcygeus identified. Then the perineal operator selected the anal site and made a vertical midline incision. A radially expanding trocar was passed up over a Veress needle in the intrasphincteric plane behind the urethra and between the two bellies of the pubococcygeus to reach the peritoneal cavity. After sufficient dilatation was achieved the rectum was grasped and pulled down to reach the surface. Then bowel was then fixed in place to the skin of the perineum by the perineal operator; the rectal wall was sutured laparoscopically to the presacral fascia to lengthen the skinlined anal canal.

In 2001 Yamakata and his colleagues added a refinement; a muscle stimulator was introduced into the peritoneum to identify the levator sling by direct stimulation.

Objective Assessment of Function

The technology of Electromanometry and Electromyography has improved greatly, and these can be used not only preoperatively and postoperatively but peroperatively. Biofeedback had just been introduced in the 1980s to improve function by the patient's own efforts; this has advanced a great deal. We will revert to this in Chapter 16.

Imperforate Anus Initiative

In an earlier era we had considered that colostomy was the cornerstone in the management of a newborn with ARM. Today every effort is made to avoid colostomy.

A great deal of research has gone on since the time of Dobbing *et al* who showed in 1973 that one sixth of brain growth occurred prenatally and five sixths in the first 6 months of postnatal life. In the latter period there was growth only of glial tissue and synaptic connections; appropriate synaptic connections developed in response to the reception of repetitive somatosensory stimuli during the critical period; thus kittens subjected to occlusion of an eye for 5 weeks lose vision in that eye permanently. Freeman recommended that reconstruction should be completed by the end of 4 months of age (1980, 1986). He based his opinion on the work of Hickmann who had found that evoked spike potentials from the anus were absent in the first 3 to 4 months of life but developed at the end of the fourth month. In 1981 Hubel and Wiesel were awarded the Nobel Prize for showing that visual experience early in life is necessary for maintenance and full development of function in experimental animals. More recent studies have shown that this applied to the somatic sensory neocortex of the brain as well and that the window of opportunity for the development of normal somatic sensory brain neocortical neurocircuitry in rats was limited to 7 days after birth (Moore, 1990).

Moore (1994) has subsequently stressed the importance of winning the race for the space allotted in the cerebral cortex for the anorectal area by early reconstruction of congenital malformations. He performs the repairs within 72 hours of birth to make possible "optimum activity-driven somatocortical neurocircuitry and neuroconnectivity between the peripheral target area (anorectal) and the somatic cortex of the brain and prevent the loss of cortical space by disuse deprivation in the all important immediate postnatal 'critical' period of neurodevelopment". He has been leading a group named Imperforate Anus Initiative whose slogan is to operate at birth and without a prior colostomy. A number of surgeons of this group have reported good results after primary reconstructions.

Note: Much of the early historic data has been obtained from the masterly survey of Webster (1971) in the book 'Anorectal Malformations' edited by Stephens and Smith and from papers of Dinnick (1934) and Pathak (1997).

CHAPTER 2

STRUCTURE AND FUNCTION

The prime object in the management of infants with ARM is to establish normal fecal continence and normal defecation. To achieve this objective, a study of normal anatomy and physiology of the region is essential.

ANATOMY

The structures that need to be studied are:

1. The gut, namely the cecum and colon and the rectum and anal canal.
2. The striated muscles of the pelvis, perineum and abdominal wall.
3. The nervous system.

1. The Gut

According to Gray's Anatomy (Williams,1996) the large intestine consists of cecum, colon, rectum and anal canal and its opening on the surface of the perineum is called anus. The anus is located in the middle of the line joining the two ischial tuberosities.

The Rectum has been unequivocally described as being continuous above 'with the sigmoid colon at the level of the third sacral vertebra, the junction being indicated by the lower end of the sigmoid mesocolon' and as being continuous below 'with the anal canal by passing through the pelvic diaphragm'. The anorectal junction has been described as being 'situated 2 to 3 cm. in front of and slightly below the tip of the coccyx; from this level which in the male is opposite the apex of the prostate, the anal canal passes downwards and backwards from the lower end of the rectum, the backward bend of the gut at the anorectal junction being termed the perineal flexure of the rectum'. The adult rectum is 23 cm. long.

The rectum is lined by a single layer of columnar epithelium with goblet cells, mucus secreting glands and crypts and is capable of absorbing water and crystalloids. The tenia coli above fuse to give it a complete coat of longitudinal muscle; its coat of circular muscle is also complete and uniform. It is concave forwards and has three lateral curves. In the adult, the upper diameter is 4 cm. wide; it then dilates to an ampulla and then narrows abruptly at its lower end. It consists functionally of two parts, the upper, free to distend towards the peritoneal cavity, and the lower, enclosed in condensed extraperitoneal tissue.

The Anal Canal has been described as 'beginning where the lower end of the ampulla of the rectum suddenly narrows' and 'as passing downwards and backwards to end at the anus'. It is surrounded over its whole length by sphincter muscle that normally keeps the canal closed. It is 4 cm. long in the adult, and shows in its upper 1.5 cm. columns, valves and sinuses. The epithelial lining at its upper end resembles rectum with a single layer of columnar cells and intestinal glands; on the other hand the lower end is skinlined with hair and sweat glands. The junctional area is the pectinate line; above, the epithelium is stratified columnar or transitional or low stratified polygonal; below, it is nonkeratinized stratified squamous. Jit (1974) has studied this lining in great detail, his findings can be summarized as follows: "A variability in the type of epithelia in this (intermediate) zone cannot be denied. The line of change over from the stratified squamous to another type of epithelium is also variable even in the same specimen. The changeover usually takes place in the sinus but may occur at the free margin or outer (upper) face of a valve or even cranial to a sinus. Interdigitation of the two types of epithelia at their junction may also be seen sometimes." Our findings are identical.

The circular muscle of the anal canal is enormously thickened to form the internal sphincter; in the adult it measures 2 x 0.6 cm.; its lower end can be palpated digitally; its upper end blends with the circular muscle of the rectum.

The longitudinal muscle of the anal canal is replaced progressively by fibroelastic bundles. These divide into septa; accompanied by some extensions from both the smooth and the striated muscles they pierce the internal sphincter and tether the mucosa to the smooth muscle; they also pierce the striated muscle mass placed subcutaneously and reach the dermis of the perianal skin.

Unfortunately, the term 'anal canal' was introduced relatively late in descriptive human anatomy, being first used to describe the last part of the alimentary tract by Symington in 1888. This part continued to be named pars analis recti by the BNA, and it was only in 1933 that the anal canal was said to begin where the rectum ended. Nevertheless, a famous textbook dealing with diseases of this region is named 'Surgery of the anus, rectum and colon' (Goligher 1985). Furthermore, even those who accept the anal canal as an independent entity, sometimes place its upper end at the site of change of epithelial lining, blood supply, lymphatic drainage, innervation and development. Thus there are 'two distinctly different definitions of the anal canal, that of the anatomist and that of many clinicians; in consequence the term anorectal junction has no meaning unless it is defined' (Hollingshead 1985) (Figs. 2.1-4).

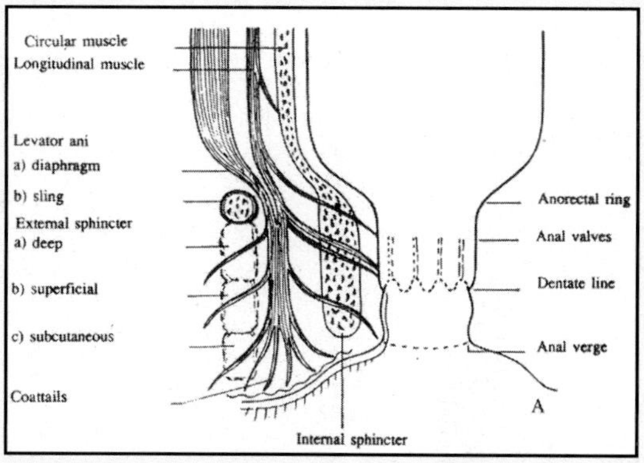

Fig. 2.1 Diagram of coronal section through lower rectum and anal canal.

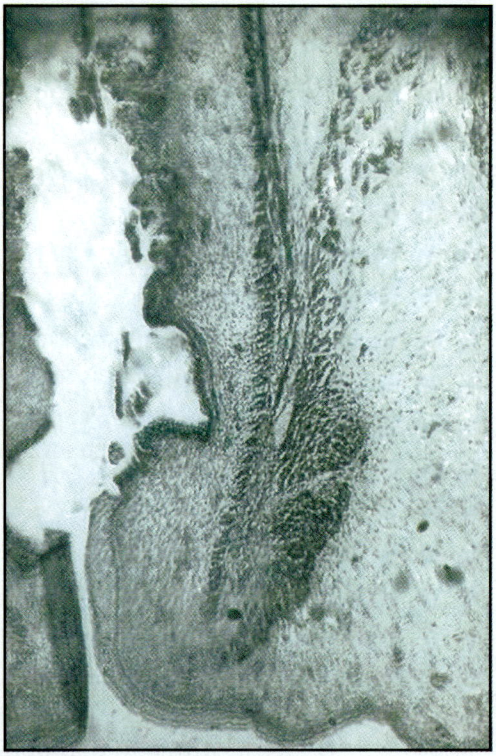

Fig. 2.2 Photomicrogram of identical section through 24 week fetus.

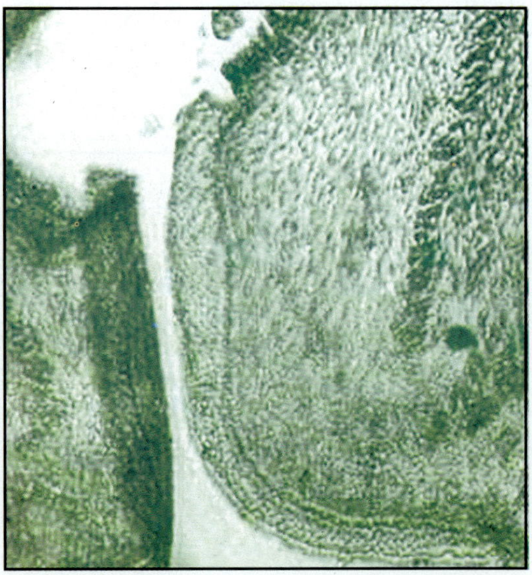

Fig. 2.3 Photomicrograph showing epithelium at lower end of same fetus.

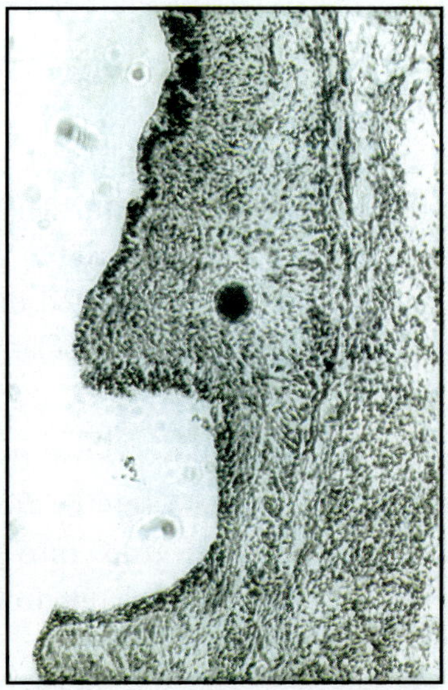

Fig. 2.4 Photomicrograph showing epithelium of same fetus higher up.

2. The Striated Muscles

The Levator Ani has been described in Gray's Anatomy (Williams *et al* 1995) as 'a broad thin muscle which is attached to the inner surface of the side of the true pelvis, and unites with the opposite muscle, to form the greater part of the floor of the pelvic cavity. The muscle's fibers pass towards the median plane with varying degrees of obliquity. The most anterior fibers sweep backwards and downwards across the side of the prostate to end in the perineal body. They constitute the levator prostatae but in the female they cross the sides of the vagina to reach their attachment and so constitute an additional and important sphincter for it, the pubovaginalis. Intermediate fibers pass backward across the side of the prostate and then turn medially to become continuous with those of the opposite side and form a muscular sling around the anorectal flexure. This relatively thick part of the muscle is termed the puborectalis. Posteriorly its fibers are inextricably mingled with those of the deep part of the external anal sphincter. Other intermediate fibers blend with the longitudinal muscle coat of the rectum and descend within the puborectal sling as the conjoined longitudinal coat of the anal canal. More posterior fibers are attached to the last two coccygeal segments and to the anococcygeal ligament or raphe' (Fig. 2.5)

The External Anal Sphincter is traditionally divided into three components; subcutaneous, superficial and deep. The subcutaneous part is a flat band 15 mm. broad; it surrounds the lower part of the anal canal; some fibers are attached anteriorly to the perineal body and posteriorly to the anococcygeal ligament. The superficial part arises from the posterior surface of the terminal segment of the coccyx and is inserted into the perineal body, after surrounding the lower part of the internal sphincter. The deep part surrounds the upper part of the internal sphincter and is a thick annular band.

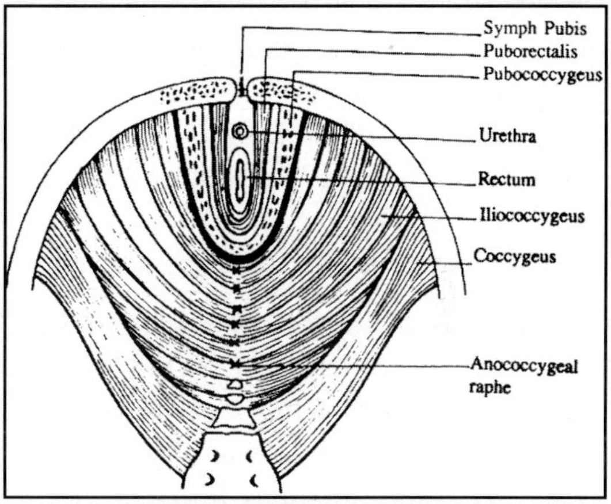

Fig. 2.5 Diagram of levator ani from above.

The fusion of the fibers of the puborectalis and the upper parts of the internal sphincter and the external sphincter at the anorectal junction is given the name 'anorectal ring'. The relationship between these muscle groups and the longitudinal muscle of the bowel has intrigued observers for years.

According to de Vries and Cox (1985), Santorini in 1824 was the first to add 'the role of rectal sphincter to the function of the levator ani muscle', and described accurately the fibers which later became the puborectalis sling. He was also the first to describe the three parts of the external sphincter. Subsequently while Cruveilhier and Roux felt that the levator and the deep part of the external sphincter could not be order separated, Robin and Cadiat, Holl and finally Thompson found that they were distinct. Subsequently, authors of the first half of the twentieth century accepted the views expressed by Thompson.

During the period 1951 to 1980, a number of investigators studied fetuses, normal fullterm neonatal cadavers and specimens of pelvis from older subjects in order to correlate structure and function. They were Fowler (1957) and Stephens (1963) in Australia, Lawson (1969) in England, Wilson (1967) in South Africa and Jit (1974) in India. None of them could clearly separate the different components.

According to Lawson, there are two main groups of muscles. 'On either side a posterolateral group forms a true diaphragm extending as far forwards as the obturator canal. The anteromedial borders of the contralateral muscles make a gothic arch, which with the bodies of the pubic bones encloses a space through which the viscera pass and are supported by a pubovisceral group of muscles.' The pubovisceral muscles, he goes on to explain 'in addition to supporting the pelvic viscera, can also by active contraction draw these viscera upwards and forwards'. The other group form a funnel through which the viscera leave the pelvis to reach the perineum. The sling surrounds the anorectal flexure and should correctly be named puborectoanal sling; how much is contributed by the levator ani and how much by the deep fibers of the external sphincter is not clear.

According to Dudowitz *et al* (1960) the striated muscles of the region contain two different kinds of fibers. Red fibers have a high myoglobin content, are small in diameter and possess slow tonic contractions; their nutrition is by Kreb's cycle and they show continuous electrical activity. On the other hand, pale fibers have a low myoglobin content, are large in diameter and have rapid phasic contractions; they metabolize glycogen by phosphorylation.

Shafik (1975) found that the external sphincter consisted of a triple loop of U shaped fibers; the top loop has a pubic origin, the middle loop arises from the tip of the coccyx and the superficial or base loop is attached anteriorly to the perineal skin. This aids in defecation by vermicular contraction and makes for watertight closure.

In October 1980, Alberto Pena reported a new approach to the management of ARM and in subsequent articles elaborated his concept of the striated musculature of the region. According to him, a funnel-like structure extends as a continuum from a pelvic insertion, namely pubic bone, pelvic rim and anterior aspect of the lowest portion of the sacrum all the way down to the skin. It is formed by the levator ani at its upper part and by the external sphincter at the lower part, but there is no way to determine the limit between the two structures. The intermediate undetermined portion is therefore named 'muscle complex'. More superficially, two varieties of external sphincter fibers have been described. In one set, the fibers are parasagittal; they run from the tip of the coccyx to the anus; they lie immediately under the skin at the anus and are separated from skin by fat as they approach the coccyx. They close the anus by their contraction. In the other set, the fibers run cephalocaudal, parallel to the bowel up to the skin. They are thus perpendicular to the fibers of the first set;

they elevate the anal skin and integrate the muscle complex. Pena does not identify any particular group of fibers as constituting a sling but admits 'although there are some horizontal fibers, most of the muscle fibers run in a cephalocaudal direction'. According to him, 'there is no predominant portion of muscle which should be considered more important than another in terms of fecal continence. The impression is rather that fecal continence depends on the preservation of the entire muscle mechanism.' The normal angle at the anorectal flexure is almost 90^0 and is accentuated when the entire muscle contracts to compress the rectum against the pubis and elevate the anus (Pena 1988).

In order to study the disposition of the striated muscle of the region, we dissected between 1972 and 1975 the pelvis of 5 neonates who had died without ARM and 45 neonates who had died with ARM. Two of these had rectal atresia, three had a low lesion with anoperineal or anovestibular fistula and 40 had the terminal bowel above the levator ani. Immediately after death the pelvis was isolated; suitable tubes were introduced through the colon from above and through the urethra, vagina, urethrovaginal canal or lower opening of the bowel, if any, and the specimen preserved for study at a convenient time. The left hipbone was removed by cutting through the sacroiliac joint and the symphysis pubis and severing all the structures attached to the left hipbone. A speck of barium was introduced into the terminal bowel from above and a true lateral Xray was taken to assess its level with reference to the right hipbone and sacrum. The relation between the levator ani and the bowel was then displayed by dissection on the intact right side and followed across the midline to the detached left side.

In 1977-78, the pelvis of two fetuses without ARM and of three neonates with ARM were submitted to serial sections; these were examined by a handlens and then under the microscope after staining.

Finally in 1983 after we had studied the initial articles on PSARP, we dissected by a posterior sagittal incision the pelvis of 4 neonates. Two had died without ARM and two with ARM. A study of these autopsy specimens as well as of patients during operation over two decades led us to postulate the following.

The striated muscle system of the levator ani and external sphincter is very delicately balanced and interwoven not only with each other but also with the striated muscles situated anteriorly around the urogenital structures and with the nonstriated muscles in the wall of the bowel. The parasagittal and perpendicular fibers of the external sphincter are easily identifiable even in the absence of a normal anus. The latter forms the stem of the funnel. However, at the junction of the funnel and the stem there is unequivocally a thickening of striated fibers that are horizontally disposed and obviously responsible for the anorectal flexure, and therefore constitute a sling (Figs. 2.6-7). (Chatterjee 1976).

The fibers of this sling originate from the back of the pubis and surround the normal anorectal flexure as described by Lawson. In some ARMs, this relationship between the bowel and the levator ani is maintained and the abnormality is confined to either the supralevator region or the infralevator region. In these situations, the sling is pubo-

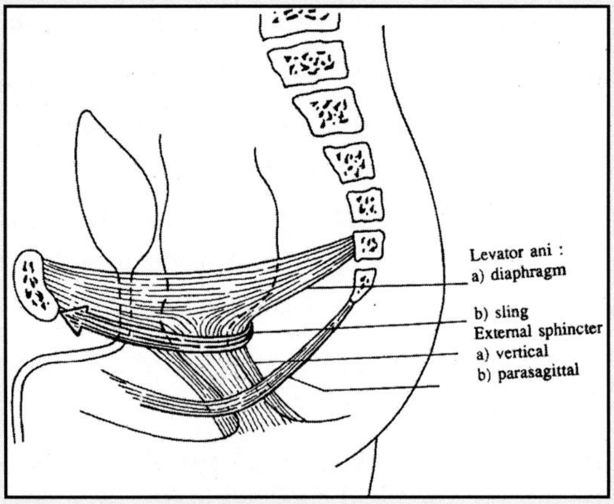

Fig. 2.6 Diagram of sagittal section through male pelvis.

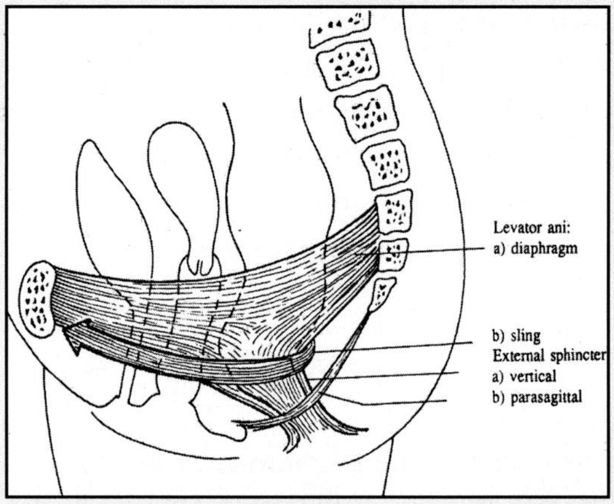

Fig. 2.7 Diagram of sagittal section through female pelvis.

rectoanal, and may be named 'puborectalis sling' for convenience. However, in the majority of ARMs, both the supralevator and the infralevator regions are abnormal. The rectum ends above the diaphragm fibers of the levator and the sling surrounds only the anteriorly placed urogenital tubes and sometimes, in addition, a fistula leading down from the bowel to either the exterior or to a urogenital tube. In these cases, the sling does not surround the rectum and should not be named 'puborectalis', the term 'levator sling' is more correct.

The other striated muscles involved in continence and defecation are the muscles of the anterior perineum or urogenital diaphragm with horizontally disposed fibers, the muscles of the anterior abdominal wall and the diaphragm. These do not merit a detailed description in this presentation.

Today, the CT scan and more particularly the MRI scan permit an accurate display of the striated muscles in region in normal and abnormal conditions in the living subject, and cadaver dissections have become obsolete.

3. The Nervous System

Three sets of peripheral nerves connect the region to the Central Nervous System (Williams, 1996). Two sets reach the neurones situated in the wall of the gut; these neurones constitute the enteric nervous system.

Somatic Nerves

These nerves do not reach the enteric nervous system. They carry both afferent and efferent impulses and have three components. The first component originates from the third and fourth sacral segments and with an occasional contribution from the fifth, passes along the upper surface of the pelvic diaphragm on either side of the rectum to supply the levator ani, the anal canal and the urogenital organs. The second originates from the second, third and fourth sacral segments and form pudendal nerves. They pass below the pelvic floor along the wall of the ischiorectal fossa to supply the undersurface of the levator ani, the external sphincters, the anal canal, the perineal skin and the urogenital diaphragm. A single nerve, the perineal branch of the fourth sacral nerve enters the ischiorectal fossa medial to the ischial spine and passes medially to supply the posterior part of the puborectalis and the external sphincter.

There is an abundance of conventional sensory nerve endings in the perineal skin and in the mucosa of the distal anal canal; afferent impulses from these nerve endings are carried to the spinal cord and brain. The mucosa of the upper anal canal and rectum do not have any nerve endings and do not appreciate any sensation.

Parasympathetic Nerves

These arise from two sources, vagal and sacral (Meier-Ruge 1974). According to classical anatomists, vagal parasympathetic fibers end at the left third of the transverse colon. However, Yhtema and Hammonds (1954) showed that in the chick embryo, neuroblasts failed to migrate into any part of the intestinal tract after the vagal neural crest was extirpated, but migrated to the pelvic organs even after the lumbosacral spinal cord failed to develop. Subsequently Okamoto and Ueda (1967) confirmed these findings in the human; migration of vagal neuroblasts into the bowel from the left flexure to the anal sphincter took place between the ninth and twelfth week of fetal life.

The nervi erigentes arise from the second, third and fourth sacral segments. Their short branches supply the rectum and upper anal canal and long branches travel on either side of the rectum above the pelvic diaphragm to reach the urogenital organs and the pelvic ganglia. When the rectum is malformed and ends high up, the nervi erigentes run close to the midline beneath the rectum to reach the pelvic ganglia and are, therefore, liable to be injured during reconstructive surgery. This is even more likely to happen if they arise from a common trunk (Fig. 2.8). There is little doubt that the nervi erigentes end in ganglia that have migrated from the neural crest along with the vagus nerves.

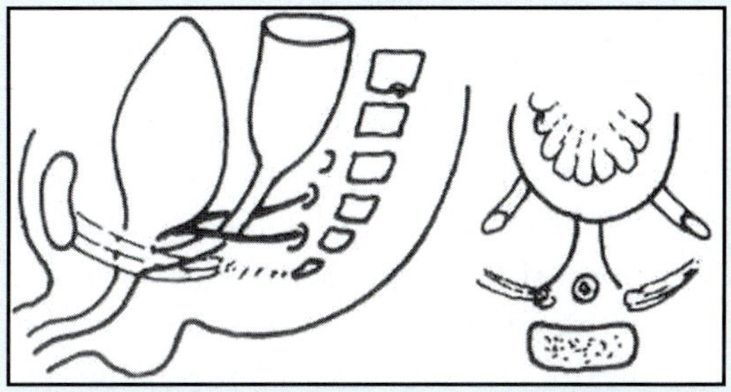

Fig. 2.8 Diagram showing disposition of somatic nerves in high anomaly.

Parasympathetic fibers are distributed to the urogenital organs and to the left colon and rectum along with sympathetic fibers. Preganglionic fibers end on cholinergic nerve cells of the gut. Short postganglionic fibers end on the smooth muscle cells of the gut and stimulate contraction; they also inhibit the internal sphincter. They also stimulate secretion of the glands in the gut wall. In addition coarse perception of rectal distension is mediated through the parasympathetic nerves conveying impulses from the muscle spindles in the rectal wall. Afferent impulses from muscle spindles situated in the puborectalis muscle and parapuborectal tissues are carried by these fibers; these are the most sensitive receptors for alterations in pressure within the rectum and are responsible for reflex contraction of the puborectalis-external sphincter complex in response to rectal distension. Hence this area has been named the 'trigger zone of continence' (Holschneider, 1976, 1988).

Sympathetic Nerves

These arise from the second, third and fourth lumbar ganglia and the preaortic plexus; they form the hypogastric plexus on either side and continue as presacral nerves to the pelvic ganglion. This is situated on the bladder base and prostate or cervix uteri and anterolateral wall of the rectum. Postganglionic fibers are then distributed along the blood vessels to the ganglion-plexuses in the wall of the bowel as well as the urogenital organs. Long branches also pass to the inferior mesenteric plexus via the hypogastric plexus and the superior rectal inferior mesenteric vessels. They are then distributed to the left colon and rectum along the branches of the inferior mesenteric vessels. Sympathetic fibers are noradrenergic. Some end on postganglionic cholinergic neurones and inhibit acetylcholinc secretion. Others end directly on smooth muscle cells, inhibiting their contraction, but stimulating contraction of the internal sphincter. Still others end on the wall of the blood vessels causing vasoconstriction.

The Enteric Nervous System

There are two major networks of nerve fibers in the gut wall up to the upper half of the anal canal, a myenteric plexus between the longitudinal and the circular muscles and submucous plexus between the circular muscles and the mucosa. As already described, they are connected to the central nervous system by the parasympathetic and sympathetic nerves, but they can also function autonomously by producing a variety of neurotransmitters. The myenteric plexus is concerned primarily with motor control whereas the submucous plexus controls intestinal secretion.

PHYSIOLOGY: CONTINENCE AND DEFECATION

Continence is the ability to prevent evacuation of bowel contents at an inappropriate time and place. This is achieved when the propulsive forces generated in the bowel can be checked by the resistance of the outlet. On the other hand, when the propulsive forces overcome the outlet resistance, defecation takes place. One of the priceless possessions of the human species is the capacity to defecate only at an appropriate time and place and to remain continent at other times and places. Without this, human civilization would not have been what it is.

The Propulsive Forces

These are of three kinds.

1. The volume of the feces

This is reduced by water absorption by the colon and rectum and by a diet with low roughage content. It is increased by exudates resulting from inflammatory bowel disease, by a diet with high roughage content, by drugs that draw fluid into the lumen of the bowel and thus act as laxatives, and by an insufficient length of functioning large intestine leading to insufficient water absorption.

2. The contraction of the smooth muscles of the colon and rectum.

The colon contracts in response to gastrocolic, ileocolic or conditioned reflexes, and thus fills the rectum. The rectum acts as a reservoir. Normally empty, it responds to distension by contracting, but later, contractions decrease. Intrarectal pressure, after an initial rise, falls, and the rectum adapts to an increase in its contents. Later a reverse pressure gradient is established and some of the rectal contents are pushed back into the colon. This stimulates further colonic contractions. The activity of the smooth muscle of the large gut can be altered by a variety of drugs; some stimulate and act as laxatives, and others inhibit and thus delay the onward passage of bowel contents. Smooth muscle activity depends greatly on local reflex arcs and function is altered by disturbance of these arcs by disease, either temporarily or permanently. The classic example of permanent loss is congentital aganglionosis, better known as Hirschsprung's Disease.

3. *The voluntary contraction of the striated muscles.*

The abdominal wall and the diaphragm contract to produce a rise in intraabdominal and hence intracolonic pressure.

The Forces of Resistance at the Outlet

Some of these work at rest, others are brought on in response to an enhanced propulsive force.

1. Those working at rest are

a) The normal angulation at the anorectal junction is the most important single factor; this develops when the infant assumes the erect posture and is brought about by a tonically contracting puborectalis with red muscle fibers.

b) The activity of the smooth muscle surrounding the anal canal, namely the internal sphincter is the second major factor. This keeps the anal canal closed. Its mucosa is folded in a star shaped manner and adjacent surfaces adhere to each other due to surface mucus.

c) The coattails of the longitudinal smooth muscles pull on the perianal skin and the anal mucosa to produce a plugging effect.

d) Congested veins at the peivic floor and anorectal junction increase the resistance further.

2. ***Those brought on in response to an enhanced propulsive force*** are the striated muscles of the region, namely the levator ani and external sphincter muscle complex. They contract physically in response to reflex stimulation. Initially the afferent impulses arise from the nerve endings in the rectal wall, the puborectalis and the para-puborectal tissues when these are stretched. The internal sphincter also initially responds to rectal distension by contraction, but this is followed by relaxation. Relaxation of the internal sphincter exposes the more sensitive receptors of the anal canal to changes in pressure, and reflex stimulation of the striated muscles is greatly strengthened. With further rise in intrarectal pressure, rectal contents actually enter the anal canal and reflex stimulation is further enhanced. The receptors in the anal canal can distinguish between flatus and feces; flatus may be allowed to escape through the external sphincter but feces is held up. While a local reflex arc mediates the rectoanal reflex, namely, the activity of the internal sphincter, reflexes involving the striated muscle initially work through spinal centers. Augmented

afferent impulses reach the higher centers as an urge to defecate. The urge can be suppressed to a greater or lesser extent by initiating voluntary contractions of the pelvic striated muscles.

Defecation

Defecation is the ability to evacuate bowel contents at an appropriate time and place. It takes place when the propulsive forces overcome the outlet resistance. This normally takes place when the higher centers decide to yield to the urge to defecate. The urge to defecate first occurs when the rectal pressure increases to about 18mm Hg. Voluntary defecation can be initiated by raising intra-abdominal wall and diaphragm with the glottis closed. It is continued by voluntarily relaxing the external sphincter. Inhibition of the tonically contracting striated muscles, and consequent straightening of the anorectal angle leads to further fall of outlet resistance. Consequent desynchronization of electrical activity in the smooth muscle causes the anal canal to open up. With the external sphincter relaxed, the rectum empties and is filled up again by colonic contractions. This continues till the contents of the left colon and rectum are all expelled. A final contraction of the levator ani and external sphincter complex clears the anal canal of feces. Defecation is thus basically a spinal reflex that can be voluntarily facilitated by external sphincter relaxation and abdominal muscle contraction (Duthie & Watts 1965, Verma & Stephens 1972, Scharli 1984, 1987).

The factors responsible for continence and defecation are shown diagramatically (Fig. 2.9).

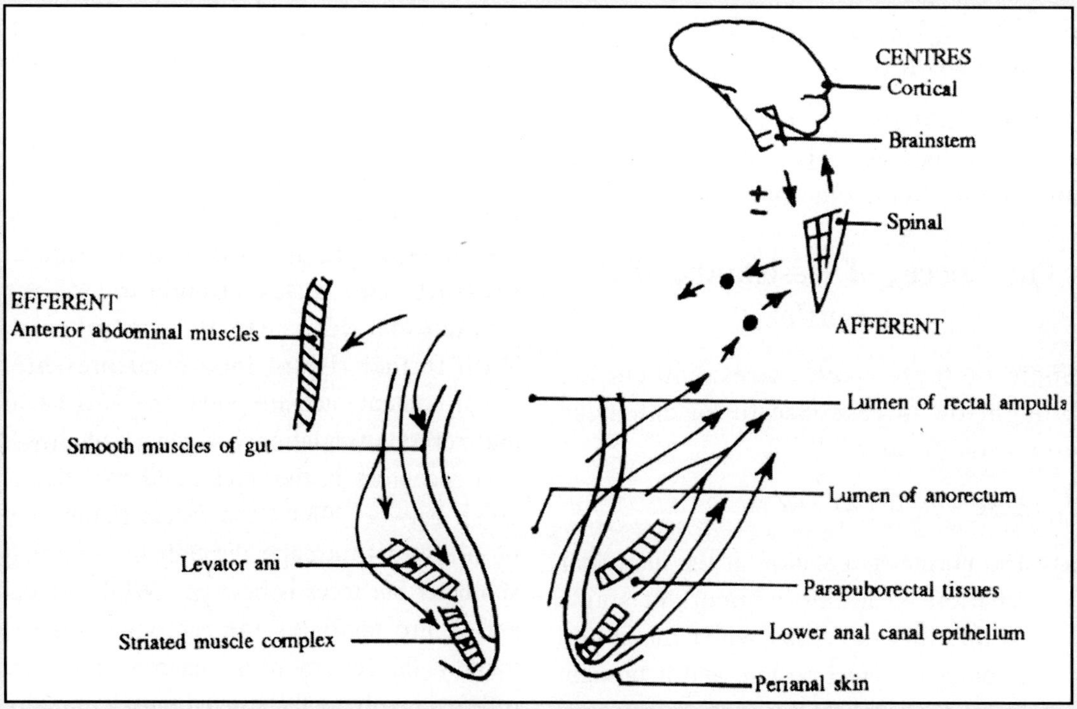

Fig. 2.9 Diagram showing factors involved in continence and defecation.

The two basic problems faced by patients with ARM are incontinence and constipation. These will be briefly discussed at this stage.

Incontinence

In infants, the spinal reflex producing defecation proceeds without either voluntary inhibition or facilitation. After the baby becomes toilet trained, the urge to defecate can be voluntarily resisted for some considerable time. In adult life the reflex can no longer be inhibited when the rectal pressure reaches 55 mm Hg. The propulsive forces then cause the rectum to empty itself involuntarily. At the other extreme is the condition wherein there is no outlet resistance and feces is passed all the time; this condition is named total incontinence. In between there are varying degrees of involuntary discharge of feces. There may be occasional staining of the underwear when stools are loose, or more regular fecal soiling even with formed stools. This involuntary emission may occur with the rectum more or less empty or with the rectum filled with moderate or massive amounts of feces. Overflow incontinence is the name given to leakage around a fecal mass.

Patients with ARM suffer from incontinence because of absence of normal resistance at the outlet and because of damage to this resistance in the course of treatment.

Constipation

This is one of the most difficult words to define. Three components are involved, namely the frequency of the stools, the consistency of the stools and the ease or difficulty in passing the stools. How infrequent should defecation be for the condition to be labeled as constipation depends on age, weight and diet However there are variations between individuals; some remain in good health passing stools every 5 to 6 days and others remain in good health passing 3 to 4 stools every day. Assessment of the consistency of the stools is easier, and constipation can be graded according to the hardness and dryness of the stool. The difficulty experienced in passing stools is probably the most important index. The difficulty may be due to local pain, to a narrow passage to the exterior or to loss of normal defecation reflexes.

The vast majority of patients who present with constipation suffer from nonorganic or functional constipation, a subject outside the purview of this book. However constipation is one of the cardinal problems faced by patients with ARM primarily because of a narrow passage to the exterior and secondarily because of absence of proper neuromuscular coordination. These problems are sometimes aggravated by treatment for the malformation. Of other causes of organic constipation, the most important are aganglionosis or Hirschsprung's disease and Hirschsprung-like disorders. Others include metabolic disorders like hypothyroidism, and chromosomal disorders like Down's syndrome. All of these can coexist with ARM.

CHAPTER 3

CLASSIFICATION, DIAGNOSIS, IMAGING

Patients with ARM clearly fall into one of two groups. Some present soon after birth as an emergency; others present after some time. The latter may come at any age, with a variety of clinical features and often with a history of management elsewhere. The proportion of patients falling into the two groups depends on the character of the institution.

A normal anus is absent in about 95% of patients with ARM. The absence of a normal anus in a neonate is as easy to determine as its sex; the person conducting the delivery should diagnose both at the same time. Such persons both medical and non-medical should be trained to look at both the anterior and the posterior perineum as soon as they have delivered a live baby (Figs. 3.1-2). Diagnosis of ARM in the 5% of patients born with a normal anus is a little more difficult.

CLINICAL CLASSIFICATION

It is based on the findings at the first examination of the perineum.

Those who have a normal anus are:

I Those who have a visible abnormal opening.

The opening may be

1. small, at the normal anal site, or
2. at an anterior site
   a) in the perineum:
   b) in the vestibule, or
3. abnormally large.

II Those who have a manifest invisible opening.

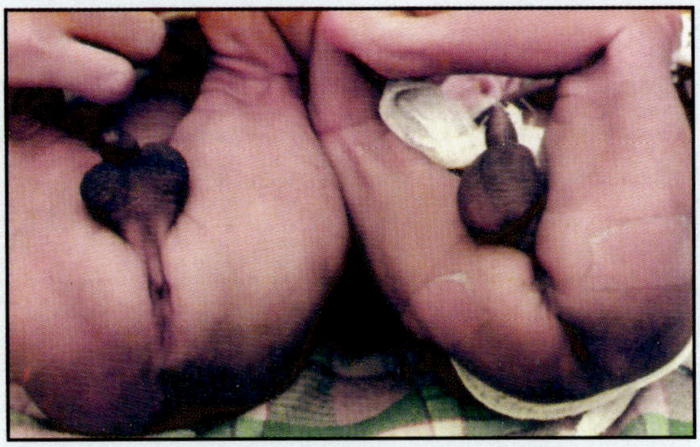

Fig. 3.1 Photograph of boys with ARM.

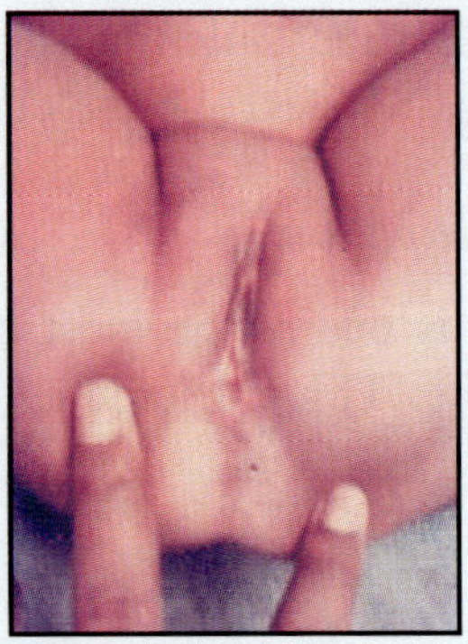

Fig. 3.2 Photograph of a girl with ARM.

The opening may be manifest by the passage of meconium through

1 the male urethra, or:

2 the vagina, or

3 the urethrovaginal canal

III Those who have two manifest abnormal openings

IV Those who do not have any manifest opening.

Those who have a normal anus are:

I Those who have an abnormal anorectum

II Those who have a normal anorectum and a manifest fistula.

A systemic clinical examination is carried out after the local examination of the perineum is concluded. This includes recording of body weight at first presentation, evidence of complications and, evidence of associated malformations.

Body Weight

In our earlier series a large number of neonates with ARM and low birth weight reached the NRS Medical College and there was a significant mortality, the mortality rate being higher in babies with lower birth weight. Since then the weight of neonates coming with ARM has greatly improved, especially in our private clinic. Pari passu, there has been a great improvement in the care of small neonates and no death can be attributed only to low birth weight.

Older patients with ARM falling below the 3rd percentile also pose a management problem; the cause is generally protein-calorie malnutrition due to the chronic intestinal obstruction that follows untreated or improperly treated ARM. They are poor subjects for major reconstructive surgery.

Complications

In the neonate these generally result from unrelieved intestinal obstruction. Abdominal distension and vomiting lead to pneumonitis, loss of fluids and electrolytes leads to renal failure; and septicemia follows. A particularly dramatic complication is perforation of the proximal large bowel resulting in pneumoperitoneum and fulminating peritonitis (Fig. 3.3). This is more likely to occur if the baby does not have a manifest opening of the bowel and if there is delay in starting surgical treatment.

Intensive therapy consisting of parenteral nutrition, antibiotics, and ventilatory support together with surgical intervention

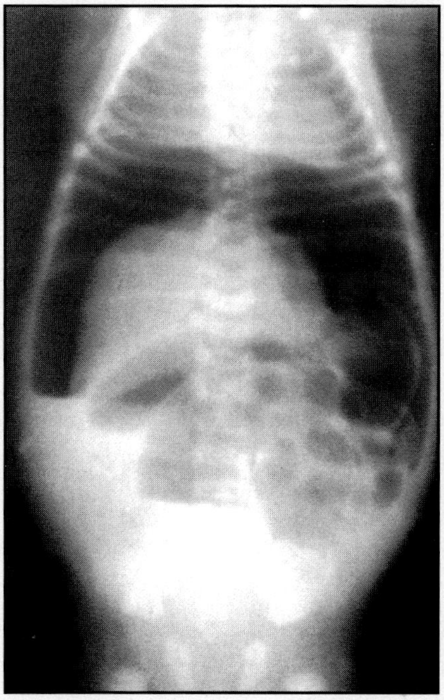

Fig. 3.3 Xray showing pneumoperitoneum in a baby with ARM.

can salvage such situations; the timing of surgery has to be carefully selected.

As mentioned above, patients not treated or incorrectly treated as neonates present in the postneonatal period with intestinal obstruction, either chronic or acute on chronic. There is accompanying protein-energy-malnutrition, anemia, intercurrent infection and enterocolitis. These problems have to be solved before definitive treatment for the ARM can be started.

Patients with urinary fistulas additionally have urinary tract infection and electrolyte imbalances and renal status has to be stabilized prior to definitive surgery. Details will be discussed later.

Associated Anomalies

These are collectively given the name VACTERL; the mnemonic stands for Vertebral, Alimentary, Cardiac, Tracheo-Esophageal, Renal and Limb. Some significantly influence management in the neonate and others in the postneonatal period; still others demand treatment on their own merit but do not influence the management of the ARM.

The precise incidence of associated anomalies can only be assessed if every patient is submitted either to intensive imaging or to autopsy. Since this was not possible in our series, many of the lesions that were asymptomatic or showed no clinical abnormalities remained undetected.

In the series of 250 patients studied in the Children's Memorial Hospital, Chicago, in 1967, 4 had five associated anomalies, 12 had four, 21 had three, 39 had two and 59 had one; thus only 115 patients (46%) did not have an associated anomaly. The number of babies who died was 49, and 44 were autopsied. In the series reported by Cook (1978) from Liverpool, the incidence of anomalies was well over 60%. Smith and Saeki (1988) have recorded an almost identical incidence. A recent study at the All India Institute of Medical Sciences has shown an incidence of 45%; 21% of these had genitourinary anomalies; cardiovascular and gastrointestinal anomalies accounted for 16% each. (Gupta and Dave, 2001). We shall discuss the following associated anomalies.

1. Tracheo-esophageal

Esophageal atresia (EA) and tracheo-esophageal fistula (TEF) take pride of place in all series. In most the esophageal lesion was diagnosed after the baby was admitted for the ARM, either by observing frothiness at the mouth, or by noting obstruction to the passage of a routine nasogastric tube. As inspired air enters the alimentary tract freely through the fistula, there is early abdominal distension and early arrival of gas in the terminal bowel. Thus useful information can be obtained by an invertogram much earlier than usual. At the same time, intestinal obstruction facilitates regurgitation of alimentary contents into the respiratory tract through the fistula. This is increased when the baby is held head down for an invertogram; the prone cross-table position is safer. We have no case of pure EA associated with ARM. Many of the babies who had both ARM and TEF also had other serious malformations, particularly cardiac and renal.

Our management policy for babies born with both ARM and TEF has changed over the years. If the baby does not have gross abdominal distension, we first close the TEF. If conditions permit an esophageal anastomosis, we would do it, otherwise we would do cervical esophagostomy and gastrostomy another day. Only in the presence of gross abdominal distension would we relieve this distension first by methods that will be described in later chapters. In all other situations, we would treat the ARM after the thoracotomy.

2. *Cardiac*

Cardiac anomalies may manifest in the neonatal period or later in life. Neonatal cyanotic heart disease may pose an immediate threat to life and may require urgent treatment, before, during and after the initial treatment for the ARM. Xray and echocardiography leads to an anatomical diagnosis. A baby with an uncorrectable cardiac anomaly is best left alone but few cardiac malformations are now uncorrectable; once intestinal obstruction is relieved, a pediatric cardiologist and a pediatric cardiac surgeon should be consulted. If cardiac surgery is indicated, a decision has to be taken jointly on whether this should be done before or after definitive surgery for the ARM. In our earlier series, we had lost two patients with untreated cardiac malformations after an excellent anorectal reconstruction. Today early cardiac surgery has saved quite a few babies and made them fit for a major reconstruction for the ARM.

It should be remembered that bacterial endocarditis is a complication that can supervene on congenital heart disease after even minor procedures on the lower intestinal or urinary tracts for example, dilatation of the neoanus or the urethra. These should therefore always be done under the protection of antibacterial drugs.

A condition that is asymptomatic but gives rise to clinical and radiological abnormalities at birth, is situs inversus. This influences immediate management of the ARM because of the unusual disposition of the colon (see Chapter 6). There are three cases in our series, two of them presented as neonates.

3. *Alimentary*

When there is a gross defect of the anterior abdominal wall, the diagnosis is obvious. Omphalocele (Exomphalos) and gastroschisis call for treatment immediately after birth. The ARM is dealt with suitably (Fig. 3.4).

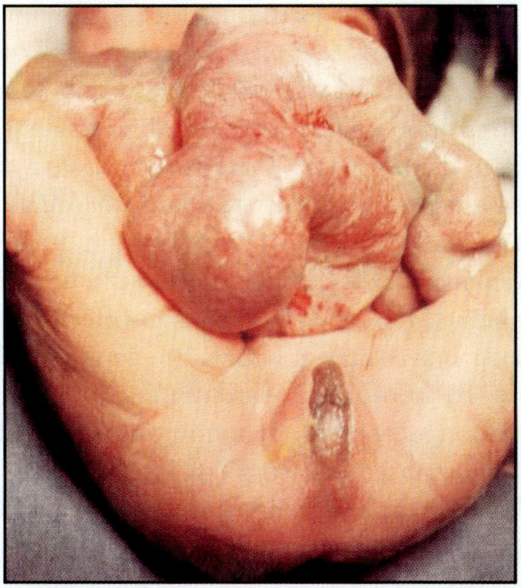

Fig. 3.4 Photograph of omphalocele with ARM.

The diagnosis of vesico-intestinal fissure is also obvious at birth (Fig. 3.5). The small bowel fistula opening between two halves of the urinary bladder allows an enormous

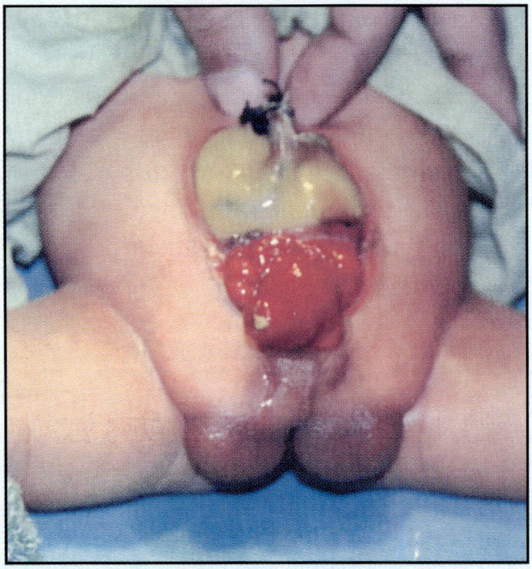

Fig. 3.5 Photograph of vesicointestinal fissure.

volume of fluid and electrolytes to escape and normal absorption of calories and protein do not take place. A second enteric fistula leads from below the first fistula to a blind loop ending at a variable distance from the perineum. There is almost always an associated omphalocele and epispadias. Generally, the sex of rearing has to be female because of the small size of the phallus. Repair of the omphalocele and a loop enterostomy at birth has to be followed up by prolonged parenteral nutrition, prolonged socio-economic support and many subsequent surgical interventions. We do not advocate more complicated procedures on the neonate.

We have a single longterm survivor; he had a small omphalocele and a phallus of reasonable size. The bowel opening between the two halves of bladder was colon. In the neonatal period, the omphalocele was repaired and a loop colostomy performed between the ileocecal valve and the colovesical junction. He was taken away and returned when 3 years old. At that time the bladder was reconstructed using the bowel between the two halves and the colon was brought out as an endcolostomy. He again disappeared and returned when 8 years old in good nutritional status and happy with his colostomy. He had total urinary incontinence; surgery was successfully done for this and readmission for anorectal plasty done for this and readmission for anorectoplasty was advised. He has not been brought back so far (Fig. 3.6).

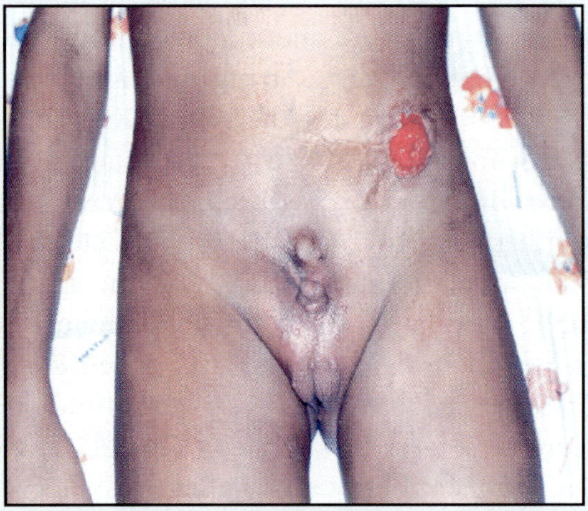

Fig. 3.6 Photograph of longterm survivor with the above.

Other lesions of the abdomen cause intestinal obstruction and can be suspected by the occurrence of vomiting earlier than is usual with an ARM alone. A routine erect straight Xray however should lead to a diagnosis before vomiting occurs. While all varieties are known to occur, duodenal obstruction due either to malrotation or atresia is the commonest. In this situation the abdomen is not distended. In duodenal atresia there is no gas below the level of the duodenum (Fig. 3.7) while in malrotation the distal bowel is relatively empty. Needless to say, the duodenal obstruction should be relieved first and then the ARM should be dealt with. However, the duodenal obstruction is sometimes detected only after a colostomy has been done.

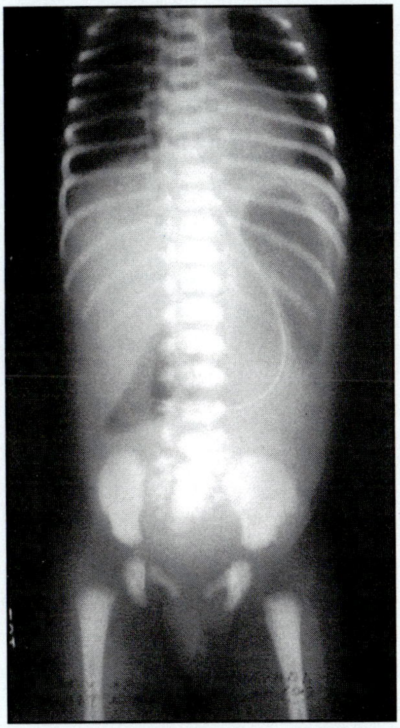

Fig. 3.7 Xray showing duodenal obstruction with ARM.

Associated Hirschsprung's Disease is uncommon; it is usually diagnosed only when investigations are carried out to find out the cause of constipation persisting after the ARM has been dealt with (see Chapter 16). However, Das made the diagnosis in one neonate who had rectal atresia and pneumoperitoneum. At laparotomy a perforation of the sigmoid was found and the bowel distal to this was narrow and thickened. Colostomy was done. Subsequently, contrast Xray and biopsy confirmed the diagnosis and the baby recovered after an abdominoperineal pullthrough.

Nonobstructive lesions of the large bowel intimately associated with ARM will be discussed in Chapter 14.

4. Urogenital

Renal lesions in the newborn can sometimes be suspected by examining the state of the abdominal wall; the abdominal muscle deficiency syndrome is almost always associated with renal dysplasia (Fig. 3.8). Ultrasonography is today the simplest method of obtaining information about renal status in the newborn and also in the unborn. Severe impairment of renal status contraindicates major anorectal reconstructions.

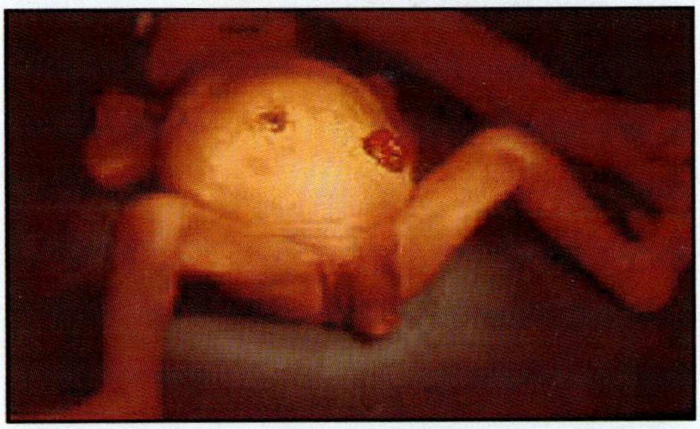

Fig. 3.8 Photograph of baby with prunebelly syndrome, megalopenis and ARM.

Urogenital malformations are of two kinds. Some are part and parcel of the ARM and are discussed in detail later. Obstructive uropathy not directly connected with ARM may affect both the upper and the lower urinary tracts, and should be relieved as early as possible; the lesions include posterior urethral valves, pelviureteric obstructions and lower ureteric obstructions. Non-obstructive lesions like vesicoureteric reflux or duplex systems can be dealt with electively.

Common associated deformities of the male external genitalia include hypospadias and undescended testes; these are electively treated. A megalopenis or a large flaccid penis is rare but very disturbing to the family (Fig. 3.8). Even more disturbing is the presence of a double penis (Fig. 3.9).

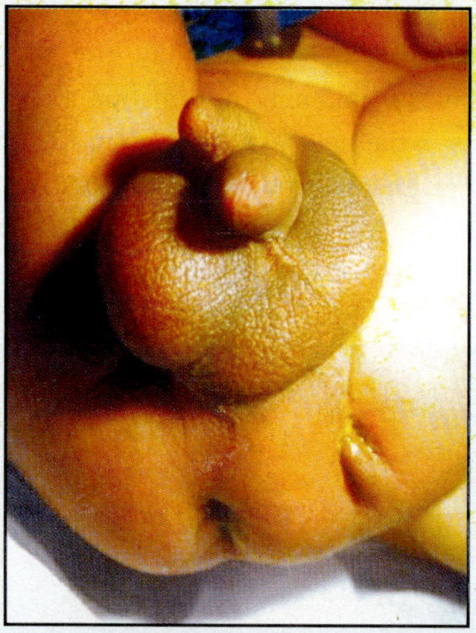

Fig. 3.9 Photograph of baby with duplex penis and ARM.

A variety of malformations of the vagina and uterus are found in association with ARM. Those that lead to distension of the vagina by secretions, urine or blood require urgent treatment; others are dealt with electively. These are further described in the section on Cloaca (Chapter 11).

Ambiguous external genitalia are found more often in babies with ARM than in the rest of the population (Fig. 3.10). Of the 12 patients in our series, 6 died and 3 were lost to followup; 9 had high lesions and major associated anomalies affecting the heart, the kidneys and the alimentary tracts, and their gonads were either absent or severely hypoplastic. Only 2 patients followed up after reconstruction are doing well; both are male pseudohermaphrodites (MPH) and are reared as boys. The last patient reared as a girl came with a perineal fistula; she had a cloacal malformation and was lost to followup.

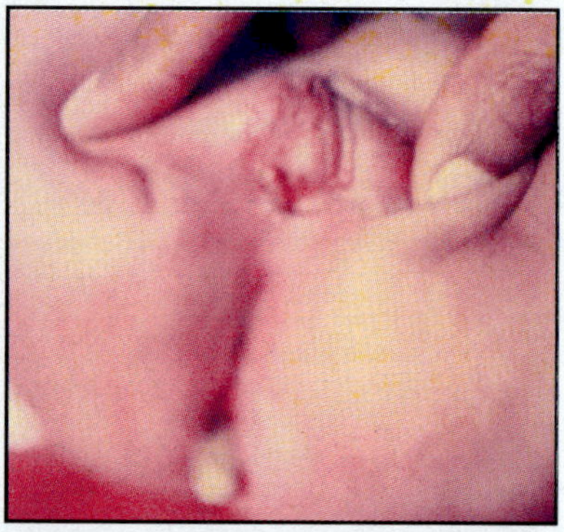

Fig. 3.10 Photograph of baby with ambiguous external genitals and ARM.

Parents in the developing world would like to rear children with ambiguous external genitalia as males and unless an adequate phallus can be developed, they tend to lose interest in having the ARM corrected .

5. *Vertebral*

The only neonatal emergency is open myelomeningocele and the management of the ARM is influenced by the extent of neurological deficit.

The commonest vertebral anomaly and one that profoundly influences the result of treatment is truncation of the sacrum; this will be described in Chapter 15.

Other lesions of the spine that are encountered are closed spinal dysraphism and multiple hemivertebra. Multiple hemivertebra in the thorax is associated with congenital absence of ribs and flail chest with reduced respiratory reserve (Fig 3.11).

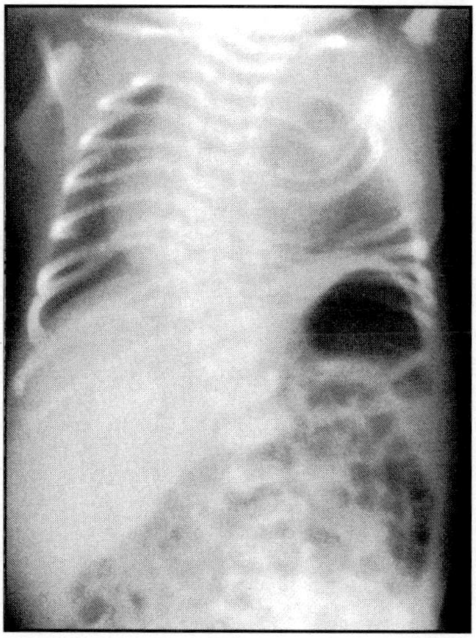

Fig. 3.11 Xray showing multiple hemivertebra and flail chest in a baby with ARM.

These call for special attention during and after operative procedures in infancy. Multiple hemivertebra producing scoliosis calls for prolonged orthopedic support throughout the period of growth. We have two patients with multiple hemivertebras and multiple urological problems who are now adults (Fig. 3.12). They have had many operations both for the anorectal and the urogenital conditions; they have learnt to adjust to the orthopedic condition and with physiotherapy lead normal lives. Our youngest patient had a massive lipomyelomeningocele with paresis, and the parents were initially reluctant to agree to surgery for this condition after perineal correction of the ARM. The operation has been done and quality of life has greatly improved.

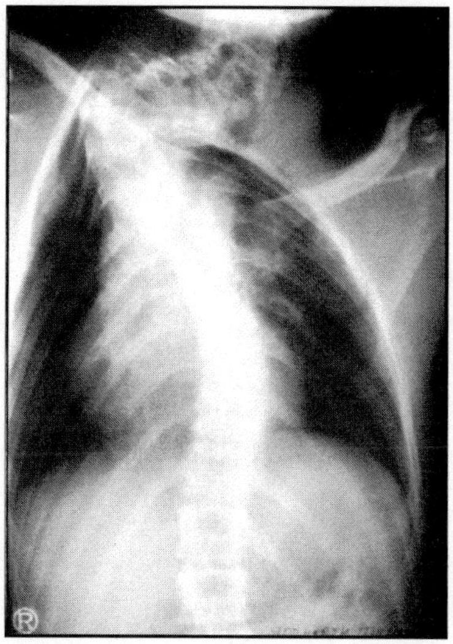

Fig. 3.12 Xray showing multiple hemivertebra with scoliosis in adolescent with ARM

The problem of tethered cord will be discussed in Chapter 15.

A rare anomaly is Currarino triad, ARM with a deformed sacrum and a presacral teratoma; we have a single case; the baby was lost to followup after colostomy.

6. Brain/ Special senses/ Endocrine

Surgically correctable disorders of the brain like hydrocephalus and cranial dysraphism do not present major problems. Uncorrectable disorders like microcephaly, leucodystrophy and Down's syndrome are the most serious obstacles to a successful cure of the

ARM. While the normal brain can overcome most disabilities; a mentally retarded child finds it difficult to use even a perfectly reconstructed anorectum.

We were initially reluctant to reconstruct babies with Down's syndrome. In 1990 we were persuaded to do so in a two-year-old boy with this syndrome by the father. When seen in 2003 after a long gap the child was reasonably toilet trained and could walk and talk, but had not had any formal education.

The blind and the deaf need special educational and emotional support. If this is available, the ARM can be handled in a routine fashion. Unfortunately, this support is hard to come by in the developing world, and ARMs in the blind and the deaf tend to get rejected. Nevertheless we do have one blind and one deaf child who have good continence after a major reconstruction.

We have two patients with hypothyroidism; this was undetected until tests were done to find out the cause of presistent postreconstruction constipation; this was cured as soon as thyroid hormone was administered.

7. Lungs

We have treated eight cases of Pulmonary agenesis (Basu et al, 2000); three of these had ARM (Fig. 3.13). Managing a baby with one lung has been difficult during a major reconstruction, and also subsequently due to recurrent episodes of respiratory infections. Nevertheless all three are doing well.

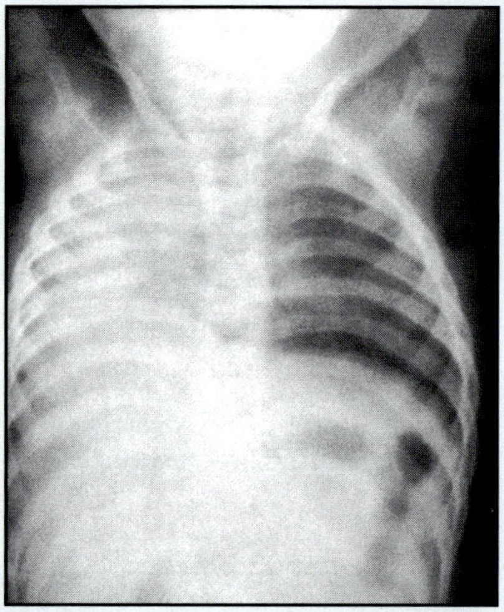

Fig. 3.13 Xray showing agenesis of lung in baby with ARM.

8. Limbs

We have three major limb lesions in our series. A boy with total absence of a lower limb was taken home after colostomy and never returned (Fig. 3.14). A boy with bilateral absence of radial shafts was presented for reconstructive surgery after living with a colostomy for 6 years. He had an uneventful reconstruction but was not brought back for discontinuance of colostomy. We were more fortunate with our third patient who was born with a grossly

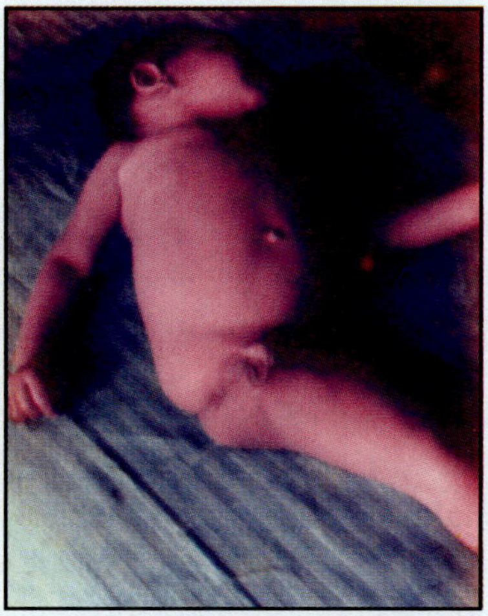

Fig. 3.14 Photograph of baby with absent lower limb and ARM.

deformed right lower limb and major urogenital malformations. He is now 10 years old, has had multiple operations and leads a normal life (Fig. 3.15).

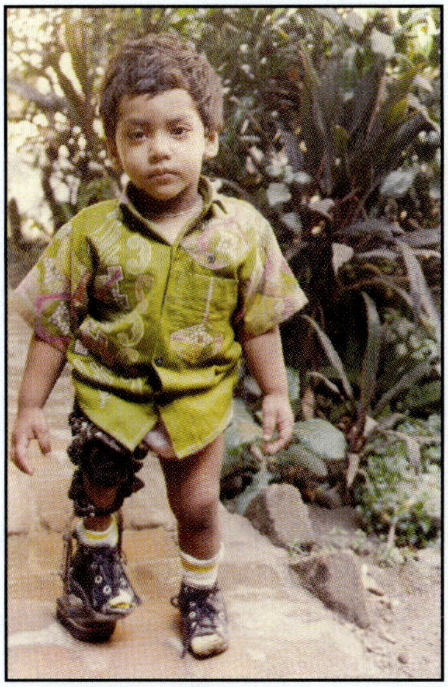

Fig. 3.15 Photograph of boy born with ARM and multiple urological and skeletal malformations.

IMAGING

The diagnosis of the anatomy of the ARM, its complications and associated anomalies is to a very large extent dependent on good imaging. Good imaging also reveals the complications of management and ensures accurate assessment of the results of treatment. Hence the next few pages will be devoted to the place of imaging of patients with ARM. The history of imaging for this condition has been described in Chapter 1. The present day scenario will be discussed here.

Xray

Invertogram has been the time-honored method of studying a newborn with ARM. Much of what Stephens had taught in 1969 still holds. However, invertograms will only show the terminal bowel after it has become distended with swallowed air. This generally takes 12 to 18 hours unless there is an associated TEF. On the other hand gas will not reach at all if there is an associated atresia at one segment or another of the gastrointestinal tract. Even without these problems, invertograms may give both falsely high and falsely low results. The gas may fail to descend if meconium cannot be dislodged from the terminal bowel, if there is spasm of the levator or if gas escapes through a large fistula. It may descend too low even below the I line if the baby presents late with huge abdominal distension and is crying and straining; the invertogram will suggest a low anomaly although the bowel has in fact terminated fairly high up. Occasionally the invertogram shows gas in the urogenital organs and the presence of a fistula is confirmed (see page 137).

Today, most centers including our own perform invertograms using the prone crosstable lateral view developed in Chandigarh. The baby is more relaxed with muscle spasm reduced and the cephalad pull of gravity on the rectum eliminated. It is claimed that the escape of gas through a fistula is much less and the level of the gas shadow reaches 1 to 4 mm lower than in the standard invertogram. Its greatest advantage is that it does not encourage reflux into the tracheobronchial tree in a patient with an associated TEF.

A neonatal straight erect Xray of the chest, abdomen and pelvis, is a fundamental tool in displaying or eliminating some major associated anomalies of the gastrointestinal tract, situs inversus, cardiothoracic malformations and spinal, particularly sacral, anomalies. The planning of the initial operation depends greatly on this examination.

Xray after instillation of contrast through the urethra or vagina has great value. A urethrogram on a boy without a visible opening of the bowel can show, on a lateral view, both the level of the terminal bowel and the nature and level of a fistula if the contrast passes through the fistula from the urethra or bladder. Similarly a vaginogram in a girl without a visible opening of the bowel may show the nature and level of a vaginal fistula and the level of the terminal bowel if contrast passes through the fistula. This examination can also show different varieties of vaginal malformations. However failure to detect a fistula does not exclude the presence of a small fistula.

Xray after instillation of contrast through an abnormal orifice in the perineum also yields useful information about the level of the terminal bowel and its caliber in both boys and girls. However this is not generally crucial to initial management.

A Post-Colostomy Distal Cologram still remains the sheet anchor in diagnosis of the majority of patients with ARM who have had a colostomy. This is generally done one week after colostomy but can be done any time thereafter. Since the contrast used is likely to enter the urinary tract, a sterile soluble organic iodine contrast is essential. Moreover, Barium encourages the formation of inextricable meconioliths and should be avoided. Before the examination the distal bowel must be washed clean with warm sterile saline through a soft rubber tube; some of the fluid is likely to emerge through the urogenital orifices. A transverse colostomy and a long interval between colostomy and washouts make things difficult. We use a soft rubber tube or a balloon catheter; if a balloon catheter is used, a fistula is revealed more easily but care must be taken not to inject the contrast forcibly; bowel ending without a fistula may be perforated. The examination is conducted under fluoroscopy. The lateral view shows the terminal bowel and delineates a fistula if present. The PA view shows the length of available bowel distal to the colostomy. When a distal cologram done through a right upper quadrant colostomy fails to show colon in the left half of the abdomen, two possibilities have to be considered. Either there is congenital absence of the left colon or a sigmoid colostomy has been inadvertently performed in the right upper quadrant. A proximal cologram is required to differentiate between the two. On the other hand, a left lower quadrant distal cologram may show the whole length of left colon if inadvertently the transverse colon had been brought down to the left lower quadrant (see Chapter 6).

For patients with Rectal Atresia the distal cologram should be carried out with a bougie in the anal canal. The gap between the two ends of bowel is indicated by the distance between the radioopaque fluid in the bowel distal to the colostomy and the tip of the anal bougie (see Chapter 12).

The Postreconstruction contrast study that is commonly performed is a Barium Enema; this shows the caliber and disposition of the reconstructed bowel. When the patient is studied during defecation, the examination is termed a **Defecogram.**

Contrast study of the urinary tract shows up associated urological abnormalities. Whether these should be done routinely in all patients or only when anomalies are suspected on the basis of ultrasonography is debatable.Whether contrast Xray should give place to isotope imaging is also debatable. The 2 standard investigations that have been carried out on a large number of our patients are the voiding cystourethrogram (VCU) and the intravenous urogram (IVU). The former delineates the urinary bladder and urethra and shows or excludes vesicoureteral reflux and fistulas into the bowel. The latter shows the structure and function of the kidneys, ureters and bladder.

Isotope Scan

This modality has been used to study the urinary tract of our more recent patients. There is greater accuracy in functional assessment and freedom from ionizing radiation.

Ultrasonogram

In our opinion, ultrasonography (USG) is the best and quickest method of determining the level of the terminal bowel of babies born without a visible opening of the bowel. It is done by the method described by Schuster in 1979. The baby is kept supine and the hypogastric region is scanned in the sagittal plane. The relation of the bowel to the sacrum, the urogenital organs and the perineal skin can be determined very soon after birth. After this is done the position and morphology of the kidneys and ureters are recorded, and the examination concluded by examining the female genitalia and the heart and great vessels. USG is totally noninvasive, causes least disturbance to a small patient, is relatively cheap and can be repeated as often as necessary. However results are observe dependent and the investigation is most valuable if the surgeon and the imaging consultant work together.

Prenatal USG can detect obstruction of the large bowel but cannot at present demonstrate its cause. It can also detect several associated anomalies.

The latest refinement of USG is anal endosonography. With a rotating endoprobe and 2 transducers, the muscles around the anal canal can be accurately mapped out. Jones *et al* (2003) have reported a study performed on 30 normal infants and children and 15 after surgery for ARM. The study was done under general anesthesia. In normal subjects it clearly delineated the puborectalis sling, the external anal sphincter and the internal sphincter. The appearance of the external anal sphincter varied in the 2 sexes; it was incomplete anteriorly in the mid anal canal level in the females. There was no internal anal sphincter in the 2 patients operated for high lesions. The anatomy was found distorted in 2 girls operated for intermediate lesions; it was restored in 1 following revisional surgery. In the other 11 patients the postoperative appearance was normal.

CT Scan

Since 1985, the CT scan had been used to show the disposition of the striated muscle complex before and after reconstructive surgery. It can also show the caliber and situation of the bowel and the presence and nature of fistulas. With the availability of spiral imaging a three dimensional view of both the malformation and the result of treatment can be obtained. In patients with a less than satisfactory result it offers clear evidence of whether the pullthrough of the bowel had missed the sphincter complex or whether the muscles themselves were too hypoplastic to be of use. It is less expensive than MRI but it does subject the patient to the hazard of ionizing radiation. It is no longer recommended for neonates.

MRI Scan

The role of MRI in evaluating patients with ARM is now unquestioned. Because of its multiplanar imaging capability and superb tissue characterization it not only allows accurate definition of the level and type of ARM, type of fistula and developmental state of the surrounding skeletal muscle but also determines associated anomalies of the spinal cord, spinal vertebrae and the urogenital system. There is no ionizing radiation and no contrast is necessary. Moreover, the high lipid content of meconium enhances the signal in neonates.

Sachs in 1990 described 10 cases, 4 before and 6 after repair; three were newborns. He found that spinal and urological anomalies were easily detected and that more detail was available in the larger patients. In 1993, Fukuys *et al* and in 1995 McHugh *et al* reported their studies on the value of MRI in patients with ARM.

In 2002, Nievelstein and his colleagues reported on 49 patients, 24 before and 25 after repair. They found that the level of the lesion was correctly recorded in 96% of patients, fistulas were correctly recorded in 5 out of 9 clinically proven fistulas. They found that 51% had associated spinal anomalies and 37% had associated urogenital anomalies.

Also in 2002, Shah from Ahmedabad described his experience of studying 11 males and 9 females with ARM. General anesthesia with Ketamine and Diazepam was given to all. A fistula was seen in 5 of the 10 cases studied prior to reconstruction. A cloacal malformation was not clearly visualized. On the other hand, the level of the bowel, the disposition of the muscles, associated anomalies and the causes of poor postoperative results were well demonstrated. A routine prenatal MRI examination has led to the diagnosis of ARM by Kuwashima *et al* in Japan in 2001.

There are three problems with MRI.

1. The cost precludes its routine use in the developing world; here its use is restricted to problem patients, affluent patients and research.
2. It is a lengthy examination and a great deal of sedation and close monitoring is necessary. Hence MRI is best avoided on small ill babies.
3. Fistulas have been missed in a large percentage of cases. It is reported that the introduction of a new modality will soon solve this problem.

At present we agree with the Bristol group (Aslam *et al* 1998) that MRI does not have a role in deciding primary therapy for ARM but is extremely useful in detecting spinal problems and locating the cause of a less than satisfactory postoperative result.

Two concluding statements have to be made:

One, the more imaging that is done the more associated anomalies will be revealed, and

Two, no amount of imaging can substitute for a good clinical examination.

CHAPTER 4

EMBRYOLOGY

Ever since the publication of the first monograph on the etiology, pathology and management of congenital malformations of the anus and rectum by Bodenhammer in 1860, there have been attempts to classify and explain the various malformations on the basis of embryology. For nearly 125 years it had not been possible to obtain direct evidence of the steps of normal and abnormal development; nevertheless a great deal had been achieved by random studies of human embryos and of a variety of laboratory animals. The specimens were examined macroscopically and by light microscopy. The torchbearers of the 19th century were Tourneux, Rathke, Retterer and Keibel and Mall; in the 20th century, Keith, (1908, 1948) Bill and Johnson (1958), Stephens (1953, 1983), and Jit from Chandigarh (1975) carried out further studies.

NEW ADVANCES

Over the last two decades, embryological studies have undergone a radical change because of three major developments.

1. The advent of the scanning electronic microscope and three dimensional computer imaging has allowed a high degree of resolution and appreciation of the structures of embryos with a degree of accuracy not dreamt of in the past. Using the very special technique that gave a three dimensional rendering of the tissues Paidas and his colleagues in Baltimore studied human specimens. In 2000 they reported their findings on twelve embryos and five fetuses from the Carnegie collection and their own Department of Pathology. Hutson's group from Melbourne also studied human embryos using material stored in selected institutions in London, Cambridge, Rotterdam and Paris (Penington and Hutson, 2003).
2. Obviously a controlled supply of human embryos cannot be organized and access to a human embryo with an ARM is unpredictable. Hence animal models were sought. The three animal models that have an embryological pattern closely resembling humans and have been extensively used are the pig, the rat and the mouse.

The first is the pig. Farmers had known for some time that ARMs are seen in newborn piglets and that this trait is hereditary. As described in Chapter 1, Van der Putte and his colleagues in the Netherlands located a herd of pigs with this hereditary trait. They studied in the 1980s 41 pig embryos and fetuses and newborn piglets with ARM and 28 with out ARM. In 1987, Lambrecht and

Lierse reported from Hamburg their study of normal and abnormal newborn piglets. A group led by Okhawa under took similar studies in Japan in the 1990s and developed a method for mass production of these anomalies. The team operated upon the malformed piglets and used them for experimental mating. Up to 1999, 108 and embryos and fetuses had been studied.

The obvious disadvantage of using a large animal with a long gestational period of 115 days led to the use of Sprague Dawley rats by Kluth and his team in Hamburg. In 1995 they reported a study of 376 normal rat embryos between the ages of 11 and 17 days. Beasley's team in Christchurch (Qi BQ *et al*, 2000 & 2003) and Hutson's team in Melbourne (2001, 2003) reported on similar studies. Next ARMs were produced in rats by administering teratogenic agents to pregnant rats on appropriate days of gestation. The drugs commonly used have been adriamycin and ethylene thiourea.

The shorttailed (SD) mouse was next studied. ARMs were found in a spontaneous mutation, and homozygous and heterozygous offspring of these mice were found to have not only ARMs but also skeletal and urogenital malformations. Apart from Kluth and Beasley, Kimmel from Toronto have reported extensive studies on these mice.

3. Recent advances in molecular biology and genetics have been mind boggling. Techniques involving recombinant DNA and FISH have shed light into the genetic basis of normal development and the precise stage at which abnormalities occur. It has been shown that embryogenesis is regulated by secretions of specific genes at specific times and locations. Deviations from the normal process occur when in appropriate signals are received. Modern day scientists can now identify molecules that secrete substancesinducing the formation, development and apoptosis or cell death of various embryological structures.

Normal Development — Basic Facts (Sadler, 2000)

The hindgut develops between the 4th and 8th week of intrauterine life, that is, between the 4 mm. and the 30 mm. crown rump stages. The process begins at the hind end of the embryonic disc; here ectoderm is separated from endoderm by unsplit mesoderm everywhere except over an area in the midline between the primitive streak and the body stalk; this area is named cloacal membrane (Fig. 4.1).

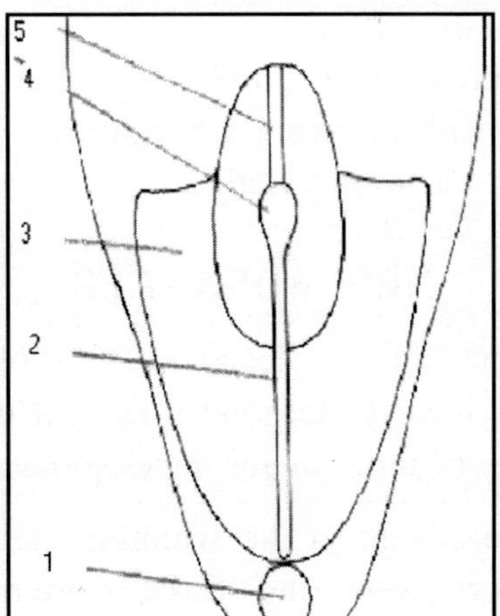

Fig. 4.1 Dorsal view of germdisc at 4th week showing cloacal membrane (1); primitive streak (2); mesoderm (3); primitive node (4); notochord (5).

At the beginning of the 4th week the embryo undergoes cephalocaudal and lateral folding, and part of the endodermal lining of the yolksac is drawn into the body of the embryo to form the gastrointestinal tract. The folding is most prominent in the head and tail. With progressive infolding its broad connection with the yolk sac gradually narrows around the body stalk to form the vitellointestinal duct. The part within the tailfold forms the hindgut. A diverticulum named allantois extends within the body stalk (Figs. 4.2-3). The cloacal cavity is the name given to the part of the endodermal cavity that is enclosed within the tail fold between the entry of the allantois and the cloacal membrane. The hindgut, the postanal or tail gut, the allantois and the mesonephric ducts open into it.

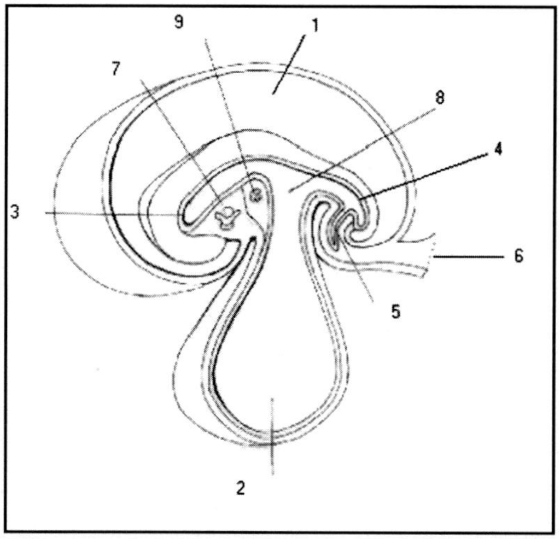

Fig. 4.3 The same at 5th week showing further folding and the appearance of midgut (8) between liver anlage (9) and body stalk.

Cephalad to the primitive streak is the primitive node. From here the definitive notochord is formed; this consists of a solid cord of cells migrating from the cranialmost part of the node. The notochord underlies the neural tube and forms the basis of the axial skeleton. Mesodermal proliferation from the node and the primitive streak forms the paraxial mesoderm, intermediate mesoderm and lateral plate mesoderm (Fig 4.4). The fundamental functions of the

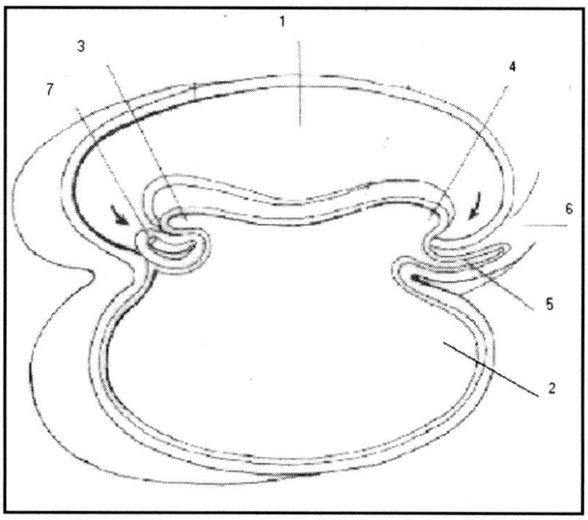

Fig. 4.2 Sagittal section of embryo at 4th week showing folding; amniotic cavity (1); yolksac (2); foregut (3); hindgut (4); allantois (5); bodystalk (6); heart anlage (7)

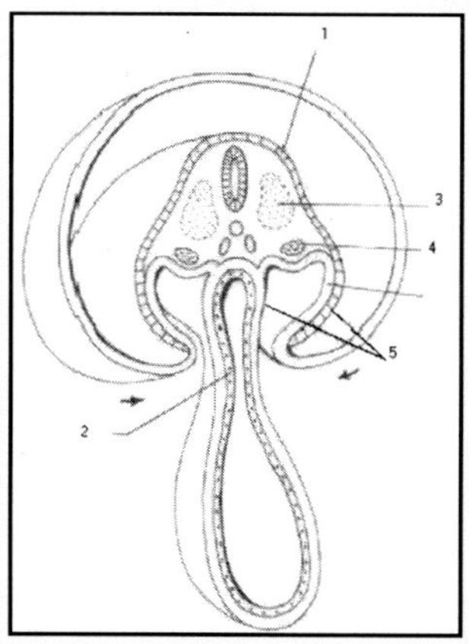

Fig. 4.4 Coronal section at 5th week showing the narrowing connection between the midgut and the yolksac, the ectodermal (1) and endodermal (2) lining and the differentiation of the mesoderm into paraxial mesoderm (3), intermediate mesoderm (4) and lateral plate mesoderm (5).

notochord during early embryogenesis are to provide craniocaudal orientation and ventrodorsal patterning and to act as a primary organizer for adjacent organs, namely the spinal cord, vertebral column, gut and urinary organs. It then separates from the ectoderm and endoderm in a craniocaudal sequence and becomes the axis of the developing vertebral column.

Extraembryonic mesoderm proliferating beneath the body stalk carries the cloacal membrane backwards. Subsequently the cloaca grows, lengthens, expands and rotates through a process called transformation. Axial growth of the neural tube contributes to this transformation and the neighboring musculoskeletal structures are also involved. Simultaneous growth of mesoderm in the angle between the allantois and the hindgut results in the formation of a urorectal septum (Fig. 4.5). This appears to descend towards the cloacal membrane.

How the cloaca develops into a ventral urogenital sinus and a dorsal anorectum has been a matter of debate for over a century. Most embryologists of an earlier era had taught that the cloaca is partitioned by the descent of the urorectal septum and its fusion with the lateral walls of the cloaca. Embryologists of a later era have shown that there is a downgrowth of the urorectal septum but no lateral folds appear; the urorectal septum has a rounded free lower edge in both sagittal and coronal sections. The separation is mainly due to the remarkable outgrowth of the cloaca in a ventral direction and rotation of the cloacal membrane. Thus the major part of the cloaca becomes the urogenital sinus and the hindgut opens into it. The tip of the urorectal septum comes to lie close to the cloacal membrane; there is no evidence to show that the two structures actually make contact. Embryologists of the 21st century (Nievelstein, 2002) believe that the dorsal cloaca is 'by no means involved in the developing anorectum' and that the whole of the cloaca becomes the urogenital sinus; in other words, the hindgut directly reaches the cloacal membrane (Fig. 4.6).

Mesodermal proliferation around the cloacal membrane results in the formation

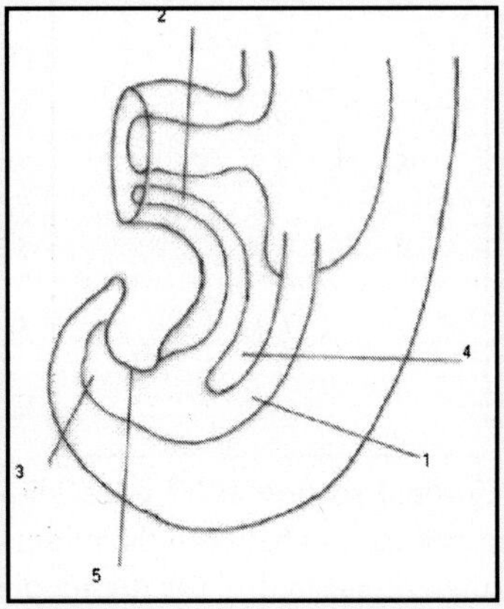

Fig. 4.5 Sagittal section of embryo at 6th week showing hindgut (1), urogenital sinus (2); cloaca (3); urorectal septum (4); cloacal membrane (5).

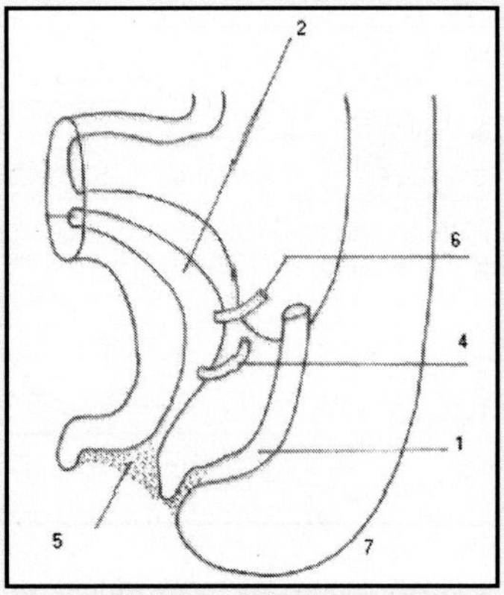

Fig. 4.6 Sagittal section of embryo at 7th week showing descent of urorectal septum to reach the cloacal membrane and appearance of the mesonephric ducts (6).

of a pair of cloacal folds. They unite cranially to form the genital tubercle; growth of the genital tubercle is associated with the ventral development of the cloaca. Caudally the folds form urethral folds anteriorly and anal folds posteriorly. Larger swellings appear lateral to the urethral folds and are called genital swellings .

Subsequently, most of the tail gut is incorporated into the embryo. Its remnant, as well as the cloacal membrane, disintegrates by apoptosis. This results in a large ventral opening for the urogenital sinus between the urethral folds and a smaller dorsal opening for the hindgut between the anal folds. The tip of the urorectal septum remains in between and will become the perineal body.

At the same time, there is proliferation of ectoderm around the hindgut opening; this protrudes into and closes the opening. Later it recanalizes to join the bowel above and forms the ectodermal part or the terminal half of the anal canal (Fig. 4.7).

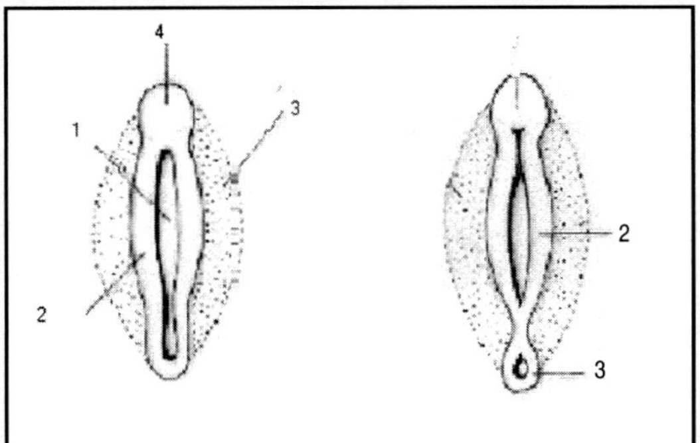

Fig. 4.7 Surface view of the perineum showing (A), at 4 weeks, cloacal membrane (1), surrounded by cloacal folds (2) and genital folds (3); these meet to form the genital tubercle (4). B), at 6 weeks, the cloacal folds become urethral folds (2) and anal folds (3) and the cloacal membrane divides into two.

The endodermal hindgut gives rise to the epithelial lining of the left third of the transverse colon, the descending and sigmoid colon, the rectum and the proximal half of the anal canal. Its musculature arises from the visceral layer of the lateral plate mesoderm. Mesoderm also forms all the striated muscles.

Next, the urogenital sinus elongates anteriorly with the growth of the genital tubercle and differentiates into 3 parts.

The upper and largest part is continuous with the allantois and forms the greater part of the urinary bladder. The allantois obliterates and remains as a fibrous cord, the urachus.

The middle or pelvic part is a narrow canal into which the mesonephric ducts open; this gives rise to the whole of the female urethra and the prostatic and membraneous parts of the male urethra. A ureteric bud arises from the terminal end of each mesonephric duct; with craniolateral movement of the ureteric buds the junctional area widens to form the trigone of the bladder and upper urethra. The ureters open superolaterally and the mesonephric ducts open inferomedially (Fig. 4.8). Since the mesonephric ducts develop from mesoderm, this area is of mesodermal origin. In the male, the mesonephric ducts become the ejaculatory ducts; they remain vestigial in the female.

The last or phallic part differs in the 2 sexes. The large ventral opening of the urogenital sinus extends under the growing genital tubercle in the male and is closed by fusion of the urethral folds that had formed on either side of the cloacal membrane. In the female, the opening becomes the vesti-

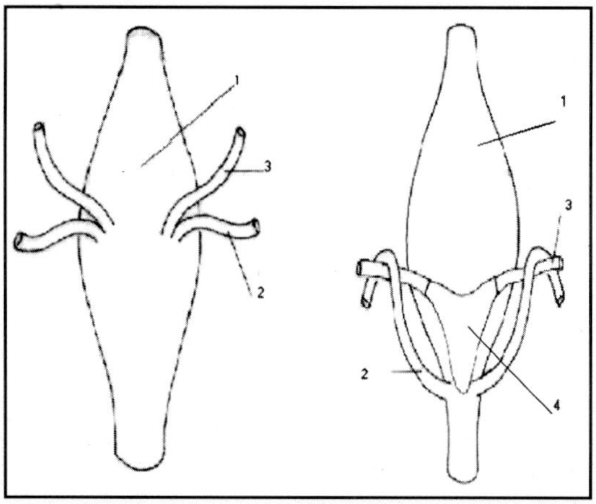

Fig. 4.8. Diagram of urogenital sinus (1); (A) it receives the mesonephric ducts (2); the ureteric buds (3) arise from their lower ends; the ureteric buds ascend and create the triangular area (4) seen in (B).

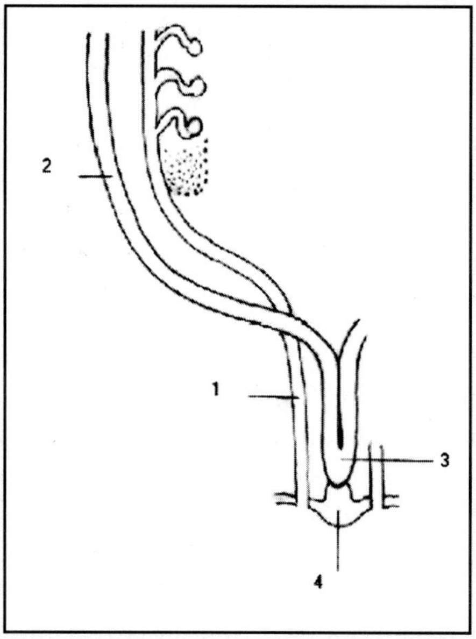

Fig. 4.9 Diagram of female embryo at 2nd month showing the mesonephric ducts (1) with renal anlage; the paramesonephric ducts (2) fusing to form the paramesonephric tubercle (3) and meeting the sinovaginal bulbs (4).

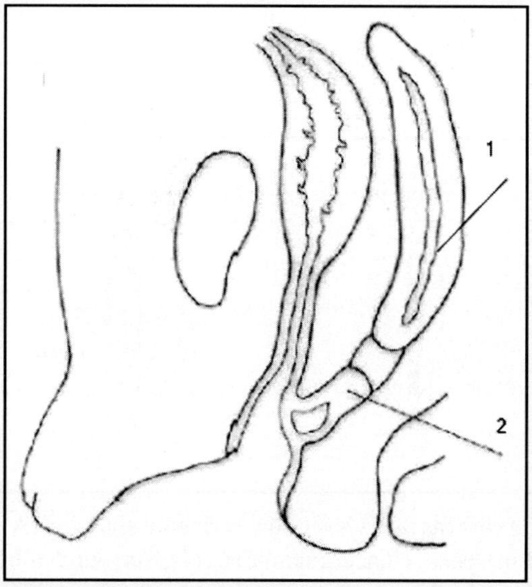

Fig. 4.10 Sagittal view of female embryo at 3rd month showing formation of uterus and vagina from fused paramesonephric ducts and tubercle (1) and sinovaginal bulbs (2).

bule. The urethra enters into it. Two ducts named paramesonephric ducts develop on either side of the mesonephric ducts and unite in the midline to form a tubercle named paramesonephric tubercle (Fig 4.9). This reaches the urogenital sinus. They are of mesodermal origin and form the uterine tubes, the uterus and the upper third of the vagina. The lower two thirds of the vagina is developed by canalization of two solid evaginations named sinovaginal bulbs that grow from the dorsal aspect of the urogenital sinus, fuse with each other and meet the paramesonephric tubercle (Fig. 4.10). Other aspects of development of the urogenital organs are not relevant to this presentation.

Abnormal Development

Van der Putte associated ARM with agenesis of the dorsal part of the cloacal membrane. When a greater or lesser part of this is missing, the dorsal cloaca does not develop and fails to reach the surface; its distance from the surface is proportional to the size of the missing segment of the cloacal membrane. The hindgut continues to open into the cloaca at a greater or lesser distance from the surface and the endoderm of the hindgut is separated from the surface ectoderm by mesoderm of varying thickness. When the defect is minimal and there is only a thin layer of intervening mesoderm, the gut reaches close to the surface and low malformations result. When the defect is large, there are progressive higher malformations. Kluth's findings are similar. Further he noted impairment of the usual caudal movement of the urorectal septum. Persistence of the opening of the hindgut into the urogenital sinus results in the formation of the various fistulas found in animal models and humans born with ARM.

Apart from agenesis of the dorsal part of the cloacal membrane, other malformations can occur. If the whole of the cloacal membrane is missing, neither the urogenital nor the alimentary tracts will reach the surface, we have a patient with this anomaly (see Chapter 14). If there is interrupted breakdown double openings result.

On the basis of his studies on teratogen induced malformations Beasley has recently postulated that the notochord plays a pivotal role in controlling hindgut development. The genetic basis of the malformations appears to be alterations in sonic hedgehog signalling at crucial periods of embryogenesis.

On the basis of MRI studies, Nievelstein *et al* have classified ARMs into two types, those occurring as a result of a disturbance during the early embryonic period and those occurring in the later embryonic period. The latter are low malformations, generally without associated anomalies. In the former, the bowel opens into the urogenital organs or is connected to them by fibrotic strands; associated anomalies of the spinal cord and spine and urogenital structures are more common.

In spite of many advances, some gray areas remain. A spectrum of clinical malformations has to be explained, and suitable animal models have not yet evolved.

Firstly, it is still not clear how precisely the opening of the hindgut into the cloaca closes, and how it acquires a new opening at the level of the cloacal membrane. Keith had written in 1948 that "in the 7th week, the rectum having reached the anal part of the cloacal membrane forms a new opening, the former opening into the cloaca becoming closed. But as we have seen the cloacal anus may persist and the true anus fail to form". Bill and Johnson in 1958 had stated that the rectum and anal canal develop "by a process of growth and caudal migration"; the growing tip was considered the opening of the hindgut into the cloaca. We had postulated that the growing tip was distal to the cloacal opening, and that a new opening at the cloacal membrane can form with the earlier opening remaining patent. With this hypothesis, it was possible to explain double distal openings of the gut, particularly when one opening was high up. Obviously, if the cloacal opening closes without the formation of any new opening, there will be a malformation without a fistula.

Secondly, the ectodermal proliferation near the hindgut opening has been shown to join the bowel above in the course of normal development and to recanalize to form the ectodermal part or the terminal half of the anal canal. If the hindgut does not reach the region of the cloacal membrane, the ectoderm remains on the surface, as Nixon had pointed out in 1968, "not agenetic but everted". We had postulated that the ectoderm around the opening of the hindgut gut is normally drawn into the body of the embryo as a result of cephalic traction on the hindgut at the time of migration of the midgut into the extraembryonic cavity. This can explain the absence of an anal pit in almost all ARM patients.

Thirdly, there are problems with low anomalies. An ectopic anterior opening of the bowel on the surface can occur in two ways. Either there has been failure of caudal migration or the opening has been covered over after migration by the fusion of the two anal folds on either side. Stenotic lesions are undoubtedly produced by insufficient recanalization of the ectodermal proliferation.

Fourthly, there are problems with high lesions. In the majority the opening of the hindgut into the cloaca is found caudal to the tissue that forms from the mesonephric ducts. If this opening fails to close, there is a fistula into the pelvic part of the urogenital sinus; namely the male urethra, or that part of the vagina that is developed from the urogenital sinus. However occasionally, the hindgut opens more cranially and this opening lies between the tissues formed from the mesonephric ducts of the two sides. Its persistence gives rise to a rectovesical fistula and the trigone and internal meatus are improperly formed. In fact all the structures that develop from mesonephros are likely to be poorly formed. This includes the ureters, the ejaculatory ducts, the seminal vesicles and the prostate. In a female with a rectovesical fistula, the paramesonephric ducts do not fuse and either a duplex or a unicornuate uterovaginal system will result.

Fifthly, there are girls with vaginal malformations. Atresia of the vagina occurs if the sinovaginal bulbs fail to develop; the upper vagina originating from the paramesonephric ducts remains as a blind pouch around the cervix. If the sinovaginal bulbs fail to fuse, a double vagina results. Also there may be a common urethrovaginal canal; this may occur in two ways. Either the endodermal vaginal proliferations arise proximally on the urogenital sinus and a common urethrovaginal channel forms after canalization, or the cells separating the vagina and urethra disentegrate and lead to the formation of a common channel.

And finally there is rectal atresia. There is universal agreement that this is due to an ischemic accident of late fetal life that disrupts the continuity of the rectum (Stone & Wilkinson, 1983). The bowel below the atresia is lined by columnar epithelium of the rectum, and stratified squamous epithelium appears only at the lower half of the anal canal (Figs. 4.11-12). However, there are patients who have a congenital ARM as well as atresia; the congenital anomaly being either a blind ending bowel or a fistula connecting the upper bowel to the vestibule.

A discussion on embryology in a recent textbook ends with the debatable sentence that "It is fortunate that satisfactory results may be achieved in the absence of clear embryological guidelines."

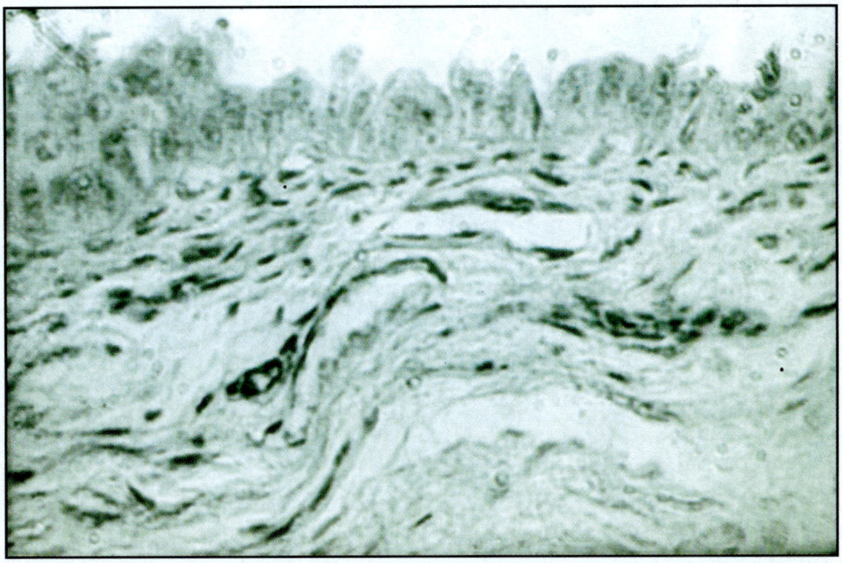

Fig. 4.11 Photomicrograph of tissue of baby with rectal atresia showing columnar epithelium at dome.

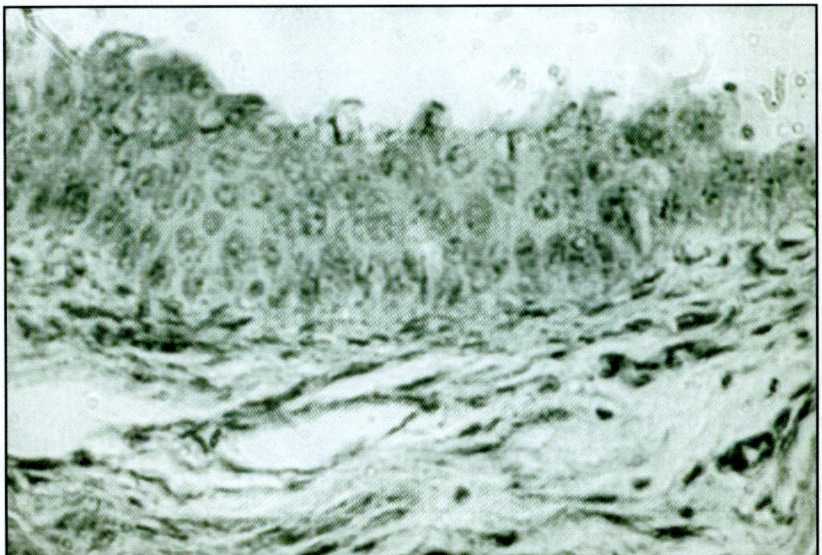

Fig. 4.12 Same, stratified squamous epithelium at anal verge.

CHAPTER 5

PRINCIPLES OF MANAGEMENT

The objectives of management are clearly three.

1. To prevent or relieve intestinal obstruction.
2. To establish normal defecation
3. To preserve or restore normal urogenital function.

The fundamental problem in management is to decide whether the three objectives can be realized simultaneously or separately. At times, a single definitive surgical procedure will realize all the objectives; at others, the latter two objectives can be realized only after intestinal obstruction has been prevented or relieved.

The decision is taken on the basis of the factors that we have discussed in the previous chapter. Before starting treatment the available data is recorded on a form that reads as follows (Table 5.1).

The two methods of preventing or relieving intestinal obstruction without correcting the prime anomaly are **dilatation of a visible fistula and COLOSTOMY**. The next chapter deals with colostomy.

The methods used for restoring normal defecation and preserving or restoring normal urogenital function can be divided into two groups: Extraperitoneal and Intraperitoneal.

We carry out extraperitoneal reconstructions whenever possible and perform an intraperitoneal procedure only if the lesion is uncorrectable by extraperitoneal procedures.

Extraperitoneal Procedures

They are either SIMPLE or COMPLEX:

The simple procedures are:

1. Y-V plasty and its extension, and
2. A limited sagittal anorectoplasty (SARP)

The complex procedures are:

1. Perineal Anal Transplant (PAT)
2. Posterior Sagittal AnoRectoPlasty (PSARP)
3. Posterior Sagittal AnoRectoVagino Plasty (PSARVP)
4. Posterior Sagittal AnoRectoVagino UrethroPlasty (PSARVUP)
5. Anterior Sagittal AnoRectoPlasty (ASARP).

Intraperitoneal Procedures

They are really necessary in about 10% of all patients with ARM. We do intraperitoneal operations only if the terminal bowel ends above the 3rd sacral vertebra, is tethered by an incorrectly performed colostomy or is malformed. The procedures performed today are:

TABLE 5.1

NAME	DATE OF BIRTH	SEX	WEIGHT

GUARDIAN	ADDRESS
PRESENTING SYMPTOMS	
PAST TREATMENT	
GENERAL EXAMINATION:	
ABDOMINAL EXAMINATION	Distension, lumps
	Scar/s
	Colostomy
PERINEAL EXAMINATION	Normal anus Neoanus Scar/s
	Abnormal opening of bowel; Its position, character
	Calibration, direction of tract leading from it
	External Genitalia.
INVESTIGATIONS	Laboratory tests: blood, urine.
	Ultrasound
	Plain Xray
	Contrast Xray
	CT / MRI.
	Endoscopy
	Others

1. AbdominoPerineal AnoRectoPlasty (APARP)
2. PSARP with Laparotomy (PSARPL)
3. PSARVUP with Laparotomy (PSARVUPL)
4. Laparoscopically assisted Abdomino-Perineal AnoRectoPlasty (LAPARP).

The crucial determining factor is the level reached by **bowel of normal or greater caliber** with respect to the levator ani muscle and pari passu to the skeleton of the pelvis.

If the level reached is at or below the lowest part of the ossified ischial bone, namely the I point, the lesion is **LOW.** It has penetrated and is surrounded by levator ani, and can be dealt with by simple perineal procedures.

If it reaches a level between this point and the lower limit of the third sacral vertebra, the lesion is **INTERMEDIATE.** It terminates above the levator ani but lies within the walls of a deepened hammock and it can be dealt with by a complex extraperitoneal procedure. It should be noted that this level is much higher than the PC line of yesteryears; this is because the new exposure allows access to structures placed as high as the 3rd sacral vertebra.

If however it is above the level of the lower border of the third sacral vertebra it is a **HIGH** lesion. It terminates above the levator ani and it can be dealt with only by an **INTRAPERITIONEAL** procedure.

In an earlier era, the gold standard for determining levels was a lateral Xray after instillation of contrast either through a perineal opening if such an opening existed or through the distal end of a colostomy. Today, MRI can determine levels but this is not generally available and in many centers colostomies are being eliminated. Treatment is often begun without determining levels. It is therefore necessary to have a relatively flexible plan and modify the approach as necessary. The level of a lesion can of course be conclusively determined during the operative procedure.

Also, in an earlier era, there was universal agreement that intraperitoneal procedures should be reserved for lesions uncorrectable by extraperitoneal procedures. Today, laparoscopy has added a new dimension to the problem and lesions correctable by extra-peritoneal methods are being treated by laparoscopy. Whether this is justifiable only time will tell.

POSITIONING THE PATIENT

It is a very important matter for all types of reconstructive surgery. The operations can be done either in the prone or supine position.

A. In the Prone Position

We use **The Spreadeagled Position** for most of the operations that we do with the patient prone.

In the 1970s, anorectal reconstructions often called for dissection in the presacral space. This dissection was generally performed with the patient in the jackknife position with the hips flexed and abducted. Dissatisfaction with this position prompted us in 1972 to position our patients differently.

The position was found so satisfactory that we used it routinely not only for procedures which called for opening up of the presacral space, but also for purely perineal anorectal reconstructions, for urethrovaginal reconstructions and subsequently for posterior sagittal reconstructions. We also used it for a massive hamartoma extending from the anus to the tip of the penis. In 1974, the position was described in detail and named 'The Spreadeagled Position' because the patient with the lower limbs splayed out resembled an eagle with outstretched wings.

The position was originally attained with the help of a padded Y shaped splint placed over the pediatric operating table with its median limb on the long axis of the table and the confluence of the Y at the foot end. A large sandbag at this site supported the pubis of the patient laid prone on the splint. The patient's lower limbs were placed and secured over the diverging limbs of the splint with smaller sandbags placed in such a way that the hips were in extension, abduction and neutral rotation and the knees were in extension. After the limbs were fixed, the buttocks were spread apart with adhesive strapping. The proximal end of a flatus tube passed down in the distal opening of a colostomy, if any, was left outside the operating fields (Figs. 5.1-2). In 1982, we designed an operating table with two ball and socket joints. This allowed the two rectangles constituting the distal third of the table not only to flex and extend as in a standard operating table, but also to abduct and rotate.

The operation begins after raising the foot end of the table; the angle of tilt is varied during the course of the operation. The surgeon sits comfortably between the patient's lower limbs and has one assistant standing on either side. The surgeon has access to the back of the sacrum and the whole of the perineum right up to the external urethral meatus of both boys and girls. At any time during the operation instruments can be passed into the urethra and/or vagina and manipulated in and out of fistulas. All structures in the region can be comfortably exposed and dealt with. The surgeon faces the perineum and the two assistants retract the tissues laterally with almost identical force; hence it is much easier to stay in the midline without the help of a muscle stimulator (Fig. 5.3).

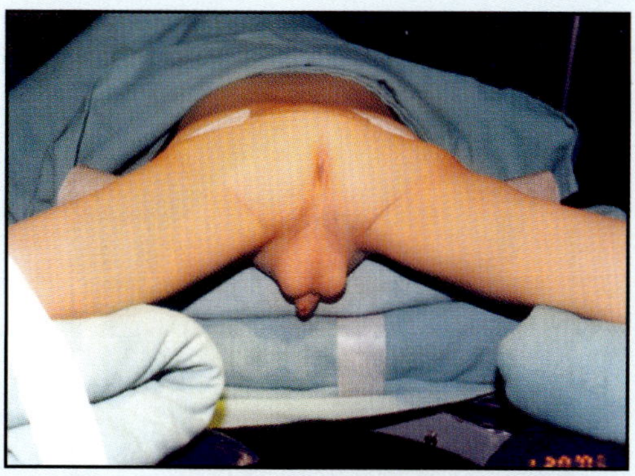

Fig. 5.1 Photograph of boy in spreadeagled position.

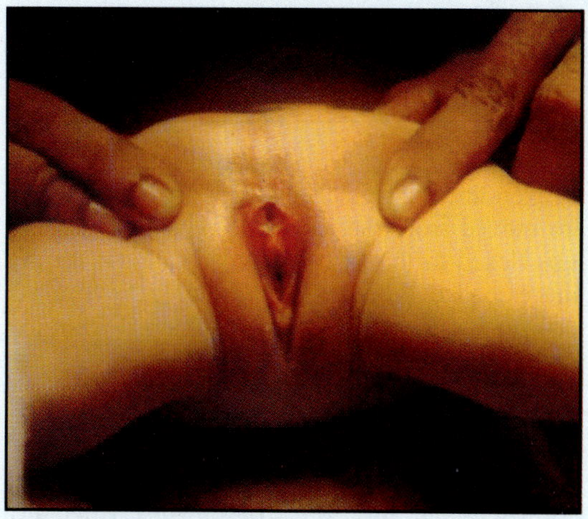

Fig. 5.2 Photograph of girl in spreadeagled position.

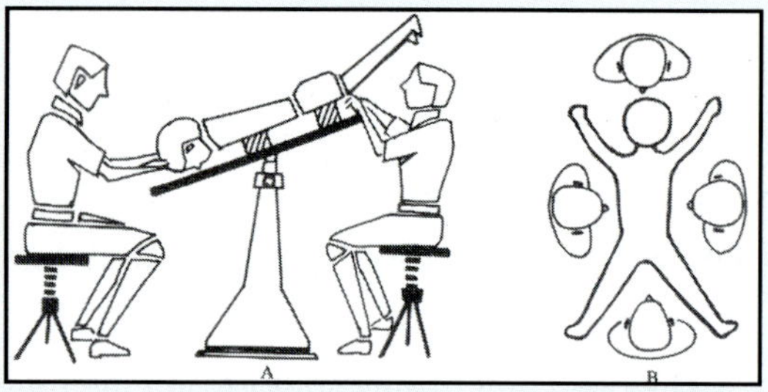

Fig. 5.3 Diagram showing position of operating team a) from the side; b) from above.

The difference between the jackknife and the spreadeagled positions have been studied by us by taking peroperative lateral radiographs. Compared to the jackknife position, the lumbar spine is more lordotic and the sacrum is tilted backwards in the spreadeagled position. The backward tilt is brought about by the stretch of the psoas muscle produced by extending the thighs. The precise geometric result of extension at the hip can be demonstrated by diagrams reconstructed from radiographs (Fig. 5.4).

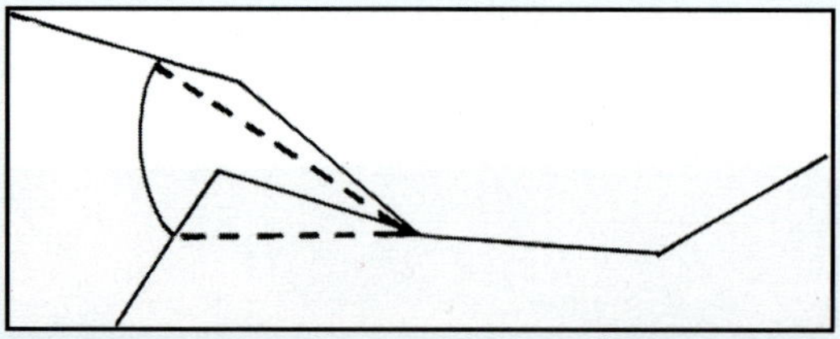

Fig. 5.4 Diagram showing how the iliopsoas muscle (broken lines) is stretched when the lower limbs are moved from the jackknife position with the hips flexed to the spreadeagled position with the hips extended; this stretch exaggerates the lumbar lordosis and the entire perineum comes within the surgeon's reach.

We occasionally use two other positions.

For small patients, the **knee-elbow position** is an acceptable alternative. It produces a similar tilt of the pelvis and affords good exposure of the perineum. The patient can be brought down to the foot end of the operating table and the surgeon can sit facing the perineum; access to the exter-nal genitalia can be arranged by suitable draping. In order to retain the position till the end of the operation, it is necessary to deploy pillows and strapping skillfully (Fig. 5.5).

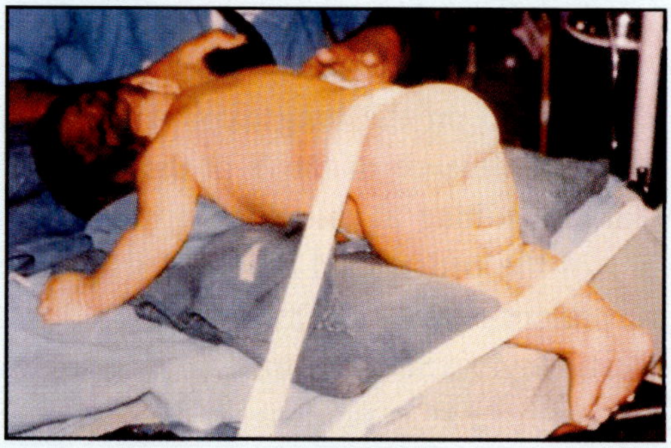

Fig. 5.5 Photograph of baby in knee elbow position.

For adults, **the position described by Hendren** (1980) has been used. The thighs are abducted and extended, the knees are flexed and the legs are suspended with adhesive tape from two sturdy stands on either side (Fig. 5.6).

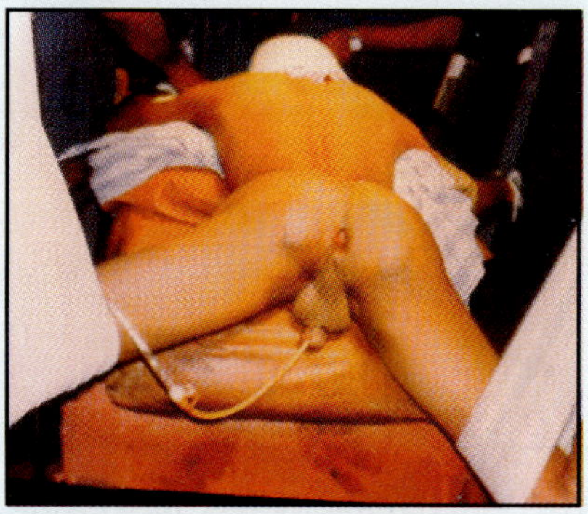

Fig. 5.6 Photograph of adult in Hendren position.

B. In the Supine Position

When we operate with the patient supine, we use **The Frog Position.**

This position is attained by having the lower limbs tucked away on either side of the trunk; the knees are acutely flexed and the hips are flexed, abducted and externally rotated. The patient is brought to the foot end of the operating table. A sandbag is placed under the sacrum and the foot end of the table is raised. Thus the perineum and the abdomen are both accessible, and laparotomy can be carried out if required without turning the patient (Fig. 5.7). We also use this position for operations for Hirschsprung's disease and have not encountered any neuromuscular or skeletal complications.

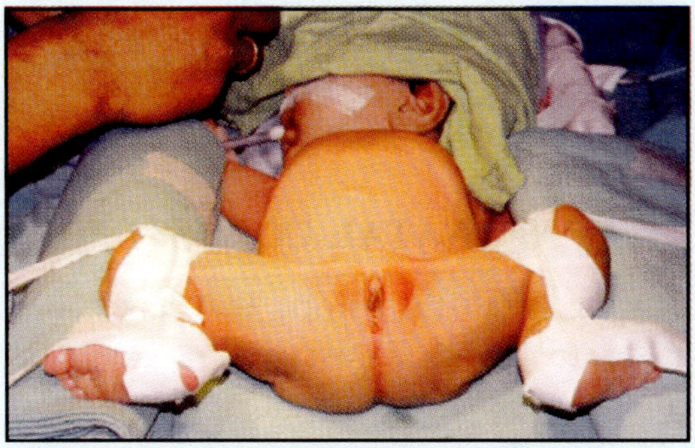

Fig. 5.7 Photograph of a baby in frog position.

CHAPTER 6

COLOSTOMY

THE NEONATAL COLOSTOMY

In spite of all the efforts that have been made to avoid colostomy, a neonatal colostomy is still mandatory if intestinal complications cannot be safely prevented or relieved by other means (Fig. 6.1).

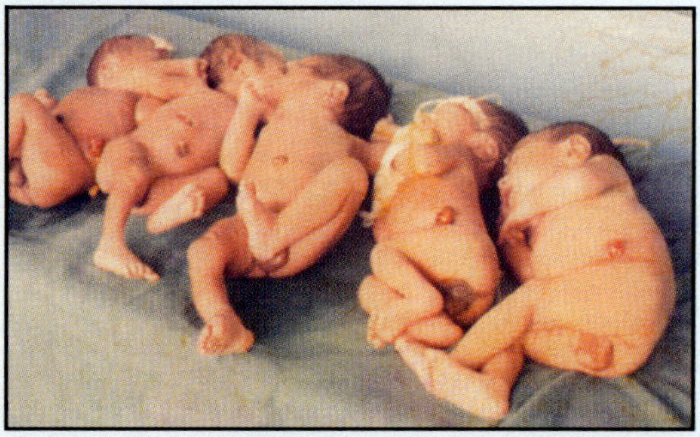

Fig. 6.1 Photograph of five babies with colostomy.

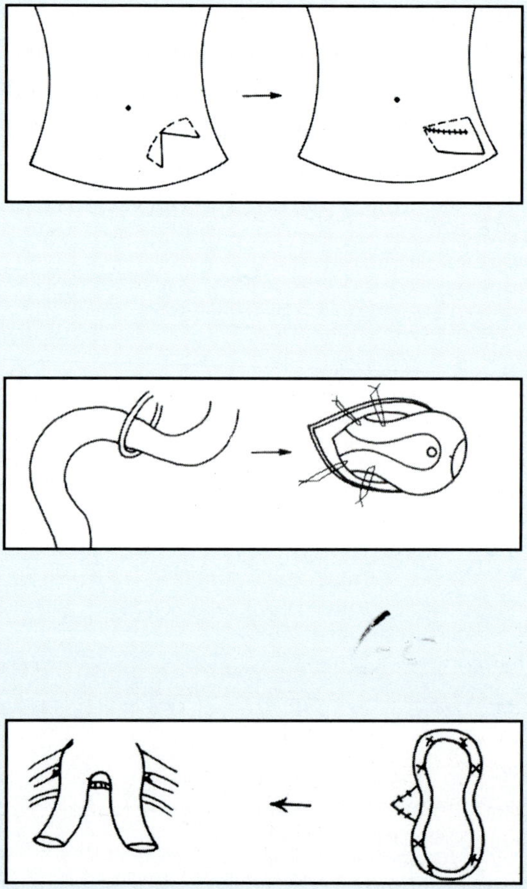

Figs. 6.2-4 Diagrams of left lower quadrant colostomy - V flap & excision of two triangles of skin - incison through flat muscles & peritoneum – exteriorization of loop with a tube – fixation of loop to margins of peritoneum & flat muscles and opening of colon – skin bridge to keep colostomy in place.

The neonatal colostomy should ideally be sited at the most proximal part of the sigmoid colon, and this is done through a left lower quadrant exposure. Before the operation begins, a nasogastric tube is inserted and a venous line is set up.

Our Technique, based on Nixon's Operation (1966) (Figs. 6.2 - 8)

A 'v' incision is made over the left lower quadrant with the base inferolaterally near the anterior superior iliac spine and the apex

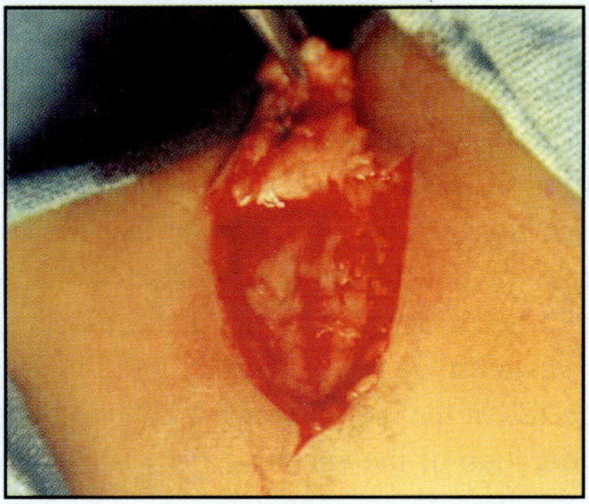
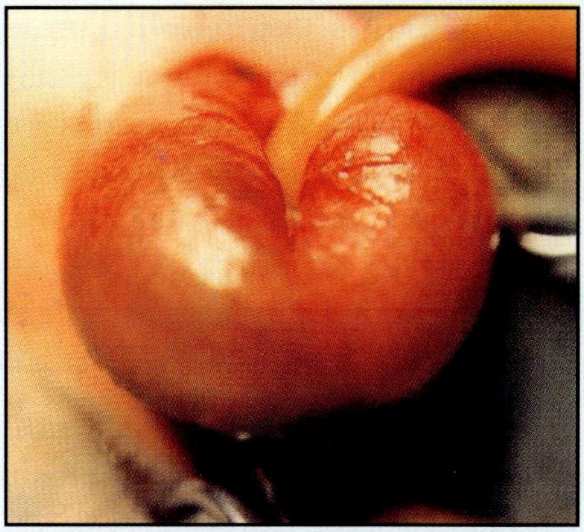
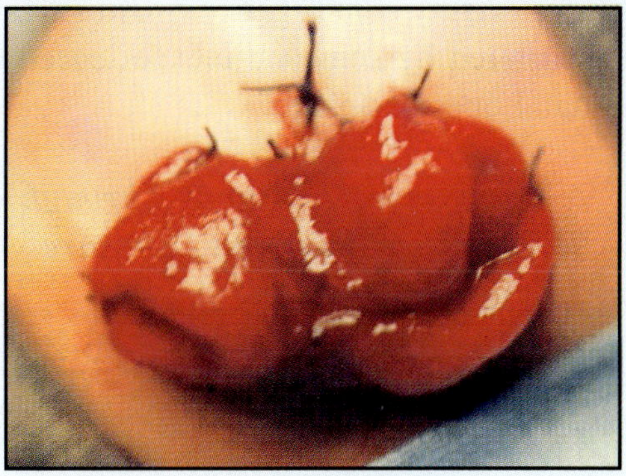
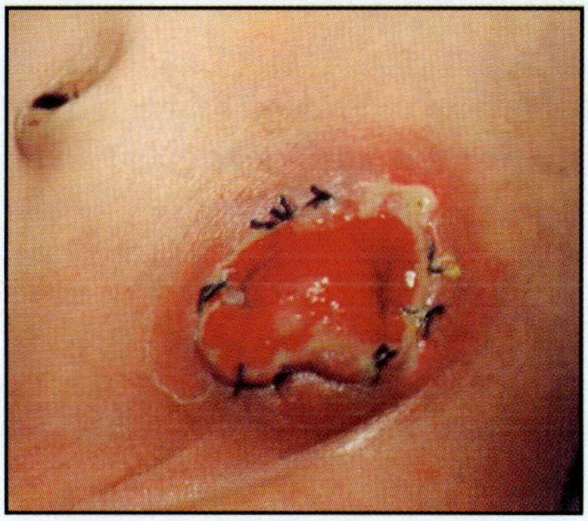

Figs. 6.5-8 Photographs to show the steps.

on the lateral border of the rectus muscle. The flap of skin and subcutaneous tissue is reflected off the external oblique and retracted downwards and outwards. All three flat muscles are divided transversely and the peritoneum is then opened by a transverse incision. The meconium-filled sigmoid loop is identified and exteriorized. It is necessary to decide which end is proximal and which end is distal; the distal loop dilates progressively. Moreover the proximal end is anchored at the left iliac region while the distal end enters the pelvis. The most proximal segment that can be conveniently exteriorized is selected for colostomy. Its vascular arcade is displayed and a soft rubber tube is passed through the mesocolon at an avascular area adjacent to the bowel. The tube is used to draw this segment outside the wound; the rest of the sigmoid is returned to the abdomen.

The cut margins of the peritoneum and the muscles are then sutured to the seromuscular coat of the emerging bowel by two rows of fine interrupted silk sutures. A cruciate incision is made over the top of the exteriorized gut and as meconium spills over, the loop collapses. The loop is then fixed in place with a skin bridge. Two medially based triangles of skin and subcutaneous tissue are excised on either side of the V flap. This is then threaded through the mesocolon along the track made earlier by the rubber tube. The tube is discarded and the apex of the skin flap is sutured in its original place to the skin in the middle of the wound. The cut margins of the colon are apposed to the skin margins on either side, thus establishing epithelial continuity.

Finally, a soft catheter is introduced first into the distal loop and then into the proximal loop. Both are gently irrigated with warm normal saline. With alternate irrigation and suction, both proximal and distal meconium filled loops are emptied and abdominal distension is relieved. The wound is then covered with paraffin gauze and a supporting binder is applied.

There is virtually no blood loss if diathermy is used. Babies operated on the day of birth can be sent back to the mother and put on breast feeds in a day or two.

The operation becomes more difficult when there is delay. The loops of small gut are distended and difficult to keep out of the operating field. It is also difficult to exteriorize the overdistended sigmoid colon. It may be necessary to open the sigmoid in situ once its proximal end can be identified; the emerging meconium has to be prevented from entering the peritoneal cavity by efficient placement of swabs and suction. The sigmoid colon once empty can be exteriorized and the operation can proceed.

Controversies

More controversies surround this operation than any other comparable procedure (Nixon 1966, Brenner and Swenson 1967, Dorairajan 1976 & 1990, Lister 1981 and Wilkins and Pena 1988).

A. *Anesthesia*

A referral institution enjoys the advan-tages of general anesthesia with controlled ventilation administered by an expert. An expert is not easy to come by in peripheral areas of the developing world, and it has been necessary to develop a technique that a surgeon can use single handed with success in the majority of his patients. Local infiltration of the operative field with 3-5ml. 0.5% lignocaine supplemented with minimum doses of intravenous diazepam affords greater safety than general anesthesia administered by someone inexperienced in neonatal anesthesiology.

B. *A Transverse Colostomy Through A Right Upper Quadrant Exposure*

This operation (Fig 6.9) is preferred by some for five reasons.

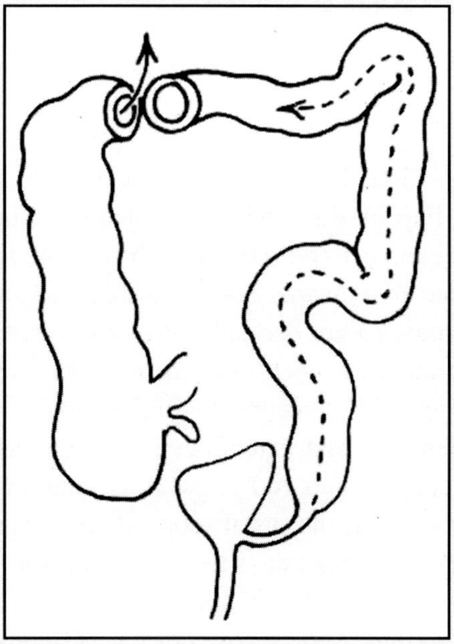

Fig. 6.9 Diagram of right upper quadrant colostomy.

i) It leaves the entire left colon undisturbed for the reconstruction.

   Enough colon distal to a high sigmoid colostomy is in fact available for standard anorectoplasties. However if there is a high cloacal malformation or an associated colonic malformation, a transverse colostomy will be a safer alternative (See Chapters 11 and 14).

ii) The greater omentum attached to the lower margin of the transverse colon protects the peritoneum against bacterial invasion

   Peritoneal contamination occurs in late cases and protection of the greater omentum can certainly be utilized if a transverse colostomy is done.

iii) It is easier to perform than a high sigmoid colostomy.

When the occasional operator performs a colostomy through a left lower quadrant incision, he tends to perform it over the most mobile part of the sigmoid and not at the junction of the fixed and the mobile part. A midsigmoid colostomy indeed results in inadequacy of bowel distal to it and serious problems will have to be solved during the reconstruction (Fig. 6.10).

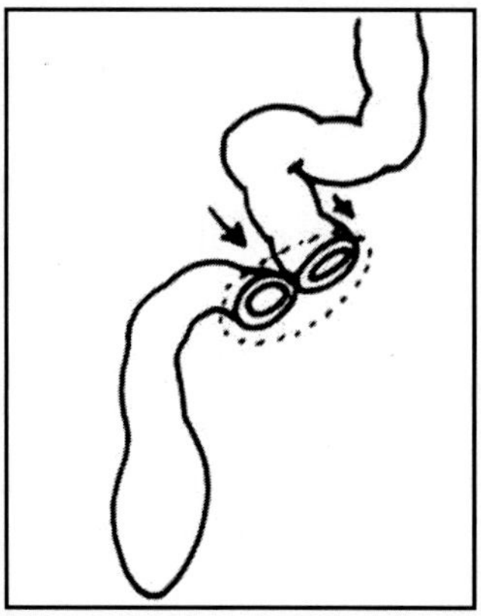

Fig. 6.10 Diagram of midsigmoid colostomy.

A transverse colostomy need not be precisely located. However after a right upper quadrant incision is made, the distended sigmoid colon may pop out first. The occasional operator often fails to notice the absence of greater omentum on this loop of colon and mistakes it for transverse colon and performs a sigmoid colostomy in the right upper quadrant. A sigmoid colon hooked up in the right upper quadrant creates very serious problems both for the patient and for the surgeon entrusted with the reconstruction (Fig. 6.11).

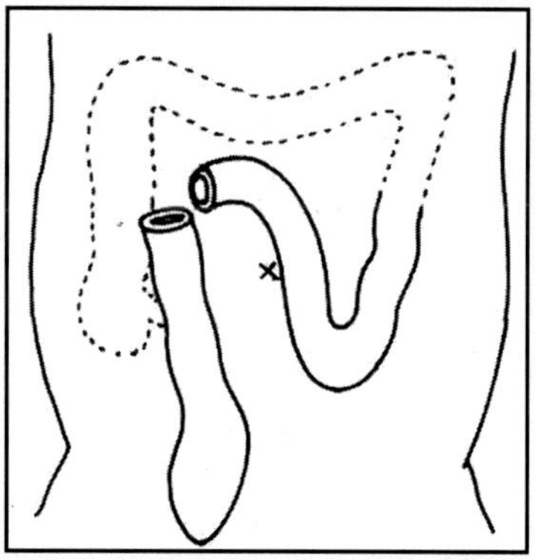

Fig. 6.11 Diagram of sigmoid colostomy in the right upper quadrant.

iv) It is easier to close than a sigmoid colostomy.

   This is indeed so but ease of performance need not be a factor in selecting the site of colostomy because the responsibility of closure lies with the surgeon who carries out the reconstruction and not with the occasional operator.

v) The surgeon who prefers to do laparoscopic reconstruction would like to have the colostomy in the upper abdomen and not in the lower.

As we have already stated, only 10% of patients require an intraperitoneal correction.

The disadvantages connected with right transverse colostomy are as follows:

i) It renders a long segment of large gut nonfunctional; fluids and electrolytes are normally absorbed in this part of the gut; without it, small poorly nourished babies in tropical countries are prone to diarrhea and dehydration and excoriation of the pericolostomy skin.
ii) If connected to a large urinary fistula, the long distal bowel readily absorbs the constituents of urine and this gives rise to hyperchloremic acidosis (see Fig. 6.9)
iii) The terminal bowel cannot be easily emptied through a transverse colostomy either during the colostomy or before the reconstruction and may be found filled with inspissated meconium during the reconstruction.
iv) The distal cologram often fails to delineate the level of the terminal bowel or a fistula leading from it because of the accumulated meconium.
v) The chances of infection following reconstruction are greatly increased because the terminal bowel cannot be easily reached either by preoperative washouts or by local antibacterial drugs.

C. A Left transverse colostomy is a hazardous undertaking if the patient has a high lesion and needs an abdominoperinal pullthrough. The pullthrough may call for ligation and division of the inferior mesenteric vessels and the pulled through bowel survives on the middle colic vessels and the marginal arcade. During closure of the colostomy, this arcade is vulnerable; if it is damaged, the distal bowel becomes ischemic and disastrous consequences follow (Fig. 6.12).

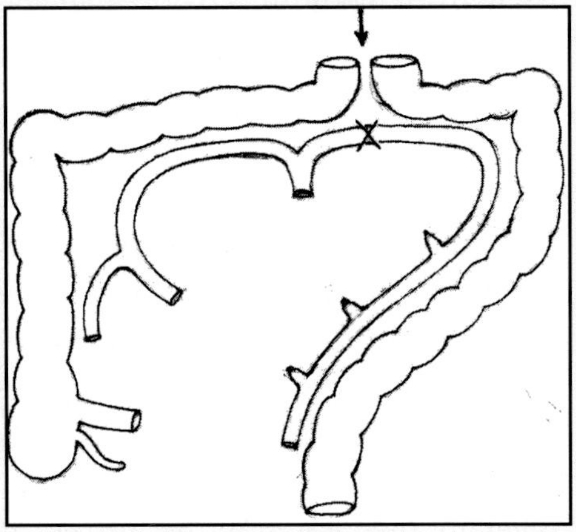

Fig. 6.12 Diagram of left transverse colostomy.

D. Exploratory Laparotomy Prior to Colostomy

This adds a new dimension to a relatively simple operation. It calls for skilled anesthetic management, and a longer period of postoperative intravenous medication. It is essential whenever there is a preoperative suspicion of associated disorders of the bowel.

If in the course of an operation through a left lower quadrant incision, additional exposure is called for, the skin, left rectus sheath and muscle can be divided transversely from the apex of the V incision up to the midline.

E. Divided Colostomy

This is one of the methods to ensure that the colostomy defunctions completely and continuously till no longer required. The mesocolon is divided partially and the bowel completely. After suturing the afferent and efferent loops to each other to form a doublebarrel, the two ends are brought out through two separate openings (Fig. 6.13). Our technique of colostomy defunctions completely and continuously without transecting the bowel, without dividing any colonic vessels, and without intraperitoneal sutures. It also permits a much easier closure.

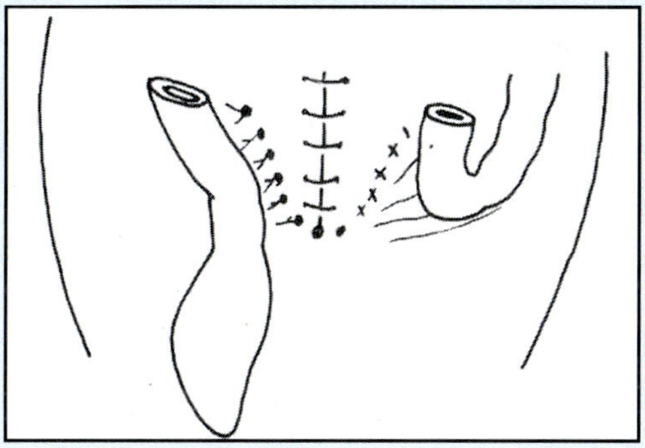

Fig. 6.13 Diagram of divided colostomy.

F. Associated Malformations

Two associated colonic malformations pose problems in the construction of a neonatal colostomy. The first is agenesis of part of the colon either in isolation or in association with a colonic pouch; this is discussed in Chapter 14. The second is situs inversus, already described in Chapter 3. This was not detected pre-operatively in one neonate in our series and the left lower quadrant incision had to be extended medially to reach colon that could be exteriorized (Fig. 6.14). The second neonate had an Xray study; after noting the position of the heart and liver shadows preoperatively, he had been submitted to a transverse colostomy. If situs inversus is diagnosed preoperatively, we would do a sigmoid colostomy in the right lower quadrant.

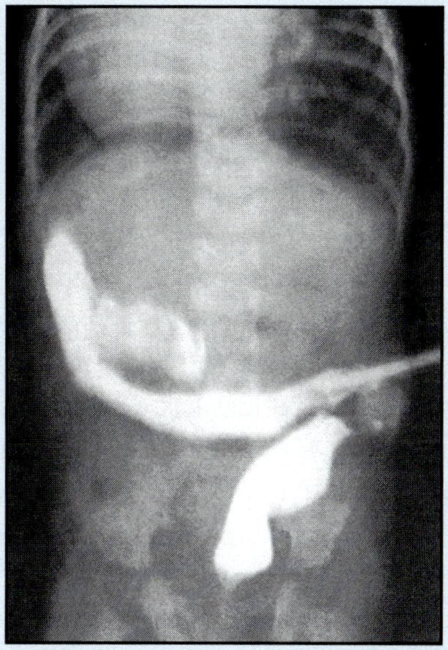

Fig. 6.14 Xray - distal cologram in patient with situs inversus.

Colostomy Care

The colostomy has to be protected from friction and injury by suitable creams and stoma appliances. Plain white paraffin is cheap and as good as anything more expensive. During the first few weeks of life, a simple dressing kept in place by a binder is all that is necessary.

If the colostomy has to be continued for a long period, standard colostomy kits that are now available in most parts of India are recommended. If not, collecting appliances can be improvised from almost anything.

Two colleagues, Banerjee & Haque (2001), have described the successful use of an indigenous dressing; namely a 'Paan' or betel nut leaf. The plant *Piper betle* Linn is widely cultivated in the 'humid' parts of the Indian subcontinent and is widely used for chewing along with lime, betel nut and catechu with or without tobacco. The lime, catechu and tobacco are undoubtedly harmful but the leaves are not. In traditional medical systems in both the Indian subcontinent and all over South East Asia they have been used as a dressing for surface lesions and after extraction of their oil, for both surface and systemic disorders. The authors have found that peristomal excoriation can be both prevented and also cured by the use of this simple and very cheap device. The leaf has a glossy side and a rough side. A central hole is made in half a leaf and this is placed on the abdomen with the glossy side up and the stoma protruding through the hole. The other half is placed with the glossy side up to cover the stoma and the whole is fixed to the abdomen with a piece of cloth. The parents learn the technique before taking the baby home (Figs. 6.15-16).

Local Complications

These occur either because the operation has been performed on a poor-risk patient with low birth weight, major associated anomalies and delayed presentation or because the operation has been performed incorrectly. Over the last 2 decades they have occurred in only 3 babies operated upon in PCC.

Immediate Complications are life threatening and include gangrene of the exteriorized bowel due to disruption of its blood supply; wound dehiscence with evisceration of either the large gut adjacent to the colostomy or of loops of small gut through gaps between the colostomy and the parietes, either because of poor placement of nonabsorbable sutures between the colon and the parietes or their

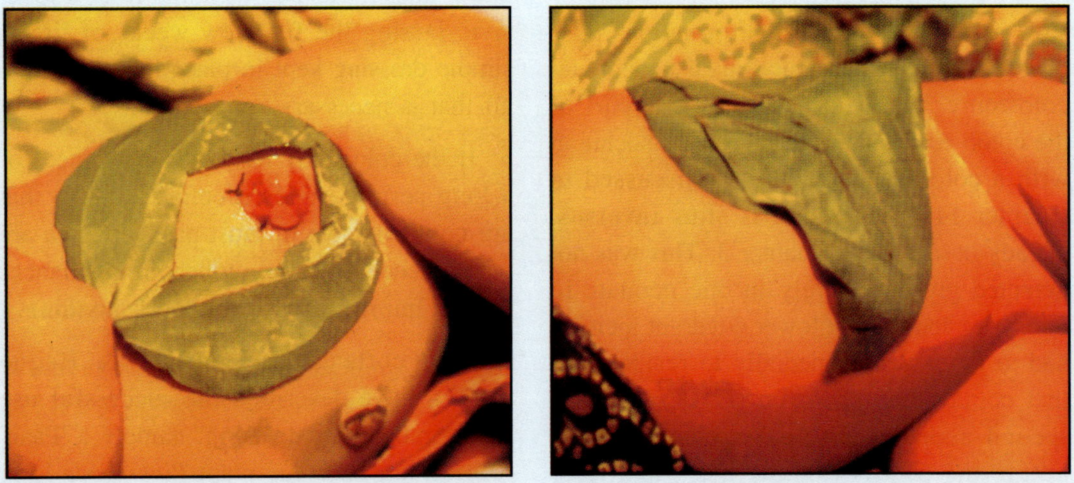

Figs. 6.15-16 Photographs of colostomy dressing with 'paan' leaf.

disruption due to increasing intraabdominal pressure; peritonitis; small bowel obstruction; septicemia and acute prolapse.

Acute prolapse occurs if the baby strains with the colostomy site unprotected by a proper dressing; the bowel may become irreducible and its blood supply may be compromised. Uncomplicated prolapse can generally be reduced after adequate sedation and retained in place by external support. Emergency revisional surgery is called for in all other situations. Babies with peritonitis, septicemia and gangrenous bowel need prolonged intensive care.

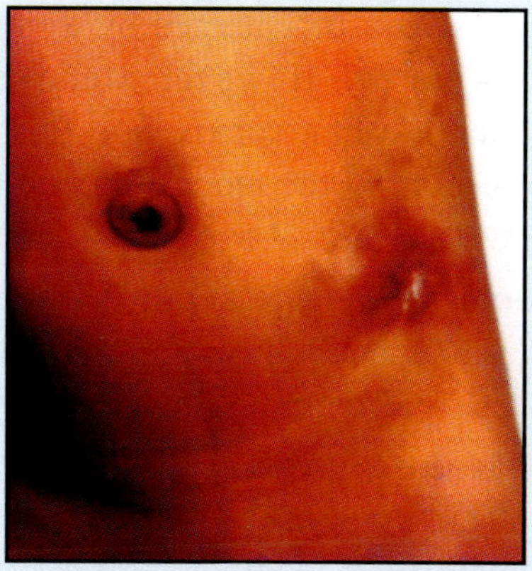

Fig. 6.17 Photograph of retracted colostomy in right upper quadrant.

Complications that develop after the first week are less life threatening.

1. **Retraction** of the spur of a loop colostomy allows bowel contents to spill over into the distal loop. Feces accumulates in the terminal loop and is likely to enter the urogenital organs if a fistula is present. The terminal loop distends and cannot be emptied properly prior to reconstruction; after reconstruction, the colostomy fails to protect the suture lines from fecal contamination. Retraction is in our opinion entirely preventable if the surgeon ensures that the colostomy is supported by a properly executed skin bridge; it occurs if temporary supports are used or if the skin bridge loses its blood supply and disintegrates. An inadvertently performed sigmoid colostomy in the right upper quadrant is particularly prone to retract (Fig. 6.17).

   A colostomy that has retracted should be revised if defunctioning is considered essential, The colostomy is mobilized sufficiently to elevate the spur and a new skin bridge is created to support it. Usually in the course of this procedure, the peritoneum is opened and several sutures are required to hold the colon in its new position.

2. **Stenosis** is a more serious complication because it results in intestinal obstruction. It occurs in both divided and undivided colostomies (Fig. 6.18). It is again entirely preventible. A stenosed

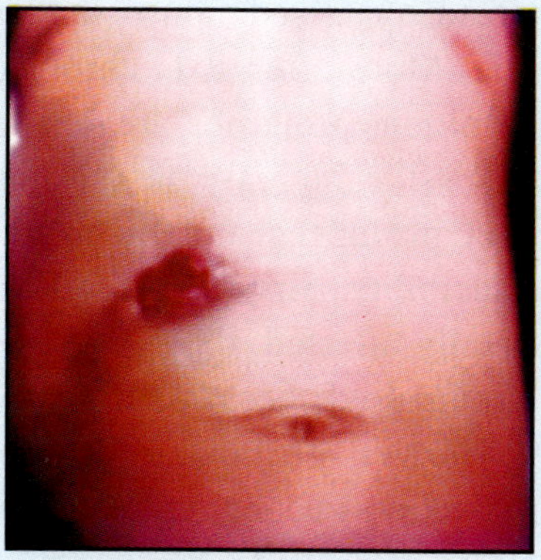

Fig. 6.18 Photograph of stenosed colostomy in left lower quadrant.

opening can be enlarged by a modified Y-V plasty. However stenosis and retraction often coexist and this needs correction by the more elaborate procedure described above.

3. **Hemorrhage** is generally chronic and leads to anemia. It can also be acute and severe and require blood transfusion.
4. **Pericolostomy hernia** is again a problem associated with protein-energy -malnutrition together with a straining factor; it can be kept under control by suitable appliances until the colostomy is discontinued.
5. **Excoriation of the pericolostomy skin** is sometimes very troublesome and leads to significant blood loss. It is generally associated with diarrhea and occurs more often around a transverse colostomy. A zinc oxide cream and control of the enterocolitis together with nutritional support brings the situation under control. We have already mentioned the role of Paan leaf in dealing with pericolostomy excoriation.
6. **Prolapse** is the commonest of all complications. Prolapse can occasionally be acute even after the first week; this calls for instant reduction either after adequate sedation or under anesthesia. More often it is chronic; small intermittent prolapses are followed by progressive increase in the length of bowel prolapsed and by progressive irreducibility. Since the distal bowel is generally affected, the passage of feces is unimpaired; occasionally the proximal bowel prolapses resulting in intestinal obstruction, and an emergency revision is needed.

Prolapse occurs when the abdominal muscles are not snugly apposed to the emerging bowel. This happens if the sutures had not been accurately placed during the operation either because the abdomen was greatly distended or the baby very ill. It also occurs if the colon was hugely dilated during the colostomy and returned to its normal size with time. Prolapse occurs commonly in patients suffering from protein-energy-malnutrition, diarrhea and respiratory infection in the postoperative period (Figs. 6.19-20).

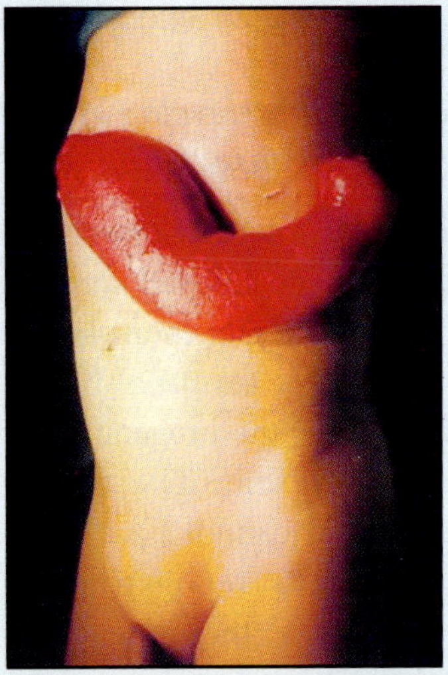

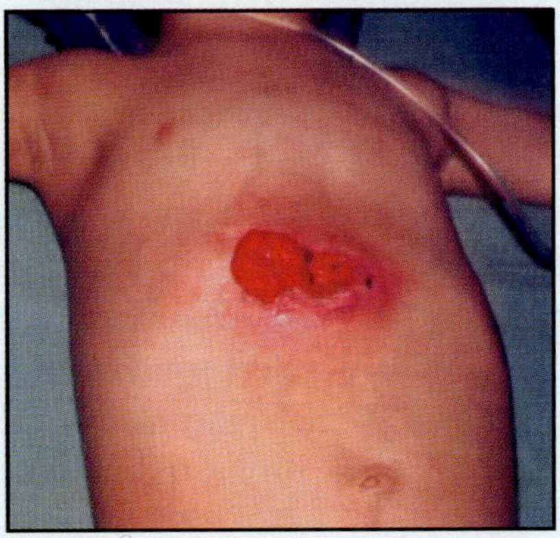

Figs. 6.19-20 Photographs of baby with prolapse of colostomy, before and after repair.

Earlier, we had recommended that the posterior wall of the colostomy be incised all the way down to the spur with diathermy but without anesthesia before the baby is sent home; this was found to prevent prolapse. We now reserve this procedure only for selected cases.

Management of Prolapse

The ideal treatment for chronic prolapse of the distal loop is to discontinue the colostomy as soon as possible by completing the reconstruction early. However if early discontinuation is not feasible, an operation resembling the one proposed by Thiersch for anorectal prolapse can be done.

The steps are as follows. The prolapse is reduced. Two small incisions are then made on opposite poles of the opening through which the prolapse occurs. A large curved needle threaded with thick suture material preferably PGA No.1 is passed from one wound to the other in the subcutaneous plane traversing a half circumference round the bowel; and then withdrawn from the second wound. It is then reintroduced and withdrawn from the wound of entry after it has traversed the other half circumference of the bowel, also in subcutaneous plane. After the needle is unthreaded, the suture material is found surrounding the bowel with a loop of thread emerging from one wound and two strands from the other. The strands are pulled so that the loop sinks; then the strands are tied over an assistant's finger to ensure that obstruction does not occur. The two wounds are then closed with fine sutures (Figs. 6.21-22).

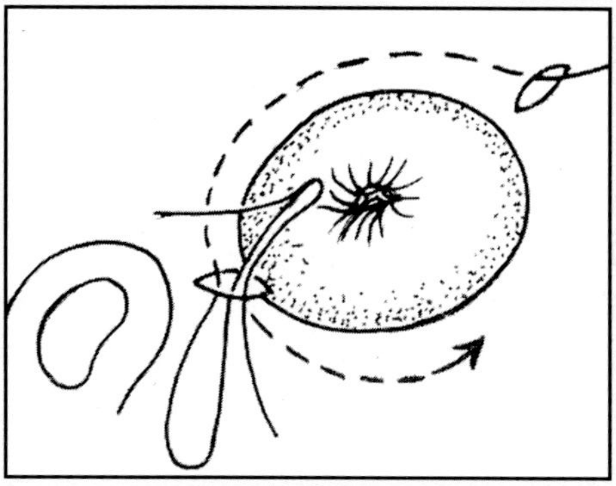

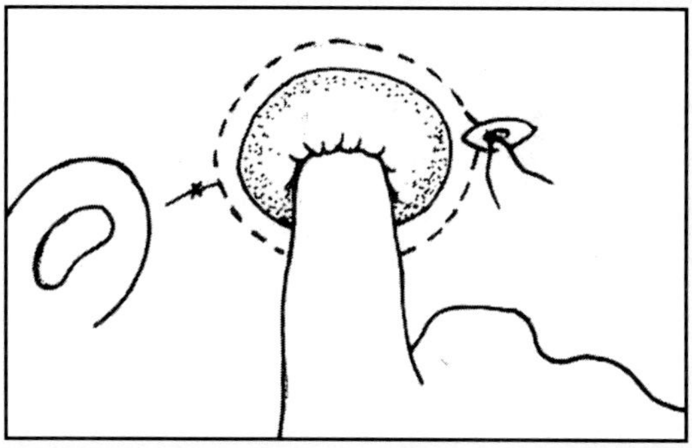

Figs. 6.21-22 Diagram of Thiersch operation for prolapse of colostomy.

Over the years we have had recurrences and do not think this is sufficient to control a large prolapse. For this we now perform the procedure recommended by Das; it is named buttonpexy (Canil *et al*, 1995). After the prolapse is reduced, two laboratory coat buttons are taken. A large needle with zero prolene or silk thread is passed through two holes of one button. The left forefinger is placed in the lumen of the bowel and held against the anterior abdominal wall. The needle held in a stout needle holder is taken inside the bowel and the bowel wall and anterior abdominal wall are pierced about 3 to 5 cm. away from the colostomy site with the left index finger as a guide. The other end of the suture is then threaded into a second needle and this needle also pierces the bowel wall and anterior abdominal wall to reach the surface close to the previous suture. The button between the two limbs of the suture is then placed inside the lumen of the bowel. The suture is then passed through two holes of the second button; this is laid on the skin surface and a knot is tied with just enough pressure to keep the buttons and the bowel in place. Care should be taken not to blanch the skin and cause skin necrosis. After about 4 weeks, the suture is cut and the external button removed. The internal button remains in the bowel and is passed out spontaneously (Figs. 6.23-25).

Unfortunately there have been recurrences even after this operation; also a more extensive dissection is required to separate the colon from the abdominal wall during closure of the colostomy.

Hence, a better option is intraperitoneal revision dividing the colostomy and bringing the two loops out through two separate openings as shown in Fig 6.9. This is particularly necessary if the prolapse is very large (Fig. 6.26).

It is necessary to remember that prolapse and retraction can coexist; the bowel prolapses when the baby is awake and crying and it retracts during sleep, thus allowing spillover into the distal bowel. If retraction can be excluded by clinical examination during sleep, early reconstruction followed by colostomy closure is the best way to eliminate prolapse. However, if the stoma retracts during sleep, this must be put right before a major reconstruction. In our very large series of PSARP, there has been only one recurrence of a rectourethral fistula; this patient had a transverse colostomy done elsewhere; there was massive prolapse but also some retraction. Because the parents were in a hurry, we had

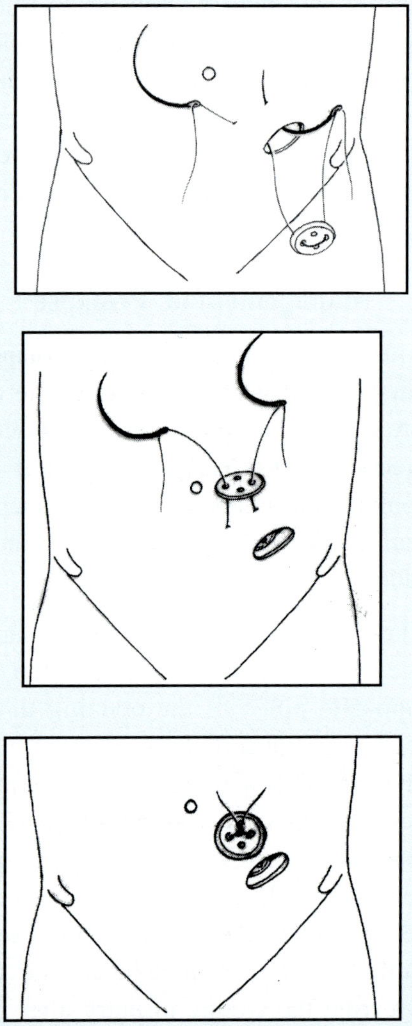

Figs. 6.23-25 Diagram of buttonpexy for prolapse of colostomy.

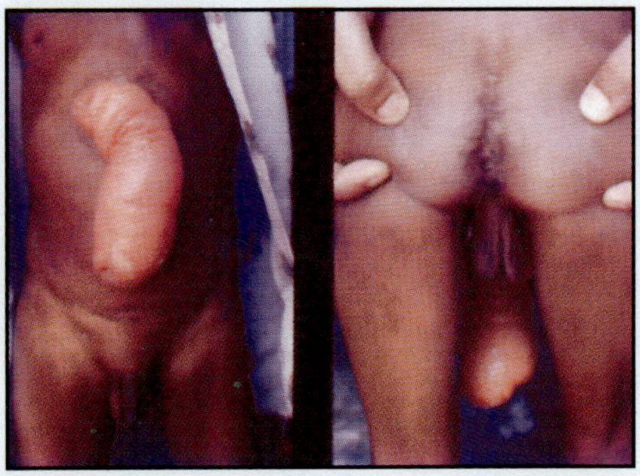

Fig. 6.26 Photographs of patients with massive prolapse.

agreed to do the PSARP without revising the colostomy and there was recurrence of the urethral fistula.

Systemic Complications

Of far greater importonce than the local problems are the systemic effects of colostomy. The two cardinal pediatric problems of any developing overpopulated country are diarrhea and protein-energy-malnutrition. While all infants below the poverty line are likely victims of these maladies, their impact on the colostomized is greater, particularly if the length of functioning colon has been reduced by a transverse colostomy. The vicious cycle of diarrhea and malnutrition leads to a third problem, poor development of cell-mediated immunity. As a result, these babies are more prone to recurrent infection and less able to cope with a major operative procedure.

The culminating disaster of all is **rejection** (Fig. 6.27). Rejection of an infant with a colostomy by the family is more likely to occur in families with poor educational as well as socio-economic status and in family with many children competing for attention. It is more likely if the baby suffers from multiple malformations. There is nodoubt at all that girls tend to get rejected more often than boys.

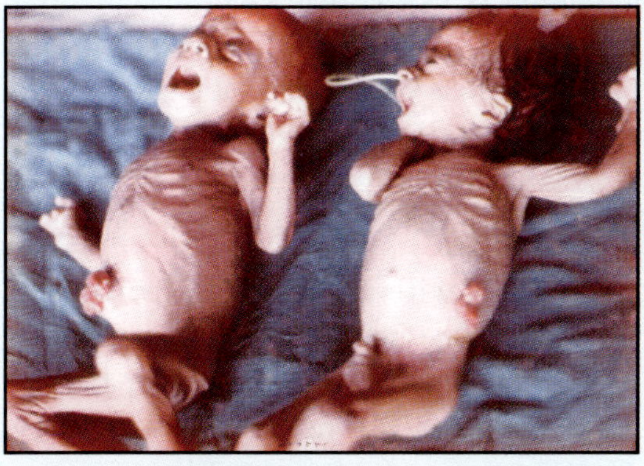

Fig. 6.27 Photograph of rejected babies.

Surgeons working in such communities have tried to reduce the rejection rate by performing fewer colostomies and by closing them earlier. As has been indicated already, a one-stage correction in the neonatal period should always be considered provided it does not lead to increased mortality and morbidity and does not compromise the final result. A neonatal reconstruction with a concurrent colostomy or a reconstruction shortly after a neonatal colostomy, with discontinuance as soon as possible thereafter is an alternative solution (Cruz 1984). The rejection rate can be reduced in a more realistic manner if the neonatal colostomy is performed as near to the mother as possible and the baby is returned to the mother in a day or two for domiciliary care and breast feeding. One of the hazards of sending the baby for surgery to a distant center without the mother is that the mother's breasts dry up by the time the baby gets back to her, and the family is burdened with a search for alternative nutrition. In India it should not be necessary for a neonate to travel to a distant center for a colostomy. In areas where pediatric surgeons are not available, many general surgeons are now able to perform a hassle-free neonatal colostomy.

The Unnecessary Colostomy

It had been our teaching 'when in doubt about the level of the lesion and the available expertise for a onestage correction, do a colostomy'. This has inevitably resulted in the performance of unnecessary colostomies because the surgeon has not examined the perineum of a neonate as meticulously as he should have. A perineal or a vestibular fistula is missed. Furthermore a low anomaly without a fistula can be corrected by a simple perineal operation once the diagnosis is made after simple imaging (Figs. 6.28-29). We have 8 cases in our series with this iatrogenic disorder; all did well after a simple perineal operation and discontinuance of colostomy.

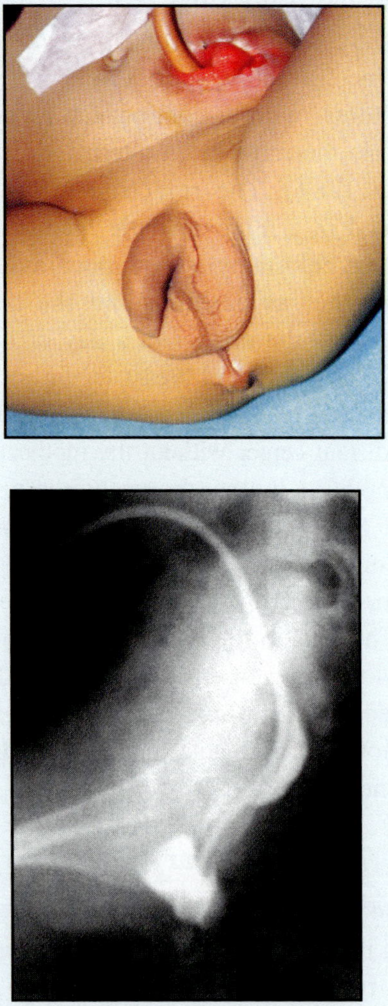

Figs. 6.28-29 Unnecessary colostomy; bowel at anal verge; Photograph & Xray - distal cologram.

THE POSTNEONATAL PERIOD

A colostomy properly performed soon after birth requires very little attention, and most babies thrive if offered the same loving care due to any normal infant. In addition, the colostomy has to be protected from injury. Attention is necessary when infants present with the complications that have been discussed earlier; some require revisional surgery, others require medical and supportive treatment.

I. ***The postcolostomy distal cologram*** is the first diagnostic procedure that is done. Details have been described in Chapter 3.

II. Timing of the Postcolostomy Reconstruction

Over the last two decades, postcolostomy reconstructions are being done on progressively younger patients for reasons that have been discussed earlier. Early reconstruction reduces the length of colostomy life and restores function to bowel distal to the colostomy. We decide on timing on the basis of weight with reference to age, hemoglobin, cardio-respiratory and urological status and the magnitude of the procedure necessary. If an intraperitoneal operation is likely, this should be delayed. Today we recommend extraperitoneal reconstructions on healthy babies in the first month of life but postpone intraperitoneal reconstructions until at least the fourth month when their weight is about 8 kg.

Patients with a colostomy performed elsewhere often present to pediatric surgeons in the developing world long after the age considered ideal for reconstructive surgery. The question to be answered here is up to what age would it be reasonable to accept patients for such reconstructions. Very little information is available about the time taken by the human brain to lose the capacity to learn the art of defecation.

Two groups of patients have presented late to us.

One group was left with a colostomy because of an associated uncorrectable or uncorrected handicap involving the brain and special senses, skeleton, external genitalia, or cardiovascular system. The parents were motivated to reverse their earlier decision to accept a permanent colostomy, either by families of successfully treated children or by the child who expressed a desire to defecate like his or her siblings or playmates. In our opinion, reconstruction of the anorectum is very worth-while, but the associated handicap must get the attention it deserves.

The other group consists of patients who had been submitted to reconstructive operations in the past but these had failed and the colostomy had either not been closed at all or had been reestablished. Some patients in this group were in their teens, and 3 were in the twenties. Whether to try again or not depends on psychological assessment to find out how well adjusted a person is to a colostomy life and whether he or she possesses the necessary motivation to take risks and learn a new and difficult skill.

Our results of reconstruction on patients over the age of 6 years have been disappointing in both groups. Some families did not carry out the dilatations and did not get the colostomies discontinued. Other children could not be disciplined to empty their bowel in response to training, and remained partially obstructed and incontinent. Our best result is in a boy, who was refused reconstruction initially because he was deaf; he was accepted at the age of 10 years after he attended a special school and learnt to speak. He now has socially acceptable continence.

III. Preoperative Treatment Prior to Postcolostomy Reconstruction

Although many of these reconstructions are done extraperitoneally, and most often without handling the bowel proximal to the colostomy, both the proximal and the distal bowel should be prepared, by mechanical cleanising and by antibacterial drugs. The proximal bowel is cleaned by oral administration of polyethylene glycol electrolyte solution, suppositories and bowel washes; the patient is put on a low-residue diet for 48 hours preoperative, is given suitable antibacterial drugs and is allowed only clear liquids for 24 hours preoperative. The distal bowel is irrigated with sterile normal saline; it must be assumed that there is a fistula through which the effluent will enter the urogenital tract; hence an antibiotic solution is periodically instilled into the distal bowel immediately preoperative.

THE POSTNEONATAL COLOSTOMY

This may be either preliminary or concurrent.

A Preliminary or Prereconstruction Colostomy is carried out when the patient is not fit for reconstruction because there is intestinal obstruction not responding to decompression, protein-energy-malnutrition and anemia that cannot be reversed rapidly and body weight too low for the proposed reconstruction.

A Concurrent Colostomy is done to protect the suture lines of a complex reconstruction till healing is complete. Today, with good preoperative bowel preparation, meticulous operative technique, parenteral nutrition and modern antibiotics, we reserve concurrent colostomy for revisional surgery on adults and on really difficult children.

The technique of performing a postneonatal preliminary colostomy is similar to that for a neonatal colostomy, only simpler; usually a tube can be introduced into the colon from below to decompress and help identification. A concurrent colostomy is required for relatively short periods, hence the skin bridge can be eliminated and a rubber tube can be left to prevent descent of the spur until the perineal wound heals. Once the reconstruction is adequately healed the spur can be allowed to descend and the colostomy discontinued.

While most postneonatal colostomies are trouble free, some prolapse and some retract; these complications are managed in the manner already described.

DISCONTINUANCE OF COLOSTOMY

From the point of view of the patient and the family, this is the most important operation, because it is this that enables the patient to defecate, perhaps for the first time in his or her life. Yet recorded information about its correct performance is minimal. Furthermore, the operation is often delegated to relatively junior members of the team. A superb reconstruction is tragically and totally wasted if an attempt at discontinuing the colostomy ends with a fatal complication.

The importance of the operation will only be appreciated if the term 'closure of colostomy' is replaced by the more correct '**resection of colostomy followed by end-to-end anastomosis**'. This is a procedure of great magnitude and calls for careful preparation, execution and postoperative care. We recently had a baby who had no serious problems during a major reconstruction but went into cardiac failure secondary to a missed cardiac malformation during discontinuance of colostomy.

A colostomy should only be discontinued when the patient is thriving and it is certain that the reconstruction is sound. Healing must be complete, there must be no fistula and the lumen of the new anorectum must be large enough to allow the free passage of feces; it should admit a little finger or a dilator of appropriate size. Too early closure has led to breakdown of the repair and to the formation of a fistula, urethral, vestibular, vaginal or cloacal. Worse, if the lumen is inadequate, feces will be retained; with rise of intraluminal pressure, the anastomosis is likely to leak. While a postoperative distal cologram is not mandatory in all cases, this should certainly be done if there is the slightest doubt about the success of the recon-struction.

Preoperative preparation must be carried out as outlined earlier for reconstructive surgery. Distal bowel washouts should emerge freely from the new anus.

Technique

Our method of discontinuing a colostomy is INTRAPERITONEAL. This is done in the following manner for a left lower quadrant colostomy.

a) A circumferential incision is made through the mucocutaneous junction and prolonged medially (Figs. 6.30-31).

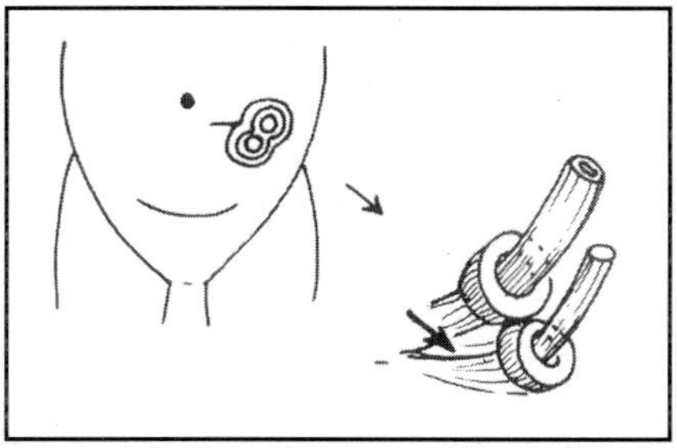

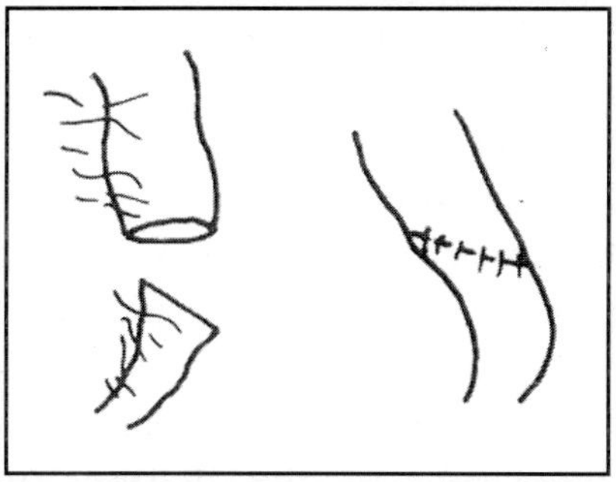

Figs. 6.30-31 Diagrams of operation for colostomy closure; incision and dissection; preparation for repair and end result.

b) After the skin flaps are raised, the muscles are divided, starting from the medial end of the wound, so that the peritoneum can be reached through an area with minimum scarring. Then with a finger in the peritoneum, the muscles are divided circumferentially around the colostomy, keeping close to the colon and taking great care not to perforate either the emerging loops of colon or any other loop of bowel which may be adherent to the colostomy. Introduction of catheters of suitable sizes into the colon loops helps to prevent injury, and diathermy is essential to minimize bleeding. When the colostomy has been completely freed, its blood supply and the diameter of the two loops are studied.

c) An appropriate resection is then carried out, to ensure that two healthy segments can be united. The caliber of the distal bowel shrinks with disuse; hence if the duration of colostomy life has been long, the incision on it must either be oblique or fishmouthed so that its caliber will match that of the proximal bowel. When there is great disparity, we perform an end-to-back anastomosis as in ileal atresia.

d) The anastomosis is performed with interrupted silk sutures passing through all the layers; this is reinforced if necessary by further interrupted seromuscular sutures also of silk. After the anastomosis is complete, the colon is allowed to drop down into the peritoneal cavity, and a drain is placed to reach it.

e) The wound is then closed in layers. While the peritoneum and muscles come together relatively easily, the skin flaps together with the underlying subcutaneous tissue need to be mobilized so that a tension-free apposition is achieved. Muscles are generally apposed with polyglycolic acid sutures. A second drain may be placed in the subcutaneous tissues, before the closure is completed.

f) It usually takes 72 hours for peristalsis to return and for stools to be passed. During this time, intravenous fluid therapy, antibacterial drugs and nasogastric decompression should be continued. Sometimes ileus lasts longer and spontaneous restoration of intestinal function is delayed.

g) After successful discontinuance of colostomy, the programme of dilatation of the new anorectum must be continued, it should be gradually tapered off and discontinued when the caliber of the bowel is normal for age.

Complications

Most complications like anastomotic leak and inadequate stoma are avoidable. The only complication that occasionally occurs and apparently cannot be entirely prevented is small gut obstruction due to adhesions and bands. This should be suspected if ileus persists for over 5 days, or if it sets in after initial passage of flatus and feces. The diagnosis is confirmed after a straight PA erect Xray; laparotomy should be carried out forthwith to relieve the obstruction.

As mentioned earlier, a transverse colostomy is easier to close than a sigmoid colostomy. A sigmoid colostomy that has been done in the right upper quadrant has its own problems. After the anastomosis, the colon drops down to its natural habitat, the left lower quadrant. When we closed such a colostomy for the first time, this was not realized and a drain was left only at the site of operation. There was postoperative peritonitis and small bowel obstruction, and another operation was necessary to put things right. On the second patient with this iatrogenic lesion, a drain was inserted in the left lower quadrant also and recovery was uneventful.

Alternative Methods

1. Extraperitoneal procedures were sometimes advised in the past to eliminate the possibility of postoperative peritonitis. They have now become obsolete for 2 reasons. One, there are often adhesions between the emerging colonic loop and loops of small bowel; these loops are endangered during a blind mobilization, but can be kept out of the way by an intraperitoneal procedure. Two, there may be a marked disparity in caliber between the proximal and distal loops and a straight forward anastomosis can not be performed.
2. Closure without resection implies preservation of the posterior or mesocolic wall of the exteriorized colon. This is possible if the colostomy has existed for a relatively short time, if there is an excess of colonic tissue with prolapse, and if the spur has sunk. Under these conditions, the colostomy can be mobilized sufficiently to permit apposition of the margins in the transverse axis of the bowel after suitable trimming. Thus the mesocolon is undisturbed and the operating time is reduced. However when this is attempted on a patient with an efficient spur and no prolapse, the free flow of bowel contents is impeded, the suture line commonly breaks down, and a fecal fistula results.
3. Discontinuance during reconstruction is done in the course of an abdominoperineal reconstruction when there is insufficient bowel distal to a colostomy done elsewhere. All the patients who had a short loop of bowel distal to a left lower quadrant sigmoid colostomy were submitted to resection of the colostomy together with bowel distal to it and to pullthrough of bowel proximal to the colostomy. If the bowel

is well prepared it is generally not necessary to carry out a proximal diversion. However it was necessary in a patient who came in 1981 with a sig moid colostomy in the right upper quadrant. SPR could not be completed because the bowel would not come down. The colostomy had to be dismantled to allow the pullthrough, and then a new colostomy was done on the transverse colon.

Transposition of colostomy is a method devised by Das to avoid discontinuance when distal bowel length is insufficient. A left lower quadrant colostomy is mobilized en bloc and displaced medially and downwards. After the abdominoperineal pullthrough is accomplished, the colostomy is fixed in its new situation and the site of the original colostomy repaired in layers. Inadvertent right upper sigmoid colostomy can also be transposed to the left lower quadrant in a similar way (Figs. 6.32-33).

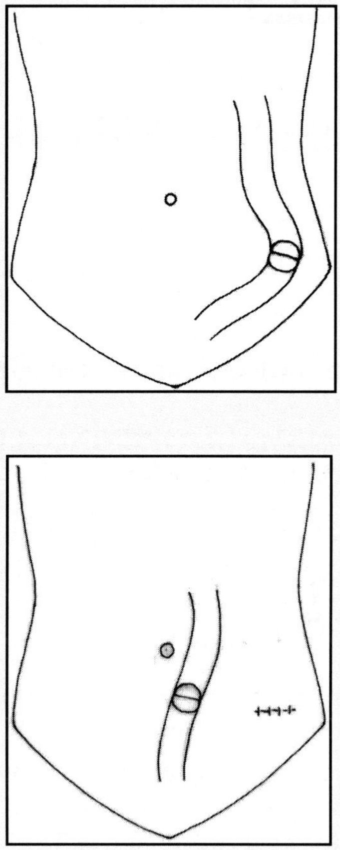

Figs. 6.32-33 Diagrams of transposition of colostomy.

CHAPTER 7

A VISIBLE ABNORMAL OPENING

Four varieties can be recognized

ONE : A SMALL OPENING AT THE NORMAL ANAL SITE

These are of three types depending on the level of the lesion.

I. Anal Stenosis

This is a **low** lesion, very common in boys, (about 16% of our cases); relatively rare in girls. The bowel opens at the normal anal site through a stenotic orifice. The rectum and anal canal are of normal or greater caliber and have passed throughout the entire striated muscle complex. The orifice may be pin point; it may give rise to complete obstruction if untreated, or it may allow the passage of some flatus and feces and produce chronic obstruction; this may become acute some time later by impaction of feces (Fig. 7.1). Patients presenting after the neonatal period with vomiting, abdominal distension, episodes of diarrhea, recurrent respiratory infection and failure to thrive are often thought to be suffering from Hirschsprung's disease by pediatricians who do not routinely examine the infant's anus.

The appearance of the orifice varies; it may be central or eccentric; it may be covered by a bucket-handle fold of skin or open on an elevated ridge, in a depression or by a perforation in a membrane covering the anus. Its earlier name was 'covered anus in situ-incomplete' (Fig. 7.2). The level of the lesion is confirmed by passing a balloon catheter into the bowel; the balloon is inflated and the catheter is gradually withdrawn; its downward passage is obstructed almost at the anal orifice.

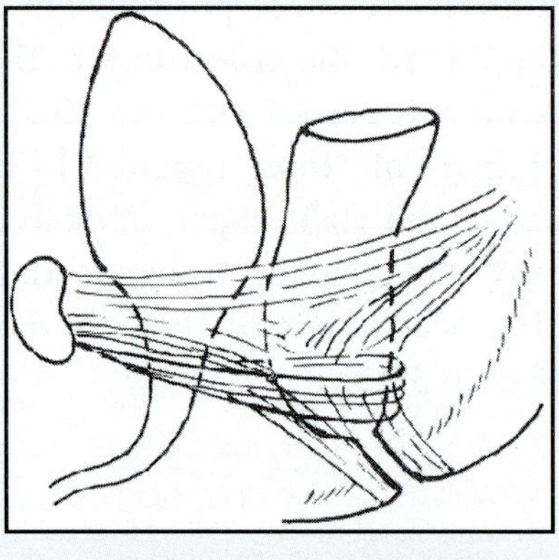

Fig. 7.1 Diagram of anal stenosis.

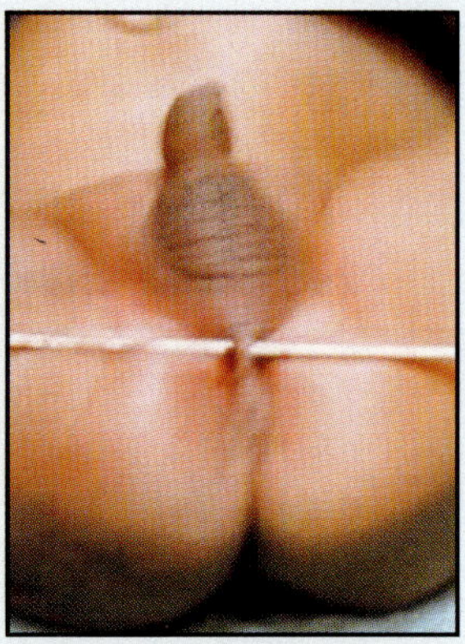

Fig. 7.2 Photograph of bucket handle lesion.

Management

In the past, a simple cutback in the midline posteriorly was the recommended operation. This was done with a pair of scissors inserting one blade in the lumen of the bowel and keeping the other blade on the surface. Neither anesthesia nor sutures were required; the opening was kept patent by periodic dilatations throughout the period of healing by granulation. Cutback has been an excellent lifesaving procedure for the peripheral surgeon but the stenosis recurred in most babies.

Today, the stenotic orifice is enlarged as soon as detected, and the epithelium of the anal canal is sutured to the skin by one of 2 methods:

1. Y-V plasty is the procedure preferred by us. A V incision is made with its apex at the posterior margin of the bowel opening. A midline incision through the full thickness of the bowel wall reaches bowel of normal caliber; this relieves the obstruction and provides space for the V skin flap. After tags if any have been excised, sutures are placed between the anal mucosa and the perineal skin and the wound is closed (Figs. 7.3-5).

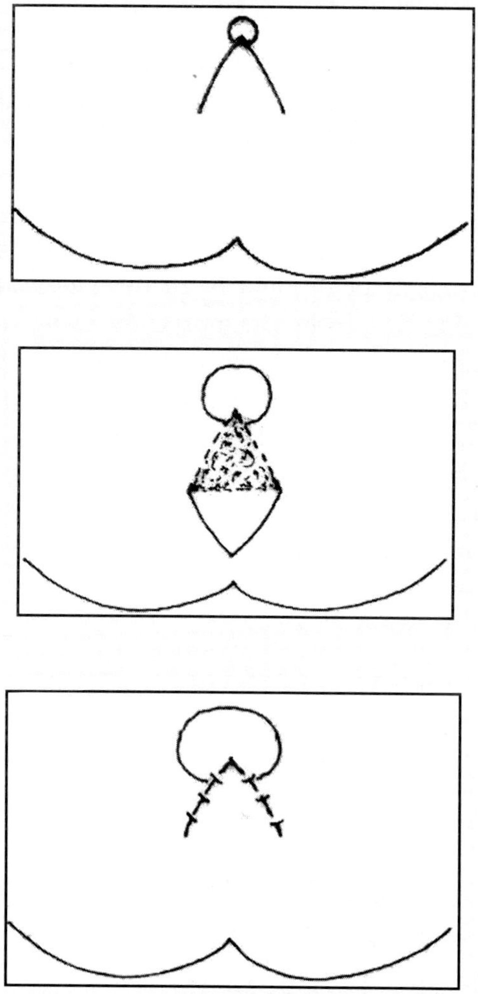

Figs. 7.3-5 Diagrams showing Y-V anoplasty.

2. Pena (1987) recommends a limited sagittal anorectoplasty (SARP). A circumferential incision is made around the stenotic anus and is extended in the midline anteriorly and posteriorly; tags, if any, are excised. The anterior and posterior limits of the vertical fibers of the striated muscle complex are marked with stay sutures. Two sagittal incisions are made on the bowel wall anteriorly and posteriorly extending up to bowel of normal caliber. The bowel is opened in the midline and its wall is sutured to the skin on either side within the limits of the vertical fibers. The wound is closed.

In the postoperative period, the neoanus should be dilated at intervals. If the repair is incorrectly performed or dilatations are not done, the stenosis recurs and revisional surgery, becomes necessary.

There have been no problems in any of the patients treated by us.

II. Anorectal Stenosis

This is the name given by Wilkinson (1972) for a condition, which resembles anal stenosis externally, but the stenosis extends upwards and bowel of normal or greater caliber is found above the long narrow zone (Fig. 7.6). It does not figure in the Wingspread list and is an **intermediate** lesion. It can be diagnosed by using the balloon catheter mentioned earlier. The balloon in this lesion is held up about 5 cm. from the anal verge. It can also be demonstrated by taking a lateral Xray after instilling contrast. The narrow tract passes through the center of a normally disposed striated muscle mass.

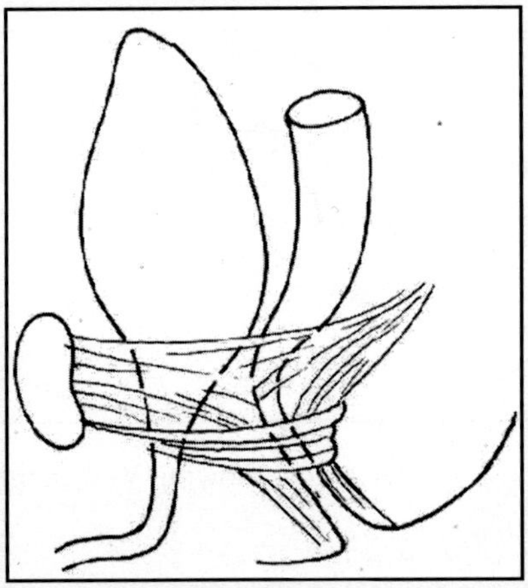

Fig. 7.6 Diagram of anorectal stenosis.

We have 7 patients, 4 boys and 3 girls, with a narrow tract 5 cm. long, and with dilated bowel lying above the levator. Three presented in the early 1970s and were treated by dilatation of the tract and Y-V plasty at the anus. They all improved but were subsequently lost to follow-up. Two presented in 1999; they improved with dilatations and did not come back. The other two, a boy and a girl, presented in 1987. The boy improved with dilatation in the neonatal period but relapsed. He was then readmitted and after bowel preparation, we did a PSARP, the tract was densely adherent to the urethra and the operation was extremely difficult. Colostomy had to be done to ensure healing. He did well after the colostomy was closed. The girl presented at the age of 3 years with severe constipation and a gluteal fecal fistula; a perineal operation had been done elsewhere. We did a colostomy; after the fistula healed we did a PSARP and closed the colostomy. She did well for some time but came back when she was fourteen with intractable constipation. The anorectum admitted a finger but there was huge megarectum on Barium enema. Revisional surgery was advised but she again disappeared. In retrospect, these patients probably deserved correction by a laparotomy.

III. Anal Canal Stenosis

This lesion falls between the two described above and is also not mentioned in the Wingspread list. The stenotic segment is about 2.5 cm. long and bowel of normal or greater caliber is found in the region of the I line (Fig. 7.7). This is determined by using the balloon catheter or by Xray as described earlier.

We have 8 patients, 6 boys and 2 girls; they were cured in infancy by a relatively simple perineal operation that can be named extended Y-V plasty. After the entire stenotic segment is opened up by a posterior midline intraluminal incision, a long posterior V flap of skin is fashioned and connected by a narrow tract to anal canal of incision so that its tip reaches the dilated bowel above the stenosis; it is then sutured in place.

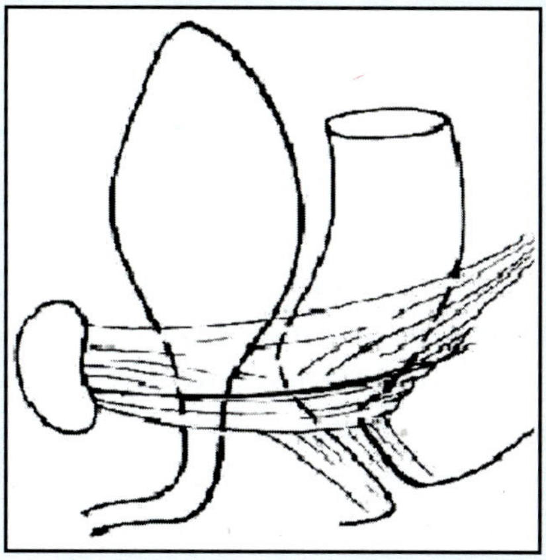

Fig. 7.7 Diagram of anal canal stenosis.

TWO: AN OPENING ANTERIOR TO THE NORMAL ANAL SITE IN THE PERINEUM

There are two types depending on the level of the lesion but there are undoubtedly shades of gray in between.

I. Anoperineal Fistula (Anocutaneous Fistula)

In this common condition (18% of our cases), there is a visible abnormal opening anterior to the normal anal site. It is equally common in both sexes. It is a **low** anomaly; there are two varieties.

1. **More commonly**, the orifice of the fistula is small and inadequate. It is normal or greater caliber situated in the normal position. The anorectum passes through the entire striated muscle complex up to the normal anal site, but fails to open at this site. The tract lies parallel to the surface (Fig. 7.8). In females, it opens between the normal anal site and the posterior margin of the vestibule. In males, it may extend as far forwards as the ventral surface of the penile shaft. In the newborn, a meconium filled tract may be visible in the midline under the perineal skin, and beads of meconium may emerge from the orifice (Figs. 7.9-10). Sometimes there is impaction and obstruction becomes complete. In the past this was named 'covered anus anterior', namely an anus covered by excessive anterior fusion of the genital folds. We displayed the anatomy at autopsy on a male neonate who died of choanal atresia.

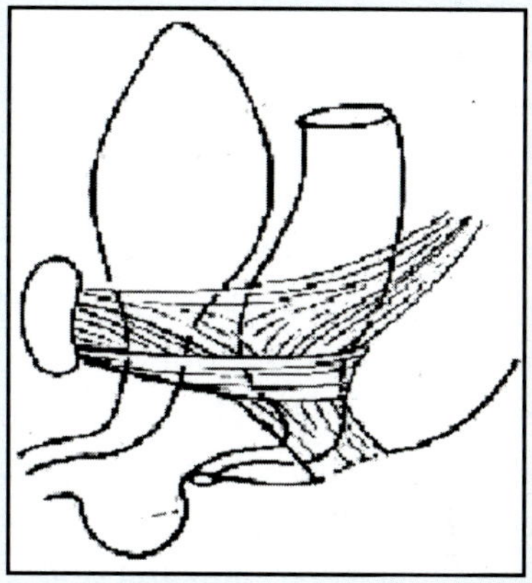

Fig. 7.8 Diagram of anoperineal fistula type 1.

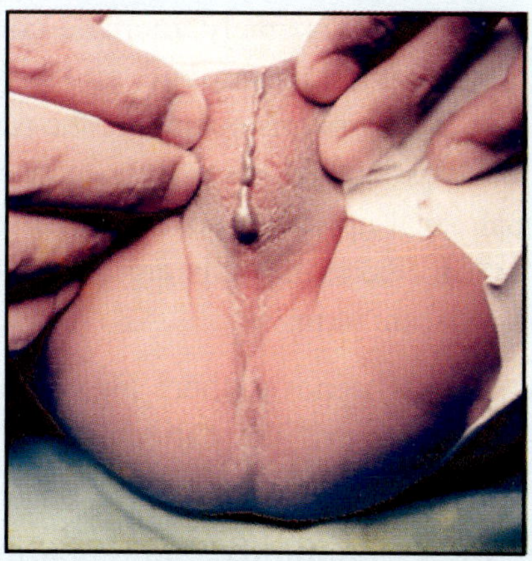

Fig. 7.9 Photograph of baby with bead of meconium.

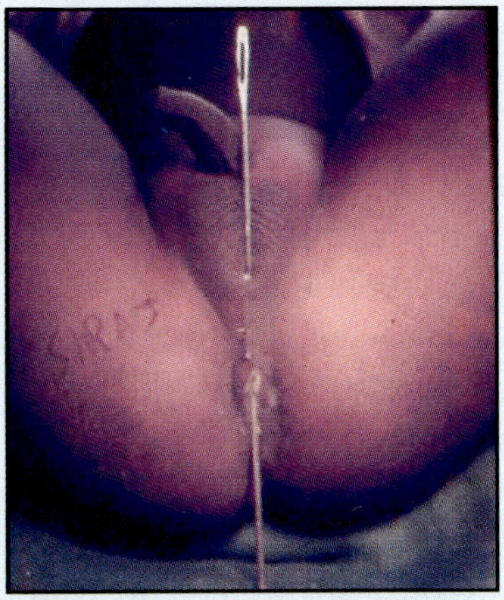

Fig. 7.10 Photograph of baby with probe in fistula.

Management

The fistula should be opened up as soon as it is detected, by a sagittal incision. A catheter introduced into the tract passes back parallel to the surface into the anal canal. The incision is continued up to the anal canal over the catheter; the operation is then completed by Y-V plasty as in Anal Stenosis. If the anterior lip of the anal canal is found deeply placed, it can be mobilized by a short transverse incision and sutured to the perineal skin.

Alternative procedures are the same as for Anal Stenosis, namely a simple cutback that we do not recommend and a more elaborate SARP. In this operation, the sagittal incision is prolonged posteriorly to open up the anal canal up to the posterior margin of the vertical fibers; its walls are then sutured to the adjacent skin.

As in anal stenosis, there have been no problems in any of the patients treated by us.

2. **Less commonly**, an opening of variable caliber is found in the midline at any point between the normal anal site and the posterior limit of the scrotum or vulva. The opening in girls may be surrounded by skin or may have red wet epithelium of the vestibule on its anterior margin A catheter introduced through it does not reach the normal anal site but passes obliquely upwards and backwards. Such an opening used to be called ‘anterior anus’ or ‘ectopic anus’, and it was thought that a normal anal canal had failed to migrate backwards. It is now established that the bowel in this condition does not in fact traverse the whole of the striated muscle complex; some striated muscle lies behind the anal canal (Fig . 7.11).

Symptoms depend on the size of the opening. If it is small and stenotic, there is obstruction; when its size resembles a normal anus there are no problems in the neonate or infant, but constipation may set in later. The diagnosis can be confirmed by the methods already described for anal stenosis, namely by using a balloon catheter; or by Xray with contrast.

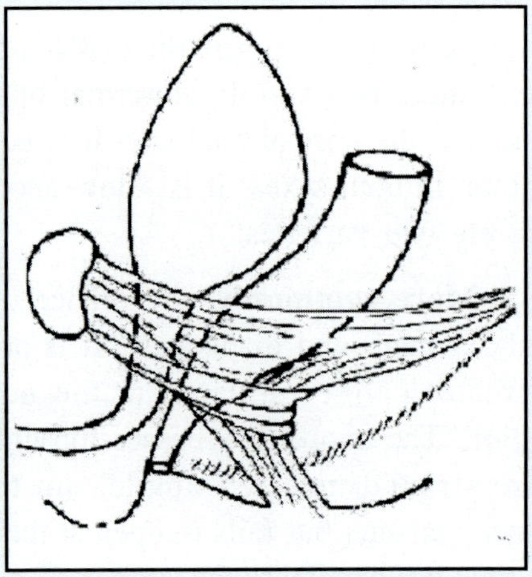

Fig. 7.11 Diagram of anoperineal fistula type 2.

Management

If there is obstruction, immediate operation is required, both for neonates and for those presenting after the neonatal period.

A limited sagittal anorectoplasty (SARP) is the operation of choice for this lesion. A circumferential incision around the fistula is continued backwards in the midline up to the normal anal site. The bowel is mobilized after dividing the striated muscle complex behind it in the midline as far as is necessary. The bowel is then placed in its normal position and the muscles repaired in front of it. The operation is completed with Y-V plasty (Fig. 7.12). The procedure enlarges the terminal bowel and at the same time introduces sensitive perineal skin into its lumen. Alternatively, a longer sagittal incision can be made and the wall of the bowel can be sutured to the skin on either side. The results are equally good. Two girls both aged 6 months had a retrorectal duplication cyst in association with this variety of APF; a more extensive exposure was necessary to resect the cyst and bring the bowel down to the normal anal site.

Two procedures done in the past are no longer recommended. A simple Y-V plasty in situ relieved the obstruction but did not bring the bowel opening to the normal site. On the other hand, a cutback divided part of the striated muscle complex and produced incontinence.

None of the patients treated by us for this anomaly have had any problems.

However, it is difficult to decide what to do for the older patient with an adequate anterior anus and habitual constipation (Fig. 7.13). Leape (1978), Hendren (1978) and Upadhyaya (1984) have suggested operative correction; they have found a posterior shelf of muscle with a bulge above. We have also clinically found a posterior shelf of muscle with a bulge above it in one boy aged 11 years and one girl aged 6 months; they are presently being treated conservatively, but it is likely that an operative correction will be needed later.

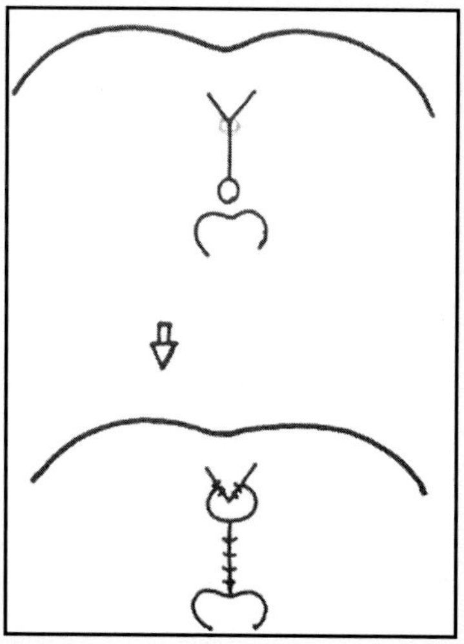

Fig. 7.12 Diagrams showing SARP.

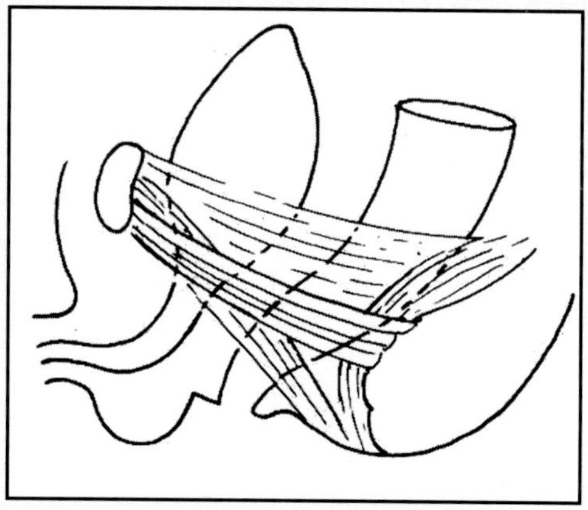

Fig. 7.13 Diagram of anoperineal fistula type 2 with large opening.

II. Rectoperineal Fistula

The external appearance of this rare lesion resembles anoperineal fistula but bowel of normal or greater caliber is found much higher up. It is an **intermediate anomaly** and does not figure in the Wingspread list.

In the 1934 Ladd and Gross classification of ARM, rectoperineal fistula is the name given to the tract that leads down from the blind rectal pouch to open on the perineum. 'The perineal openings usually appear just behind the perineoscrotal angle, but in one case, there was a more anterior location into a bifid scrotum. We have had no case similar to those in the literature in which the rectal fistula opened on the undersurface of the penis.' In their series there were 20 boys and 10 girls; in the latter, the fistulas were 'from the fourchette to the anal dimple', hence vestibular fistulas were probably included.

Wilkinson in 1972 described rectoperineal fistula as a variety of anorectal malformation where 'the rectum ends blindly above the levator ani muscular diaphragm and communicates with the exterior by a fistula which passes between the limbs of the puborectalis sling of the levator ani to the perineum'.

On the other hand, Stephens and Smith in 1971 had equated the term with anocutaneous fistula, a low or translevator malformation, finding 'no record of a true rectoperineal fistula alone, that is, a high rectal dysplasia with a long fine fistula to the perineum'.

This anomaly should in our opinion be named **'AGENESIS WITH PERINEAL FISTULA'**.

Seventeen patients with this malformation were described in our earlier book; 4 more have been subsequently studied. In the 19 boys, the opening was at the perineoscrotal junction in 9, on the scrotum in 5, and at the penoscrotal angle in 4 (Figs. 7.14-15). In one there was penoscrotal hypospadias, severe chordee and penoscrotal transposition; the bowel opened just behind the urethra and the posteriorly placed penis. One boy had an uncomplicated hypospadias and another had chordee without hypospadias. In one male pseudohermap-hrodite (MPH) the bowel opened between the two halves of empty labioscrotal folds just behind the perineal urethral orifice (Figs. 7.16-17). The only girl in our series had a small opening just behind the vulva.

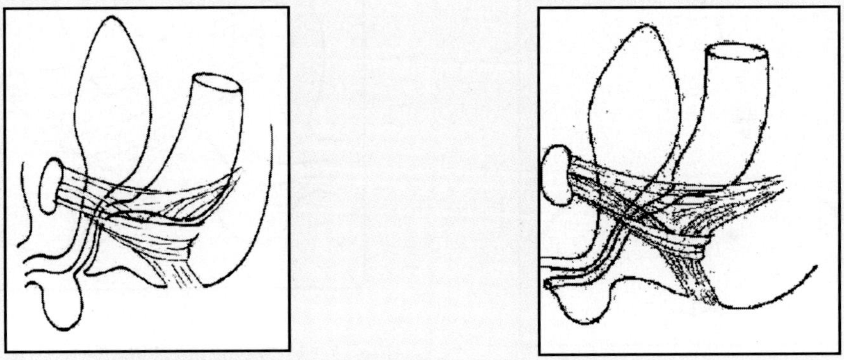

Figs. 7.14-15 Diagrams of rectoperineal fistula.

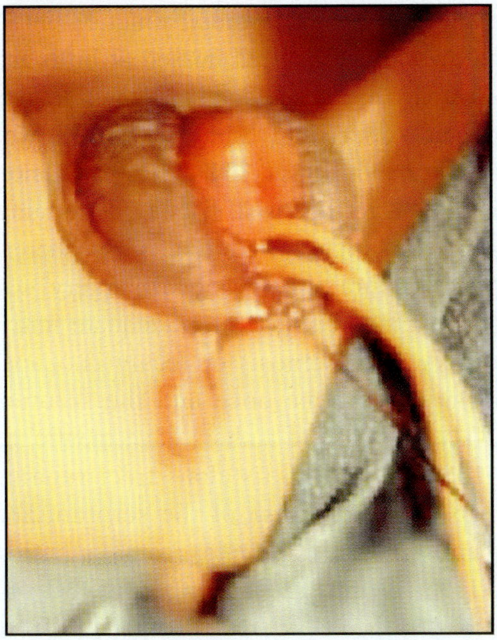

Fig. 7.16 Photograph of baby with MPH and rectoperineal fistula.

Our patients fall into two groups:

A. Thirteen patients had presented without previous surgery on the perineum.

1. Four of these, including the MPH presented as neonates. Examination of the area between the penis (phallus) and the posterior limit of the scrotum (or labioscrotal folds) revealed either an opening through which meconium emerged or a bluish blob or band covered with thin skin which when nicked, allowed meconium to flow out. A catheter passed vertically up from the opening; by using a balloon catheter the length of the fistula could be measured. A lateral Xray after instillation of contrast fluid showed the tract to be parallel to and very close to the posterior urethra, and bowel of normal or greater caliber to be high up (Fig. 7.18).

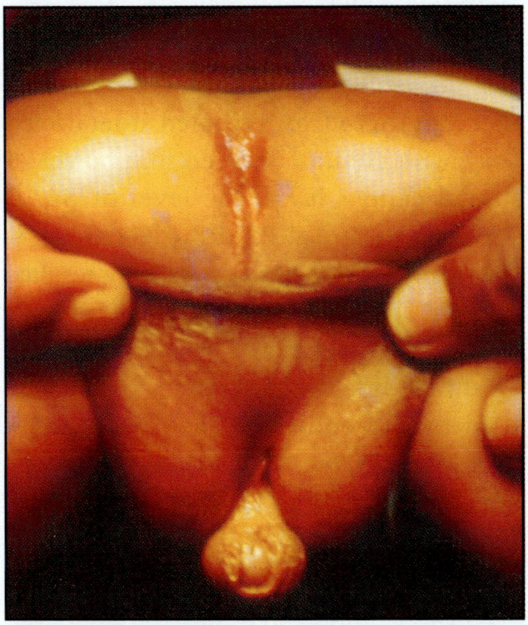

Fig. 7.17 Photograph in prone position; fistula opening at penoscrotal junction.

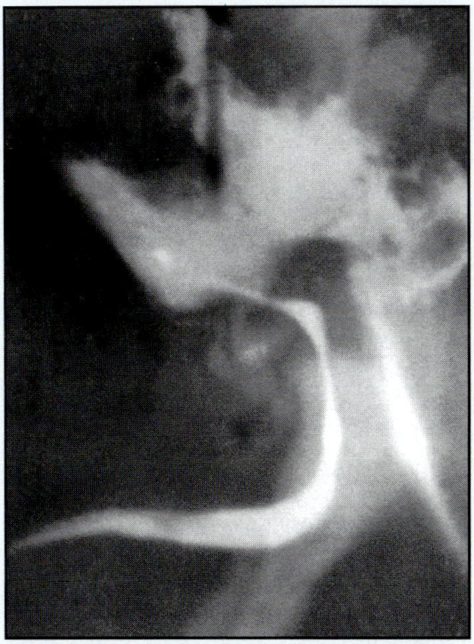

Fig. 7.18 Xray with contrast in bowel and urethra.

2. Two of the 9 patients who presented after the neonatal period had had a neonatal colostomy elsewhere. In one, there was a mound of meconium covered by thin epithelium; this had been missed. In the other, the opening at the penoscrotal junction was thought to be a urethral fistula. The others, 6 boys and one girl presented with chronic intestinal obstruction and passed stool with difficulty through the fistula. Some passed stools only after dilatation or after insertion of a catheter and a bowel wash. As in the other group, a catheter inserted into the fistula passed vertically up and the diagnosis was confirmed by taking a lateral Xray with contrast. One patient was found to have multiple urological anomalies including a vesical diverticulum, bilateral hydroureteronephrosis and a dysplastic kidney.

B. The remaining 8 patients had been misdiagnosed as anoperineal fistula and submitted to one or more perineal operations elsewhere. One had had a cutback through the entire thickness of striated muscle and was incontinent. In the others, the bowel had been opened at the normal anal site but the fistula had been left undisturbed. They had varying degrees of obstruction because the new opening stenosed and they defecated incompletely either through both openings or only through the fistula.

The condition has been encountered by a number of surgeons in the recent past and given different names. In an article entitled 'Translevator anal anomalies with cutaneous fistulae passing deep to the scrotum'. Fitzgerald *et al* (2002) described 9 cases collected from 4 centers; all had a fistula opening at the penoscrotal junction. In 2, the diagnosis had been missed at birth and colostomy had been done. In 3, the tract was indeed superficial and the fistula was therefore anoperineal. The others had almost certainly a rectoperineal fistula, the terminal bowel was high up, the tract was adherent to the urethra and revisional surgery was required in 4 because of inadequate initial surgery, anal stenosis or fecaluria. Laparotomy was done once and the scrotum bivalved in 2. The authors have mentioned a 10th case with a fistulous tract running deep above the base of the scrotum and opening near the penoscrotal junction (Aleem *et al* 1985). Fitzgerald did not include the 3 cases described from Rotterdam by Shanbhogue *et al* in 1994; in these boys, the diagnosis was not made at birth and all 3 had a colostomy before the anomaly was recognized.

Basak (2002) has reported a boy who had a perineoscrotal fistula and a Y-V plasty as a neonate; intractable constipation had been controlled by repeated dilatations. Xray with contrast showed that bowel of normal caliber lay at the level of S4. A colostomy, a formal PSARP (see chapter 8) and finally closure of the colostomy resulted in cure. The patient described by Sripathy and his colleagues from Chennai (2003) was somewhat different. The fistula was missed at birth and colostomy had been done. Subsequently feces was seen to emerge from the penoscrotal junction; probing and distal cologram showed the fistula which they labeled 'perineal canal' They have performed anoplasty and closed the colostomy 'without excising the tract in its entirety'. It is likely that a cyst will develop in due course.

Management

Today, patients with Rectoperineal fistula should be offered onestage reconstruction as soon after birth as possible. The bowel can be decompressed adequately by dilating the fistula and giving laxatives and bowel washes. The operation can be performed either in the spreadeagled position or the frog position and is named Anterior Sagittal AnoRectoPlasty (ASARP). Colostomy is not necessary.

The operation begins by passing a balloon catheter into the bladder. Then a circumferential incision is made around the fistula and a posterior V flap is made at the normal anal site; these are joined by a sagittal incision. This incision is deepened to divide the muscles up to the anterior half of the striated muscle complex. The extent of the exposure depends on the site of the fistula; if it is at the penoscrotal junction, the scrotum has to be split. The bowel is then dissected off the striated muscles on its posterior and lateral aspects, and then from the posterior wall of the urethra. If the bowel and the urethra share a common wall, the dissection may have to proceed in the submucous plane in the midline to avoid injury to the urethra. The bowel is then tapered, if necessary, and placed in front of the undivided posterior half of the striate muscle complex. The anterior half of the muscle mass is then repaired in front of the bowel and the perineal muscles are repaired behind the urethra. The wound is then closed introducing the V flap of skin on the posterior surface of the bowel (Fig 7.19).

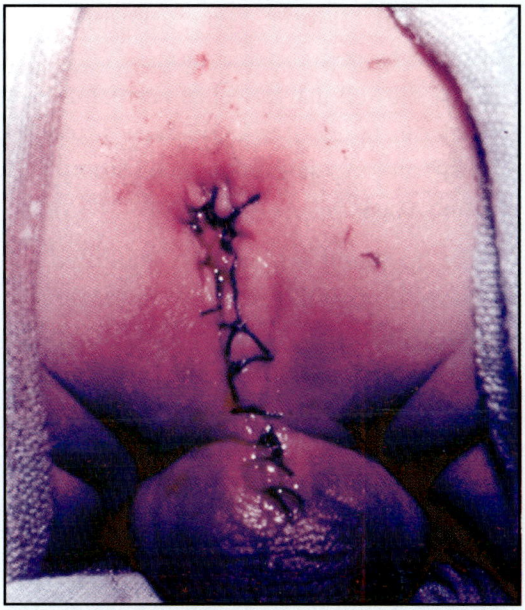

Fig. 7.19 Photograph after ASARP.

We have done this operation on 2 boys in 1989 and on 3 more recently. Our first patient was aged 3 months; he had a penoscrotal fistula, chordee without hypospadias and a colostomy. During separation of the bowel from the urethra, the latter was opened and it had to be repaired. Healing was uneventful and the colostomy was closed 3 months later. The second was one month old and had a perineoscrotal fistula; he had had periodic dilatations and washouts. Separation from the urethra could be carried out more easily and colostomy was avoided. Again, healing was uneventful. Both patients are now normal. The third patient had penoscrotal hypospadias, severe chordee and penoscrotal transposition; he also had arthrogryposis, sacral agenesis and a severe deformity of the right lower limb. ASARP was done without colostomy soon after birth. There was uneventful healing. Subsequently, he has required a few dilatations of the neoanus and several operations for his urological and orthopedic anomalies. He has no bowel problems. Our most recent patient came at the age of 3 weeks with a penoscrotal fistula; constipation was controlled by periodic dilatations. Xray with contrast showed that bowel of normal caliber was at the level of S4. He was cured by ASARP splitting the scrotum; colostomy was not necessary.

The operation was suitably modified for the girl; the fistula had to be meticulously separated from the entire length of the vagina before the perineal body was reached; this was then repaired and the anorectoplasty was successfully completed.

Prior to 1989, we had done Perineal Anal Transplant (PAT) without colostomy on the infants who had not been operated upon earlier. A circumferential incision around the fistula and a posterior V flap at the normal anal site were made and the two were joined by a sagittal incision dividing skin and subcutaneous tissues. The tract was dissected free from the posterior surface of the urethra and from the surrounding muscles. The muscular sling was then stretched and the dilated rectum above was gently delivered out. It was then brought to the normal anal site and fixed in place, accommodating the V flap of skin on the posterior wall of the bowel. The wound was then closed. Two neonates and 3 older boys had been cured with this operation. However, this limited exposure does not suffice if the fistula is placed far anterior and adheres densely to the urethra for a considerable distance.

The 8 patients who presented after previous surgery elsewhere had all presented before ASARP was devised. They had intestinal obstruction, perineal scarring, discharging sinus, dysuria and damaged striated muscles. One patient who presented in 1975 at the age of 6 weeks died of enterocolitis after Y-V plasty. Another who came in 1982 at the age of 7 weeks has required two revisions to correct anal stenosis and prolonged treatment for a urethral stricture. In the other 6, the fistula could be closed and intestinal obstruction relieved but normal continence was not achieved. None came back for follow up.

THREE: AN OPENING IN THE VESTIBULE

This is the commonest ARM seen in females (16% of all our cases).

The bowel opens in the fossa navicularis of the vestibule. It is surrounded by red wet epithelium and may vary in size from near normal to a pinpoint. The symptoms depend greatly on the size of this opening. It can almost always be dilated to allow the passage of a catheter through which the bowel can be initially decompressed.

In the Wingspread List, Vestibular fistulas are separated into Rectovestibular and Anovestibular.

The typical Rectovestibular fistula is an **intermediate** anomaly. A catheter passes almost vertically up, parallel to the back of the vagina. Bowel of normal or greater caliber is situated in a hammock formed by the levator ani. The fistula traverses the sling fibers of the levator to reach the back of the vagina, but misses the striated muscle complex entirely. At operation, the fistula is found to be intimately adherent to the posterior wall of the vagina almost up to the peritoneal reflection; in fact the bowel and the vagina often share a common wall for some distance (Figs. 7.20-21).

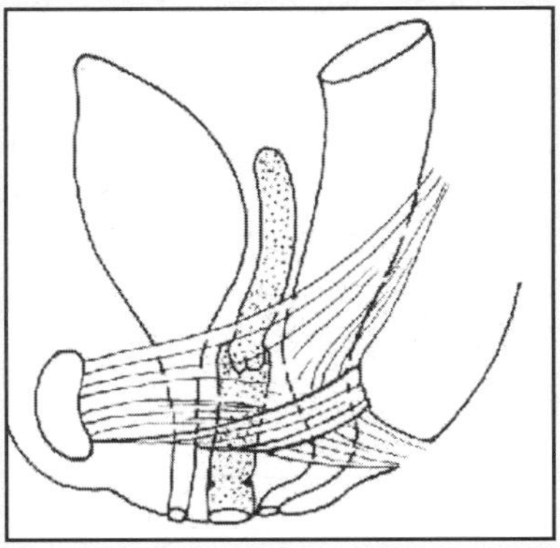

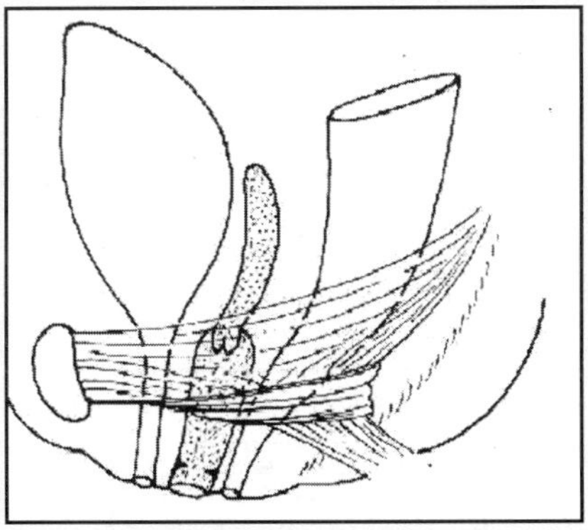

Figs. 7.20-21 Diagrams of anovestibular and rectovestibularfistulas.

On the other hand, the typical Anovestibular fistula is a **low** anomaly. The catheter passes almost horizontally backward parallel to the surface, and normal bowel is found under the skin at the normal anal site; the bowel has traversed most of the striated muscle complex. At operation, the fistula separates easily from the vagina.

Between the two typical forms, there are fistulas with varying grades of obliquity ending in bowel at varying levels. The length of the fistula can be measured by using a balloon catheter and drawing it out; it can be delineated on a lateral Xray taken after instilling contrast (Fig. 7.22).

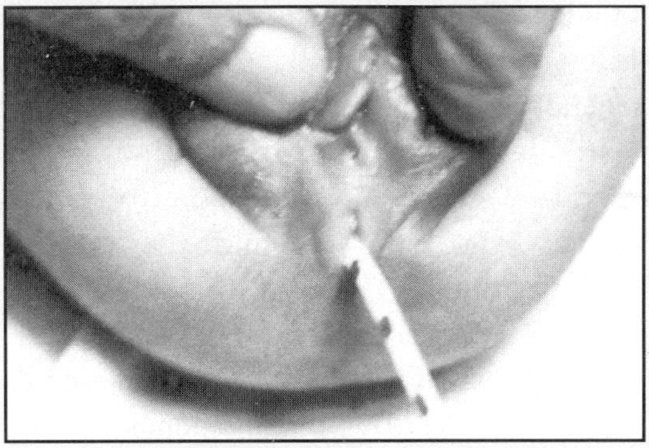

Fig. 7.22 Photograph with catheter in bowel.

In an earlier era, autopsy studies on 2 babies who had died with esophageal atresia and Vestibular fistula confirmed the anatomical arrangements described. In one, the fistula was Rectovestibular and hugged the back of the vagina before reaching normal howel. In the other, it was Anovestibular and the bowel had reached below the I line.

The condition should in our opinion be named AGENESIS WITH VESTIBULAR FISTULA to distinguish it from a lesion which though not included in the Wingspread List is nevertheless common in our series, namely Vestibular fistula with an otherwise normal anorectum.

Management

One-stage reconstruction in the neonatal period is the treatment of choice. This can be carried out provided the baby is otherwise healthy, that is, she weighs more than 2.5 kg. has no major associated anomalies, and no intercurrent infection, and her bowel can be completely evacuated by dilatation of the fistula and washouts.

At one time we attempted to distinguish between Anovestibular and Rectovestibular fistulas on the basis of preoperative radiological investigations and offered them different management plans. At present we generally perform the same operation on all vestibular fistulas though the findings at operation vary a great deal between the typical Anovestibular and the typical Rectovestibular. The operation performed for this for over 30 years is PERINEAL ANAL TRANSPLANT (PAT) (Chatterjee & Banerjee, 1999). PAT became popular in the United States due to the work of Potts *et al* (1954), Swenson and Donnellan (1969) and Santull (1962). Pathak and his colleagues from Chandigarh (Nainan *et al*, Saxena *et al*) reported good results from this procedure in 1975. Out of their 57 patients, 15 were neonates. In the neonate, the operation did not need the protection of a colostomy since there were no intestinal sutures in the depth of the wound and no muscles were divided. Surgeons who have reported good results after PAT without colostomy include Zivkovik et (1991) and Demirbilek and Atayurk (1999); both have avoided the operation on neonates. We first described our experience in 1976; at that time it was performed on infants above the age of 6 months. It has been done on neonates since 1980.

Our Present Technique of PAT

Until recently, this operation was performed with the patient prone either in the spread-eagled or in the knee chest position. We have now changed to the frog position; the anesthesiologist finds a neonate much easier to handle if kept supine. The steps of the operation are the same (Figs. 7.23-29).

a) A balloon catheter enters the bladder through the urethra. A metal bougie is used to demonstrate the lumen of the vagina.

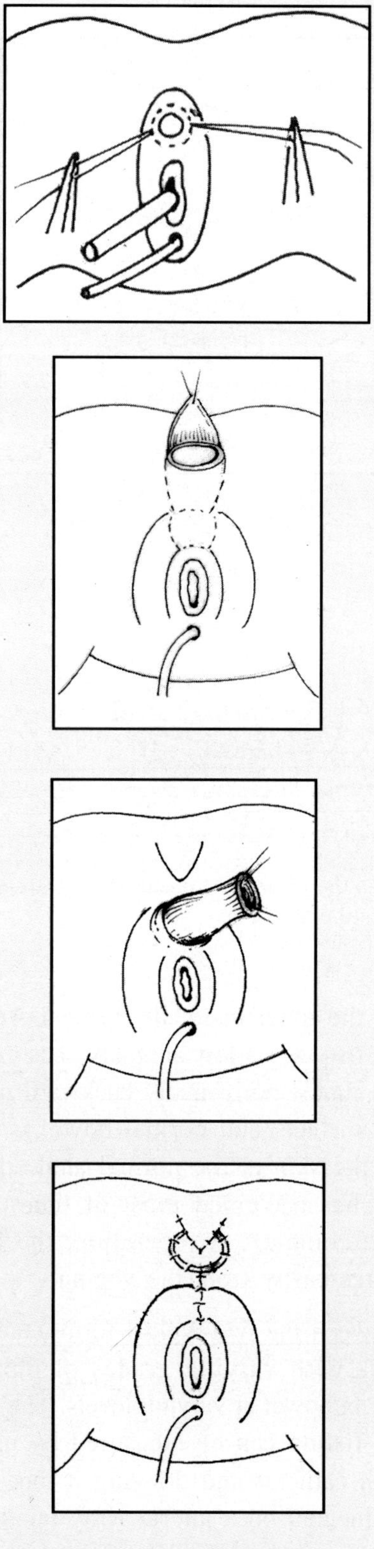

Figs. 7.23-26 Diagrams showing operation of PAT.

b) A circumferential incision is made round the orifice of the fistula and its margins are held up with 4 stay sutures. The dissection of the tract is then begun. It is separated from the striated muscles surrounding it, first on its posterior and then on the lateral aspects; sharp instruments are used and meticulous hemostasis is ensured. Anterolaterally on either side there is a large vessel that can be identified and coagulated before it is divided. Dissection then continues anteriorly to separate the fistula from the back of the vagina. As mentioned above, this may be very easy or very difficult. If a plane of cleavage is not readily found in the midline, the posterolateral margins of the vaginal orifice are held with stay sutures and a wedge of common wall is taken with the bowel. At a higher level, a plane of cleavage reappears and the bowel can be separated from the upper vagina, if necessary right up to the peritoneal reflection; this can be seen.

c) The dissection continues upwards until bowel of normal caliber is reached and sufficient length is available for it to reach the normal anal site. It is then drawn down through the levator sling. A V shaped incision with its apex pointed anteriorly is then made on the normal anal site. The skin flap is reflected to reveal the striated muscle complex; this is split in the midline and a tunnel is made through it up to the anterior wound. The bowel is then pulled through the tunnel up to the anal site carefully placing it within the striated muscle complex. Subsequently, the muscular coat of the bowel is sutured to the muscle complex. The V flap is

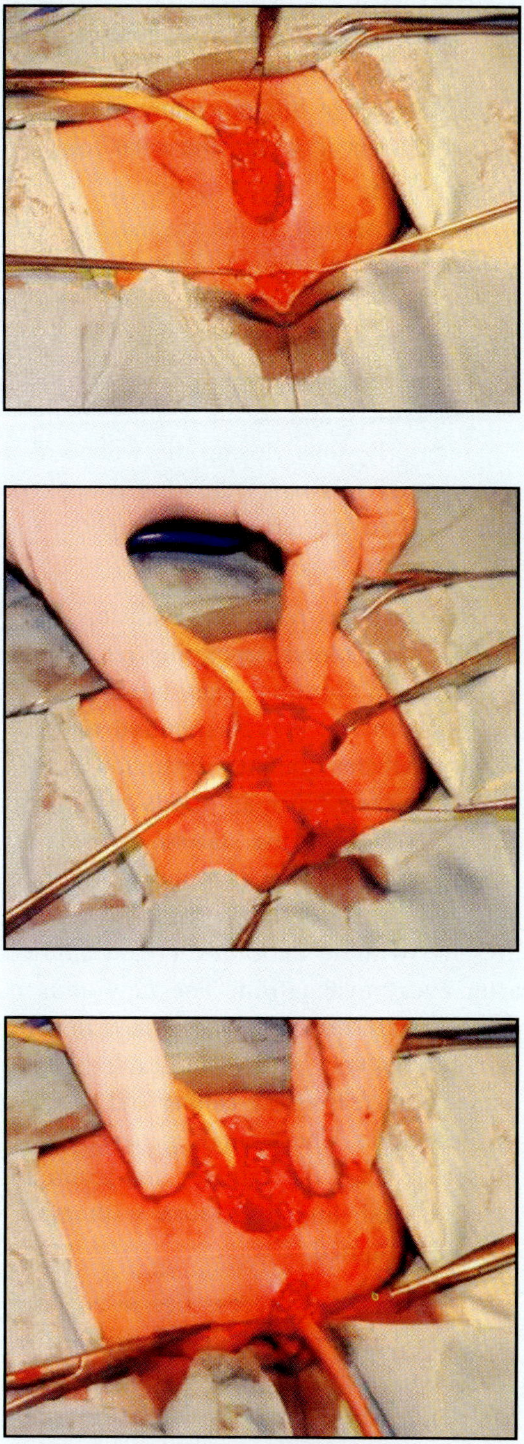

Figs. 7.27-29 Photographs of operation of PAT.

accomodated in a small midline vertical incision on the posterior bowel wall; then skin and bowel mucosa are sutured. At the end of this procedure, the bowel should recede within the natal folds.

d) Attention is then focussed on the anterior wound. If the vagina has been opened, it is repaired. Then the striated muscles on either side are apposed to reconstruct the perineal body. Finally the skin flaps are sutured to each other posteriorly and to the vaginal margin anteriorly, thus closing the wound as a reversed T; a bulky dressing is applied. Vicryl sutures are used throughout the operation.

Some patients require transfusion of 60 to 100 ml of blood depending on volume lost, age and nutrition. They are all nursed supine with the legs suspended and the urinary catheter draining continuously into a receptacle. Normal feeds and oral antibacterial drugs are started. A watchful eye is kept on bowel movements; the new anus has to be gently cleaned and a fresh dressing with an antibiotic cream applied after every evacuation. The new anus is dilated gently from the second day, initially using a relatively narrow malleable bougie, gradually increasing the caliber and stiffness of the bougie. The wounds generally heal in a week; then the catheter and restraints are removed, and dilatation with metal bougies is started.

The secret of success lies in ensuring that the baby passes stools of proper consistency. If she is allowed to evacuate hard stools, the suture lines will be subjected to strain; on the other hand, watery stools are likely to leak and cause infection in the perineal tissues.

The baby is generally sent home within 8 to 10 days after the operation with a dilator and asked to report at intervals for follow-up (Figs. 7.30-31).

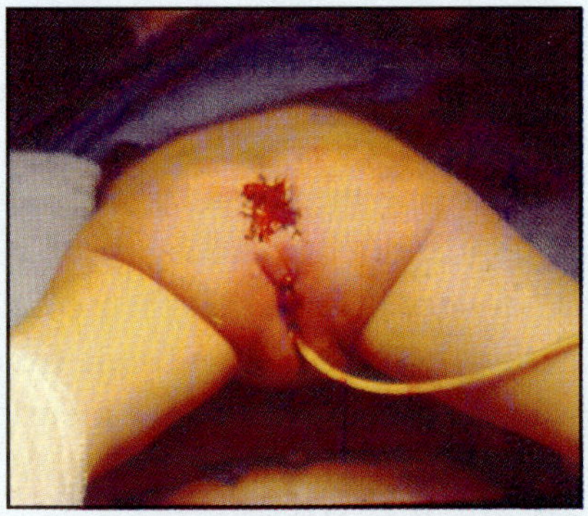

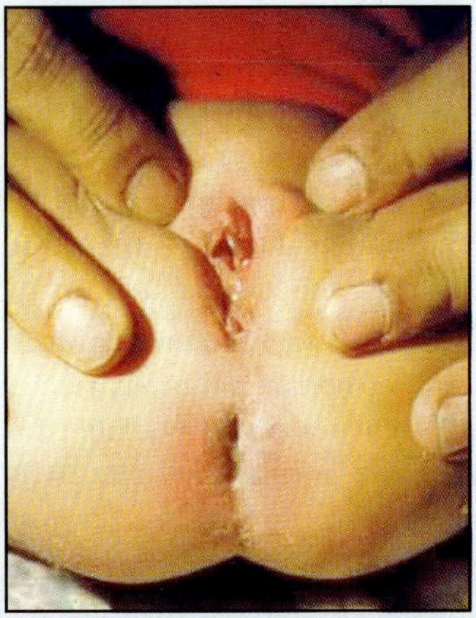

Figs. 7.30-31 Photographs of results.

Our results have been excellent. Of the 51 patients we reported earlier, one had a recurrence requiring operative closure and 2 had minor problems with wound healing. Constipation requiring treatment for about 2 to 3 years occurred in 12 patients but none of these were operated in the neonatal period. All were continent. We have subsequently done this operation on 33 more girls with even better results. A rare complication that followed untreated constipation is fistula in ano (Fig. 7.32). The obvious advantages of PAT over the alternative operation, namely SARP are preservation of the levator sling and the skin bridge between the fourchette and the neoanus.

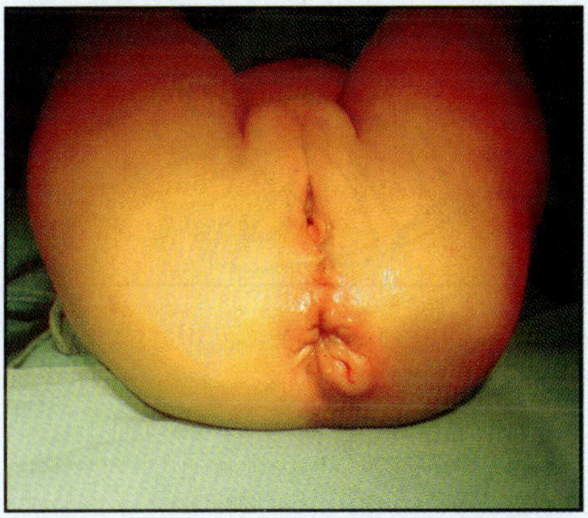

Fig. 7.32 Photograph of complication of PAT, fistula-in-ano after constipation.

Other management options are as follows:

1. In the 1970s, we advised **expectant treatment** with dilatations and washouts as an outpatient till the baby weighed 5 kg. The overall results were unsatisfactory. Success depended on the educational and socioeconomic status of the family and their ability to reach a good medical center. During the waiting period, many babies either became acutely obstructed or developed enterocolitis; others failed to thrive and did not reach 5 kg. even at the end of one year. At present we offer expectant treatment to small neonates, who are inpatients, to bring their weight up to 2.5 kg. and to correct complications; we then proceed to PAT.
2. **Cutback** is a time-honored operation that has saved innumerable lives. It divides tissues between two blades of a pair of scissors, one inserted in the bowel and the other on the surface. As mentioned earlier, no anesthesia is necessary and no sutures are given, but postoperative dilatations are necessary. More important, an inadequate cutback does not relieve obstruction and an extensive cut back results in incontinence.
3. **Y-V plasty** is a refinement that ensures epithelial continuity, and incidentally allows better visualization of the abnormal bowel. We perform Y-V plasty for Anovestibular fistula only when PAT is contraindicated because of a major associated anomaly, low birth weight and failure to thrive.
4. We recommend **Colostomy** if the bowel cannot be adequately decompressed through the fistula, if there are major associated anomalies, if birth weight is below 2 kg. and there is failure to thrive. PAT is done later. In 1988, Pena recommended PSARP after a preliminary colostomy as the treatment of choice for this condition irrespective of the level of lesion, and considered colostomy to be an acceptable price to guarantee uneventful healing of the perineum.
5. Other surgeons, notably Ahluwihare (1990), Okada *et al* (1992) and Wakhlu *et al* (1996), have performed **ASARP** on neonates without a colostomy. Das has done 19 out of 27 recent cases without colostomy with success. Pena himself now dispenses with the colos-

tomy but puts the baby on parenteral nutrition in the postoperative period. We have done ASARP with a concurrent colostomy on 4 adolescent patients and results were excellent.

Our technique of ASARP is as follows.

The operation resembles our procedure for Rectoperineal fistula. After a circumferential incision is made around the orifice of the fistula, a V incision is made at the normal anal site and the 2 are joined by a sagittal incision. The vertical fibers of the striated muscle complex are displayed and the muscle complex divided in the midline from the back of the fistula to the posterior limit of the vertical fibers. The bowel is then dissected free from the striated muscles on either side and from the vagina in front as described earlier until sufficient length is available for it to reach the normal anal site. The bowel wall is then sutured to the striated muscles all round and the muscles repaired in the midline. The V flap of skin is introduced into the posterior wall of the bowel and the wound closed.

6. We have done **PSARP** once on a 6 month old girl who had a vestibular fistula, a retrorectal mass and a postanal dimple with a discharge. The cyst was visualized by USG. At operation, a duplication cyst adherent to the rectum was found and removed and the bowel was placed in its correct position (Fig. 7.33). Recovery was uneventful (Basak *et al*, 1995).

Patients who present after a neonatal colostomy are obviously easier to handle; fecal contamination does not occur and the lower limbs do not have to be kept suspended in the immediate postoperative period.

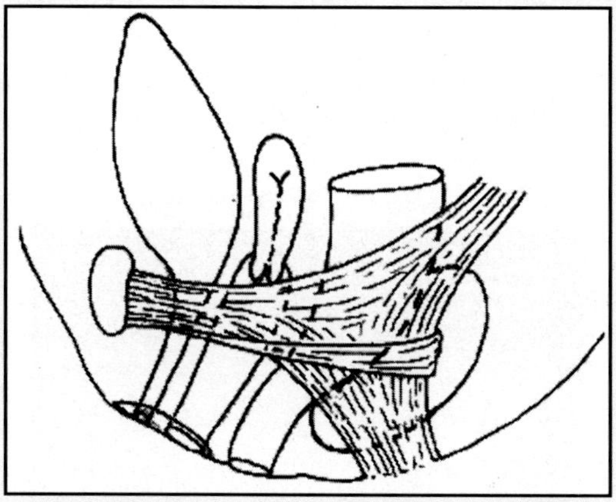

Fig. 7.33 Diagram of vestibular fistula with duplication cyst.

Most girls with agenesis and a vestibular fistula have an inadequate opening and present in infancy or early childhood. However, some girls with small fistulas are left untreated for years until a complication develops. A 5-year old girl was brought in 1989 with chronic intestinal obstruction; she survived by passing small quantities of stool through a gluteal opening and was taken away as soon as we advised colostomy (Figs. 7.34-35)

Girls with large vestibular fistulas without obstruction also tend to get neglected and families decide to seek treatment for them only after they reach the age of menarche. Worse, some girls have been brought to us by their husbands, one of them after the birth of a baby!

We perform PAT without colostomy on girls under the age of 5 years if they do not have protein-energy malnutrition or mega-

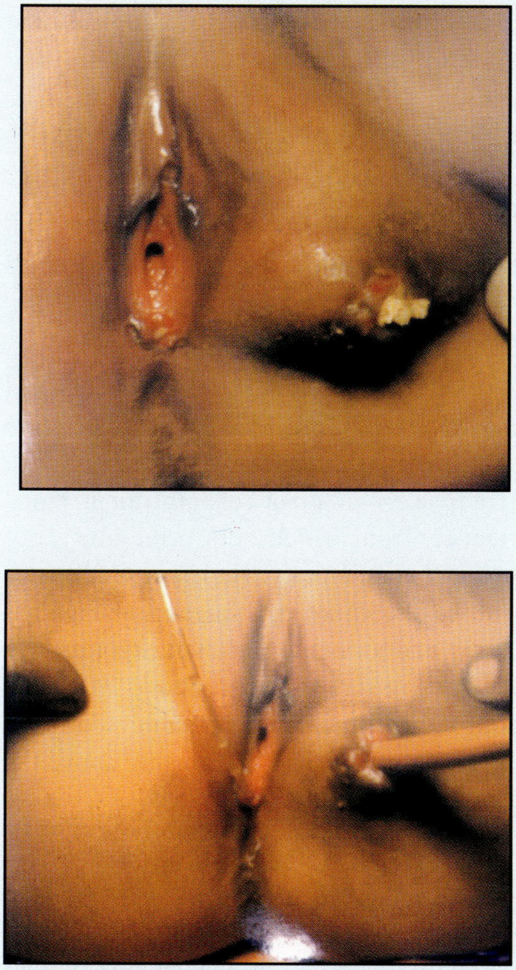

Figs. 7.34-35 Photographs of girl with untreated vestibular fistula and gluteal fistula.

rectum and their bowel can be completely decompressed by enemas and washouts. All other patients need a colostomy; in favorable situations, the colostomy may be done concurrently with the reconstruction. In the followup, there have been no problems other than constipation for varying lengths of time.

A large number of girls have come to us after incorrect management of vestibular fistula. They fall into the following categories:

1. **Continent shotgun perineum** is the expected end result of cutback or Y-V plasty. It can also be the end result of a poorly performed PAT or SARP with inadequate mobilization of the bowel from the vagina. Hence the anterior wall of the bowel returns to lie adjacent to the posterior wall of the vagina. The bowel is surrounded by the levator sling but is anterior to the trajectory of the striated muscle complex. The perineum has the appearance of a double-barrel gun (Fig. 7.36). It can be successfully managed by a revision of either PAT or SARP with or without a concurrent colostomy.

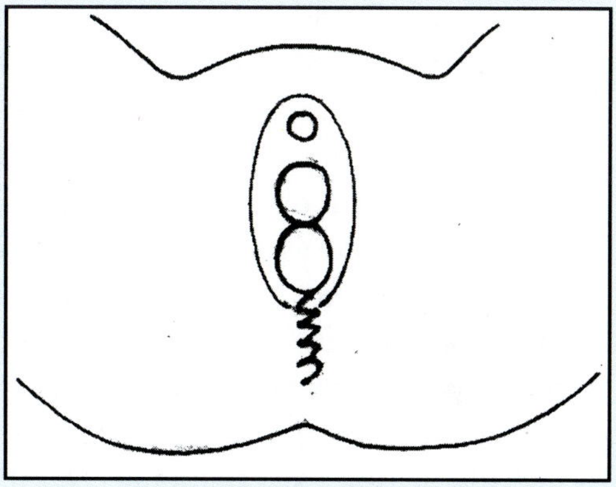

Fig. 7.36 Diagram of shotgun perineum.

2. **Incontinent shotgun perineum** results if the levator sling is damaged by previous surgery; it is treated by PSARP with colostomy protection; the operation will be described later.
3. **Recurrent vestibular fistula** is a less severe form of disruption of the anterior wound; bowel of normal caliber remains at the normal anal site but the anterior sutures have given way and feces leaks into the vagina (Fig. 7.37). This can be revised relatively easily.

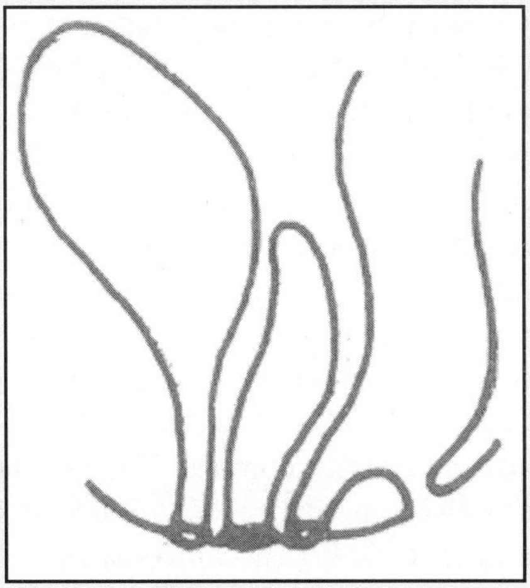

Fig. 7.37 Diagram of recurrent vestibular fistula.

4. **Obstruction** is the commonest and most serious complication.

   Obstruction following cutback is relatively mild and can be easily revised. However when bowel is brought to the surface under tension and retracts, it undergoes partial ischemic necrosis; the muscle complex is damaged; there is infection and subsequent scarring and progressive narrowing of the lumen of the bowel. Small amounts of feces emerge from the neoanus or the vestibule; fecal impaction converts a chronic obstruction into an acute one. Urgent colostomy is lifesaving. After the obstruction is relieved, the infection controlled and the patient's nutritional status stabilized, a formal revision by PSARP can be done.

   Although major associated anomalies are rare in patients with vestibular fistula, some have truncated sacrums and urinary incontinence. One girl treated by Chakravarti had a normal spine but nevertheless she had neurogenic bladder and bilateral vesicoureteral reflux. Neoureterocystostomies and CIC were necessary.

FOUR: AN ABNORMALLY LARGE OPENING

Two very unusual patients have been seen and followed up from birth for 27 and 19 years respectively.

Case 1 came in 1975 from a small town 500 km. away, when he was 6 weeks old and weighed 2.25 kg. He had a single large opening in the anterior perineum with prolapse of mucosa resembling urinary bladder, from which both urine and stool emerged continuously. He had a small penis with severe chordee, a huge right inguinal hernia and an empty left hemiscrotum. He also had severe arthrogryphosis affecting both lower limbs and moderate scoliosis. There was no clinical abnormality above the level of the umbilicus.

Plain Xray revealed almost total sacral agenesis, lumbar scoliosis, dislocated hips and other anticipated deformities in the lower limbs. A barium enema was normal except for some hold up at the anus.

We felt that the hernia posed an immediate threat to life and this was repaired. The perineum was then examined under anesthesia. When the prolapse was reduced, the opening admitted an index finger. Bowel formed its posterior quadrant and urinary bladder formed the anterior three quadrants; here the trigone and ureteric orifices could be identified (Figs. 7.38-39).

Treatment to separate the two streams was postponed and he was referred to an orthopedic colleague. Operative procedures were carried out on the lower limbs between 1975 and 1978; after he became ambulant

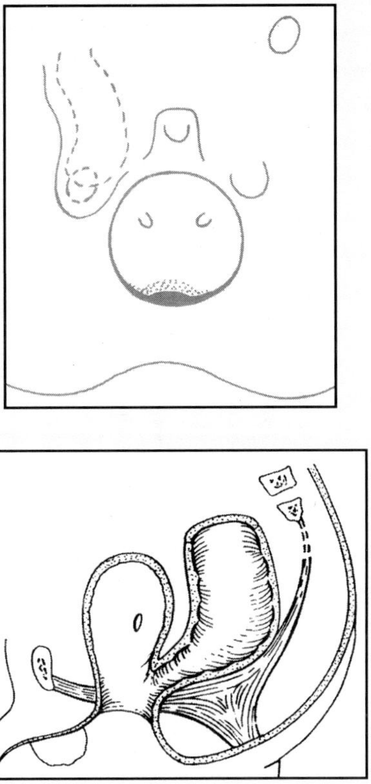

Figs. 7.38-39 Diagrams of rectovesicoperineal fistula.

with appliances, he came back for the management of urinary and fecal incontinence.

Investigations carried out showed crossed renal ectopia with both renal pelves on the right side and no renal tissue on the left (Fig. 7.40).

When he was 5 years old, the alimentary and urinary tracts were separated by a perineal operation. A circumferential incision was made around the opening of the bowel into the posterior wall of the vesicourethral canal; this term is used because it was impossible to identify a vesicourethral junction. The ureteric orifices were easily identified and kept out of the way.

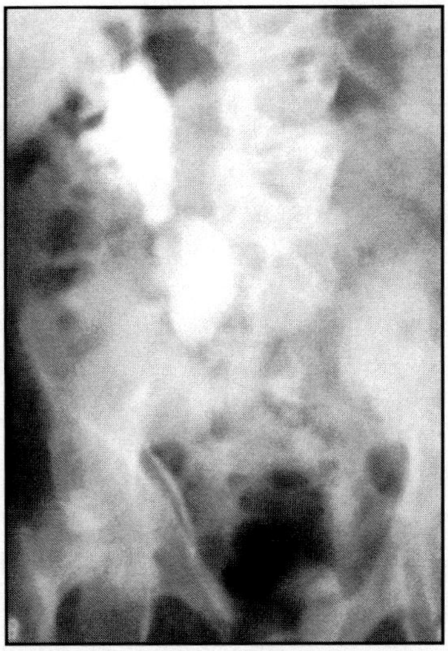

Fig. 7.40 Xray IVU of rectovesicoperineal fistula.

The bowel was mobilized and brought to the surface. A cruciate incision was made at the normal anal site, and the terminal bowel pulled through into this posterior wound as in Perineal anal transplant for rectovestibular fistula. The bowel was sutured in place at the normal anal site; then the anterior wound was closed by suturing the cut margins of the urothelium to the skin, leaving a balloon catheter in the bladder (Fig. 7.41).

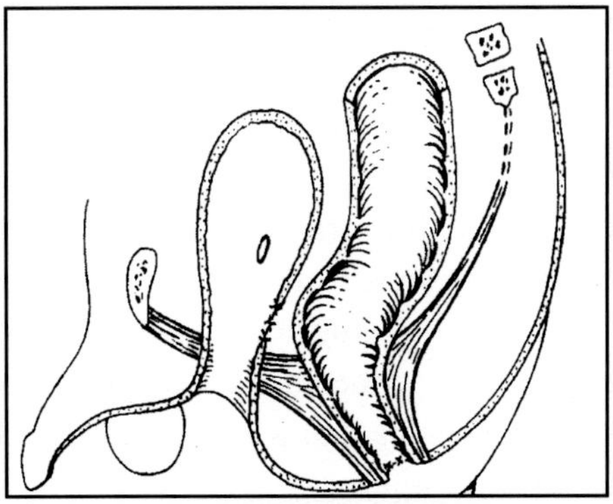

Fig. 7.41 Diagram showing postoperative state.

Recovery was uneventful and fecal continence was established. Histological examination of the junctional epithelium showed the character of large bowel changing to that of urinary bladder.

He returned 3 years later at the age of 8. He was going to school and walking with appliances and elbow crutches. He had excellent fecal continence but total urinary incontinence; this did not improve in spite of several operations on the urogenital organs. When he was 13, he and his family agreed to urinary diversion and this was carried out using the vascularized appendix as a conduit from the ureter of the lower moiety; the ureter of the upper moiety had earlier been anastomosed to the pelvis of the lower moiety. The stoma was placed in the right lower quadrant of the abdomen. He was fitted with an appliance and the postoperative intravenous urogram showed good function. The need for close followup was emphasized; the family cooperated up to 1990 and all was well.

He then disappeared for 12 years and returned in 2002 at the age of 27; a science graduate and a schoolmaster in his hometown. He was grossly overweight; he used crutches and not the appliances prescribed. He had complete fecal continence in spite of a small mucosal prolapse at the anus (Fig 7.42). Urine drained through the stoma in his right loin into diapers. Recurrent bouts of urinary infection were controlled by selfmedication with antibacterial drugs off and on. The state of his anterior perineum was as it was; there was a small penis and a single testis in the right hemiscrotum.

He agreed to undergo some investigations. These showed that his blood urea and

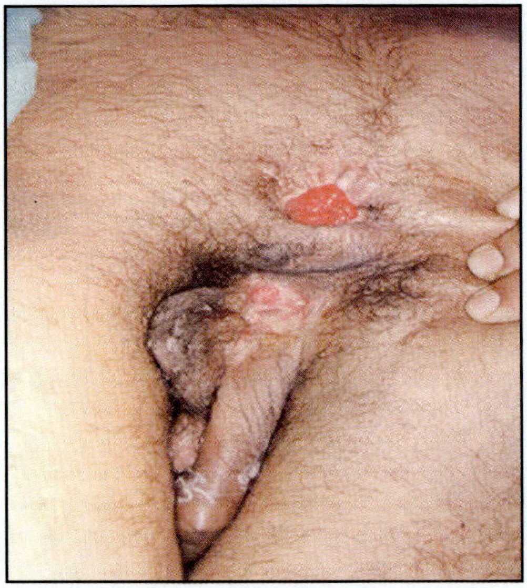

Fig. 7.42 Photograph of same patient, postoperative.

creatinine levels were normal and his urine contained plenty of pus cells but no microorganisms. USG showed gross hydronephrosis of both kidneys. Xray showed a dislocated left hip and almost total sacral agenesis. He was advised to consult his orthopedic surgeon and get proper appliances. He was also advised to undergo studies to show the functional status of the kidneys and practice clean intermittent catheterization through the stoma. He was put on longterm antibacterial drugs. He and his parents were warned that his renal status was unsatisfactory. He was not concerned about his sexual inadequacy.

Case 2 came in 1984 from a small town 400 km away; he was 4 months old and weighed 5 kg. He had a single patulous opening in the anterior perineum through which he passed both urine and feces and through which mucosa prolapsed. The anterior quadrant of the opening was taken up by the urethra and the posterior and lateral quadrants by bowel (Figs. 7.43-44). The epithelium that prolapsed had all the characteristics of large bowel lining. In addition, there was penoscrotal transposition and severe chordee. Defecation and micturation was normal for age, and the opening easily admitted an index finger. There were no skeletal abnormalities and no upper urinary tract problems.

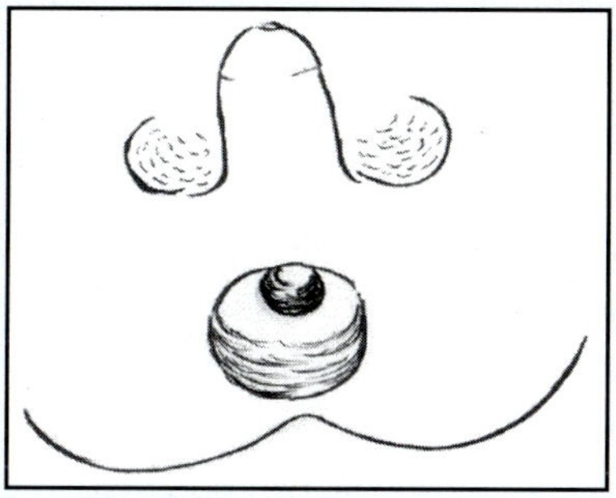

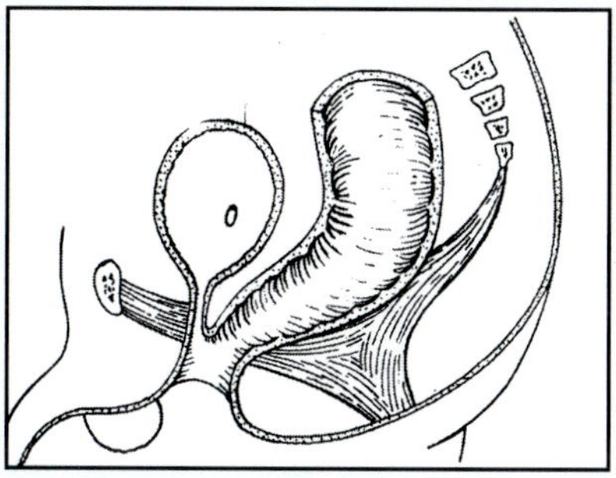

Figs. 7.43-44 Diagrams of rectourethroperineal fistula.

We decided to separate the urinary and fecal streams, With a balloon catheter in the urethra, a transverse incision was made through the junctional mucosa; the incision was continued through skin on either side as two V flaps. The anterior half of the anorectum was separated by sharp dissection from the back of the posterior urethra and bladder; it was then infolded to form a channel large enough to accommodate a number 12 dilator. The striated muscles were then repaired in front of the bowel and behind the posterior urethra and the V flaps apposed to form a Z. Healing was uneventful.

When seen two years later, there was partial recurrence of prolapse and poor fecal and urinary continence. A revisional operation was carried out at the anus excising the prolapse and transposing the anus further back. The muscles were apposed snugly in front of the bowel. Further revisions were necessary to achieve fecal continence and control prolapse. A series of operations were then carried out to ensure normal urinary continence and a reasonable contour of the external genitalia. He was doing well when seen in 1989.

He then disappeared and reported for followup 14 years later in 2003 at the age of 19. He had normal urinary and fecal continence. His anorectum appeared normal except for a small mucosal prolapse (Fig. 7.45).

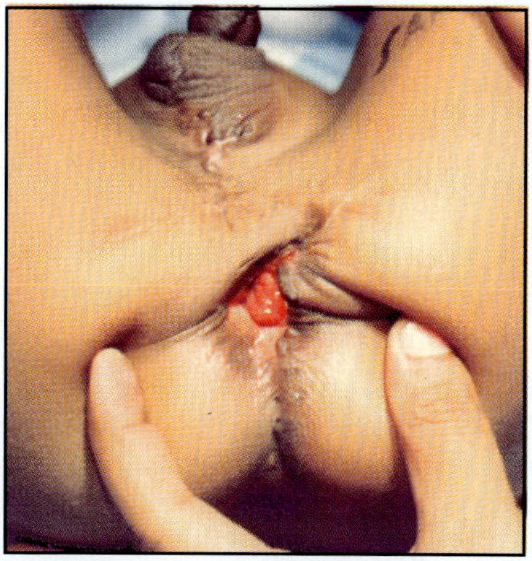

Fig.7.45 Photograph of same patient, postoperative.

There was residual chordee; the urethra ended at the base of the glans and there was a fistula more proximally. In the course of the operation to correct these deformities, a cystourethroscopy was carried out; no abnormality was detected. A satisfactory urethroplasty has now been done and he looks forwards to a normal sexual life.

We consider that the basic embryological defect in both cases is similar. The bowel terminated in the urinary tract, as a rectovesical fistula in the first case and a rectoprostatic urethral fistula in the second. Subsequently, the distal part of the urinary tract failed to develop and opened on the surface of the perineum. The deformity in the second case could be considered to be an extension of incontinent perineal hypospadias, complicated by the rectoprostatic urethral fistula and can be named **rectourethroperineal fistula.** The deformity in the first case is more profound and resembles the mermaid syndrome described by Duhamel as early as 1961. There is not only a **rectovesicoperineal fistula** but also severe skeletal and renal anomalies.

Both patients are now adults and lead more or less normal lives. Both have satisfactory fecal continence. Case 1 has a severely truncated sacrum and is unlikely to have either pelvic splanchnic or somatic nerves; bowel function appears to be dependent on vagal and lumbar sympathetic nerves. Such a superior functional result has probably resulted because reconstruction was carried out with minimum dissection in the perirectal area. Urinary continence has been achieved in Case two by reconstructing the urethra and external urethral sphincter, but diversion was the only option in Case 1. If we were consulted today for patients with similar malformations, we would surely have suggested surgery by the posterior sagittal approach.

CHAPTER 8

A MANIFEST INVISIBLE OPENING

The opening is manifest by the passage of meconium through the urethra or vagina or common urethrovaginal orifice. They differ in the two sexes.

ONE: AGENESIS WITH URETHRAL FISTULA

This is the commonest ARM seen in males (16% of all our cases) (Fig. 8.1).

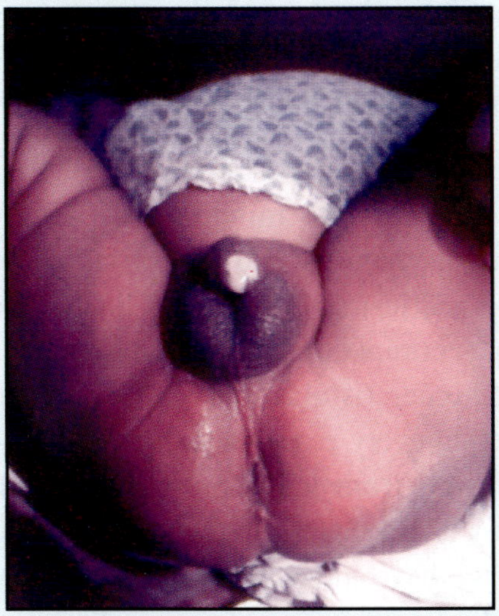

Fig. 8.1 Photograph of neonate with meconium at urethra.

According to the Wingspread Classification, if the terminal bowel is above the P-C line and the fistula is into the prostatic urethra, the lesion is a **high** one and is named ANORECTAL AGENESIS WITH RECTO-PROSTATIC URETHRAL FISTULA (RBUF). On the other hand, if the terminal bowel is between the P-C line and the I line and the fistula opens into the bulbar urethra, the lesion is an **intermediate** one and is named ANAL AGENESIS WITH RECTO-BULBAR URETHRAL FISTULA (RPUF) (Figs. 8.2-3).

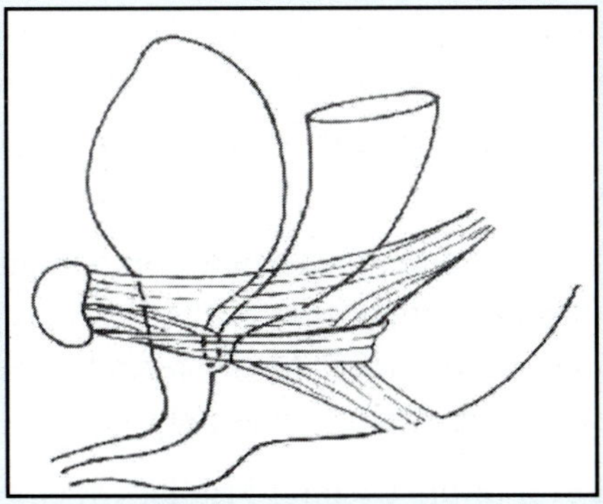

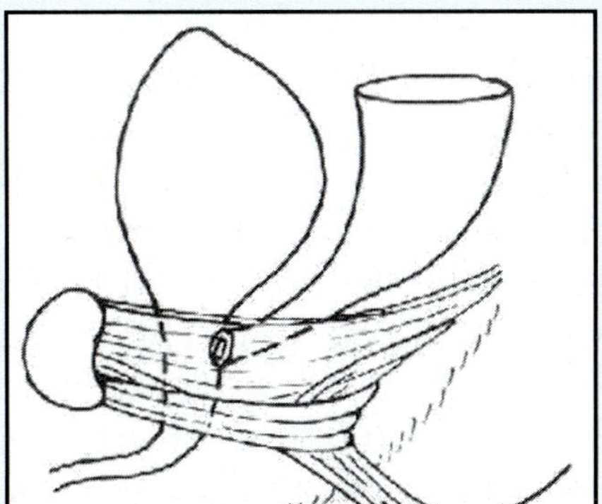

Figs. 8.2-3 Diagrams of rectobulbar urethral fistula and rectoprostatic urethral fistula.

The size of the fistula varies greatly. It can be very large and allow passage of not only meconium but also flatus and feces through the urethra. When large, a catheter introduced through the urethra easily enters the bowel but does not enter the bladder. A baby with a large fistula may survive without treatment for days. One baby survived for three months defecating and micturating through the external urethral meatus. He had been submitted to a perineal operation elsewhere only when he developed complete intestinal obstruction. He reached us two weeks later with the neoanus occluded.

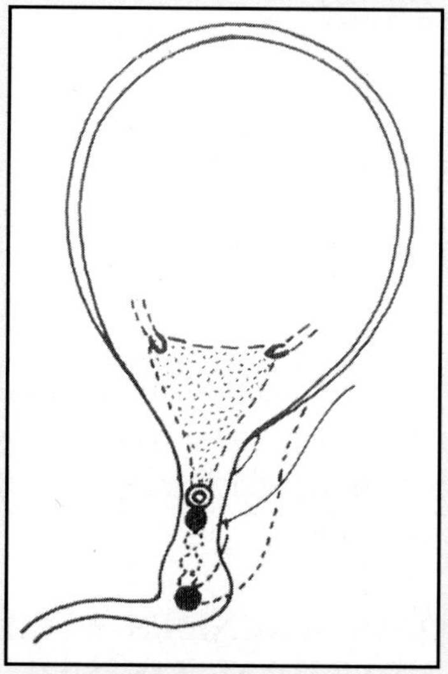

Fig. 8.4 Diagram showing sites of opening of urethral fistulas.

On the other hand, the fistula might be very small and not clinically manifest. If microscopic examination of the urine shows intestinal columnar epithelial cells, a fistula between bowel and urinary tract can be confirmed.

In our opinion, the two components of the lesion, namely the level of the urethral fistula and the level of the terminal bowel must be considered separately.

Level of the Urethral Fistula. On embryological grounds, the fistula must be in that part of the urethra that arises from the urogenital sinus, that is the part between the verumontanum and the bulb. While the majority of fistulas are indeed clustered at either the upper end or the lower end of this urethral strip, the orifice can be found anywhere along the strip (Fig. 8.4). It is intriguing to find that there has over the years been a distal shift in fistula level. Even in the early 1970s, the fistula was generally found to open in the prostatic urethra, but today in most centers, including our own, the rectobulbar fistula is more common. Also, three fistulas clearly demonstrated by clinical observation, Xray and endoscopy soon after birth could not be found later either by pre-reconstruction endoscopy or during the actual reconstruction.

Level of Terminal Bowel. In our series, the bowel has terminated as high as the sacral promontory and as low as below the I line and just above the anal line. Although higher terminations are generally associated with higher fistulas and vice versa, this is not so in every case. The shape of the bowel may vary from a sledge to a retort (Figs. 8.5-6). It is because many are retort shaped that we have numerous patients who had a simple perineal operation elsewhere at birth and who presented later with a urinary fistula but no bowel obstruction. In a large Japanese series reported in 1992, there were 420 patients with ARM and a urethral fistula; in 23 the bowel ended high up but the fistula entered low down.

In an earlier era we had examined at autopsy 14 neonates and 1 infant dying with

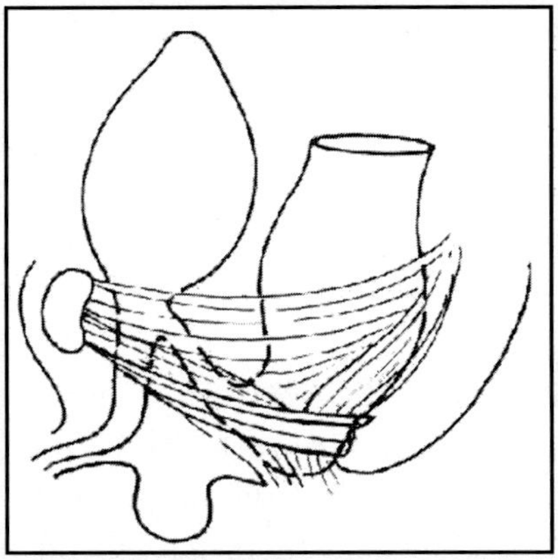

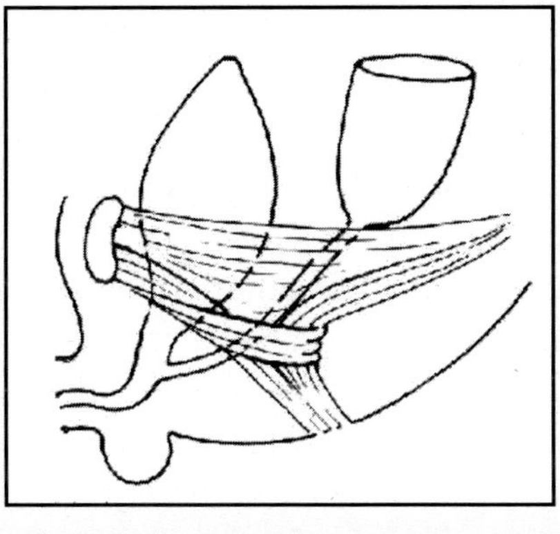

Figs. 8.5-6 Diagrams showing high and low levels of termination of bowel.

Rectourethral fistula. The bowel terminated in the prostatic urethra in all; high up above the P-C line in 9, between the P-C line and the I line in 3 and below the I line in 3; in the last 3, the rectal pouch was within 5 mm of the perineal skin. It sat in a basket formed by striated muscle of the pelvic diaphragm; the fistula emerged from its anterior surface and passed upwards and forwards to reach the prostatic urethra above the levator sling. One boy had survived for one year after a perineal operation done soon after birth for absence of anus had partially relieved intestinal obstruction. He passed small amounts of stool both from the urethra and from a stenotic perineal opening. When he reached us, he was very ill and had gross abdominal distension. Xray with contrast introduced through the perineal opening revealed a retort shaped bowel ending in a high urethral fistula. He died shortly after colostomy was done. He had pyonephrosis of a solitary kidney; the distended rectum was placed low down in the perineum and was connected to the prostatic urethra with a long wide fistula.

Management in the Neonate

The investigations that we carry out on a neonate at the time of first presentation are USG, erect straight Xray of the chest and abdomen, prone cross lateral Xray if the baby comes after 12 hours and urethrogram. Although MRI scan can show the entire anatomy of the region it is not usually affordable in our setup. Urethrography is more easily done; contrast instilled through a urethral catheter will pass through a large fistula into the bowel and a lateral Xray will show the fistula and the level of the terminal bowel (Fig. 8.7).

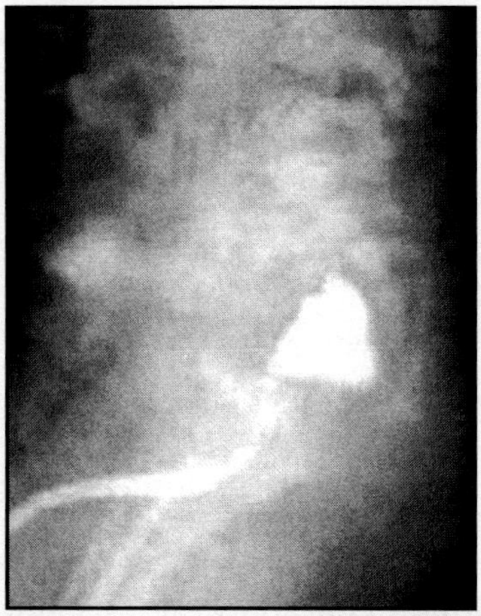

Fig. 8.7 Xray - urethrogram of baby with rectourethral fistula.

The most conclusive method of visualizing fistulas, large or small, is endoscopy; a cystourethroscopy at the start of any operative procedure yields rich dividends.

Earlier we did not recommend too many investigations on the neonate to find out levels, because irrespective of the level of the terminal bowel and of the fistula, we performed a **colostomy** as soon after birth as possible. This is the operation with the highest success rate and should be done everywhere except in centers of excellence.

We believe that reconstruction can certainly be carried out without colostomy provided safety is not compromised. This is possible in an institution with a limited number of neonatal emergencies and with everything under the control of the surgical team. In the setup of an average busy Indian Hospital like the NRS Medical College Hospital, Kolkata, colostomy is still the procedure of choice. The large number of emergencies that need to be handled, the late presentation of the neonates and the difficulties in rapidly organizing the necessary investigations and operating facilities for a major operation do not usually allow a safe primary reconstruction. The setup in the PGI Chandigarh is a lot better; even here a study by Mishra *et al* in 2000 has revealed that primary PSARP has a significantly higher mortality and morbidity than a staged procedure. There were 4 deaths out of 14 primary cases, as against 3 out of 20 staged cases. Functional assessment at the end of 1 year was not significantly different.

The procedures for **primary reconstruction without colostomy** are as follows:

1. **Sacroperineal reconstruction (SPR)** was successfully performed by us on a number of neonates 2 decades ago if they were fit for a major operative procedure and the level of the lesion permitted correction by this route. While results in some neonates have been excellent, there have been disasters in others.
2. **Primary PSARP** has now many advocates. Moore (1990) and Goon (1990) first recommended this procedure and there have been favorable reports from Bianchi and Albanese. In India Gopal and her colleagues in Varanasi perform the operation under local anesthesia and intravenous sedation with diazepam and ketamine (2001). It is done under general anesthesia in other Indian centers including Chennai and our own; we now have 8 cases. The question that has to be answered is what should be done if the bowel cannot be brought down by this approach. The alternatives are to turn the baby over and complete the pullthrough intraperitoneally or to settle for a colostomy.
3. **Primary perineal rectourethroanoplasty** has been advocated by Ahluwihare of Kandy for many years. In 1989 he reported 27 successful neonatal reconstructions by a wide perineal exposure and stretching of the levator sling. Only 4 neonates required an additional laparotomy to bring the bowel down. We would name this procedure Anterior Sagittal Ano Recto Plasty (ASARP); we have one case.
4. **Abdominoperineal reconstruction (APARP)** was done in the 1940s. At that time the structure and function of the muscles and nerves of the region had not been properly studied and methods

for establishing continence had not been developed. We have had some early successes with this but failures outweighed successes and the operation was abandoned by us in the 1960s. Pellerin of Paris, one of the few supporters of this operation, reported his results on 82 neonates in 1984; he had 23 deaths, all before 1974. Subsequently, by excluding neonates with major associated anomalies and low birth weight; he eliminated mortality but had a complication rate most surgeons would not accept.

5. **Laparoscopic assisted APARP** is being done on neonates in a few centers around the world (Georgeson 2000, Yeung 2001); its safety and long term results need to be studied. However, there is no doubt that it facilitates the dissection in the approximately 10% of ARM patients who need a laparotomy. It hastens the perineal dissection by mobilization, ligation and grabber thrusting of the distal rectal pouch toward the sphincter area of the perineal dissection and the perineal operator can then deliver the bowel easily. Details are described later.

Management in the Postneonatal Period

In the postneonatal period, most babies have reached us with a colostomy. However, some have come after they had been submitted to a perineal operation by a peripheral surgeon. The bowel had been decompressed and the emergency tided over but the urethral connection remained (Figs. 8.8-9) According to many peripheral surgeons, a perineal operation, however incomplete, saves more lives than a colostomy. Many boys have presented to us with normal fecal continence but with urinary infection and the passage of urine through the anus and flatus and feces through the urethra, A few had in addition, features of incomplete intestinal obstruction and fecal incontinence. In these boys, the anatomy of the region was displayed by contrast Xray and endoscopy.

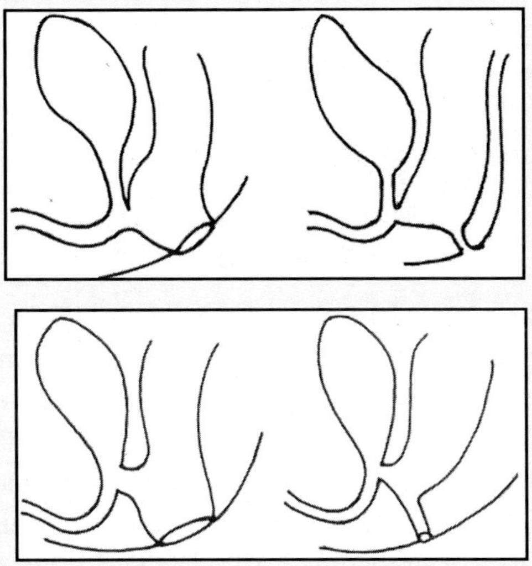

Figs. 8.8-9 Diagrams to show persistent urethral fistula.

Relatively easy cases not requiring bowel mobilization were cured by a limited perineal operation using an anterior based V flap of skin. Most have required a formal PSARP; if the bowel could be emptied by washouts through the neoanus, preliminary colostomy was dispensed with. A concurrent colostomy was added if the operation proved difficult. Things were particularly difficult in a 9 month old boy who had a large perineal opening through which he passed both urine and stool and had in addition perineal hypospadias and penoscrotal transposition. We did a preliminary colostomy and then carried out a very difficult PSARP and repaired the hypospadias before we closed the colostomy. Thomas and Molenaar had reported their study of this problem in 1979. Much earlier, in 1957, I had reported successful closure of a persisting rectourethral fistula in a 27 year old who had normal fecal continence after a perineal operation done soon after birth for absence of anus. In 2000, Kulshrestha *et al* reported successful closure of rectourethral fistulas, including one on a married 32 year old who came for infertility, he was passing all his urine and semen through the fistula.

Management after a Colostomy

The method of reconstruction is decided upon after a distal cologram is taken. This imaging device accurately reveals the level of the terminal bowel and the urethral fistula. The distal cologram on a lateral view may show a complete fistula (Fig. 8.10), or only a beak suggesting a fistula. The longest fistula in our series is shown in Figs. 8.11-12. The length of colon between the ostomy and the terminal bowel is shown on a PA view (Fig. 8.13).

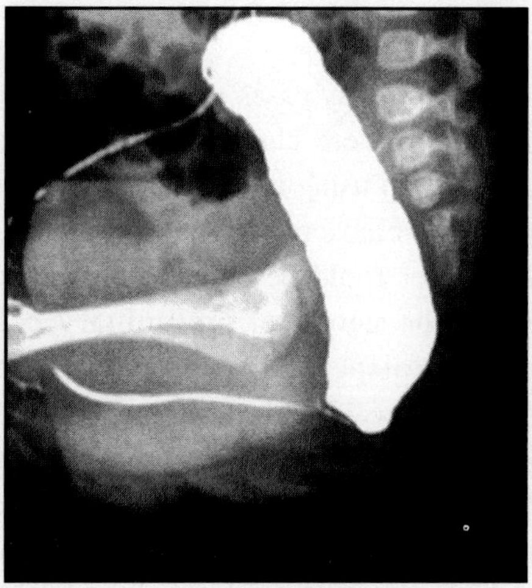

Fig. 8.10 Xray - distal cologram showing standard fistula.

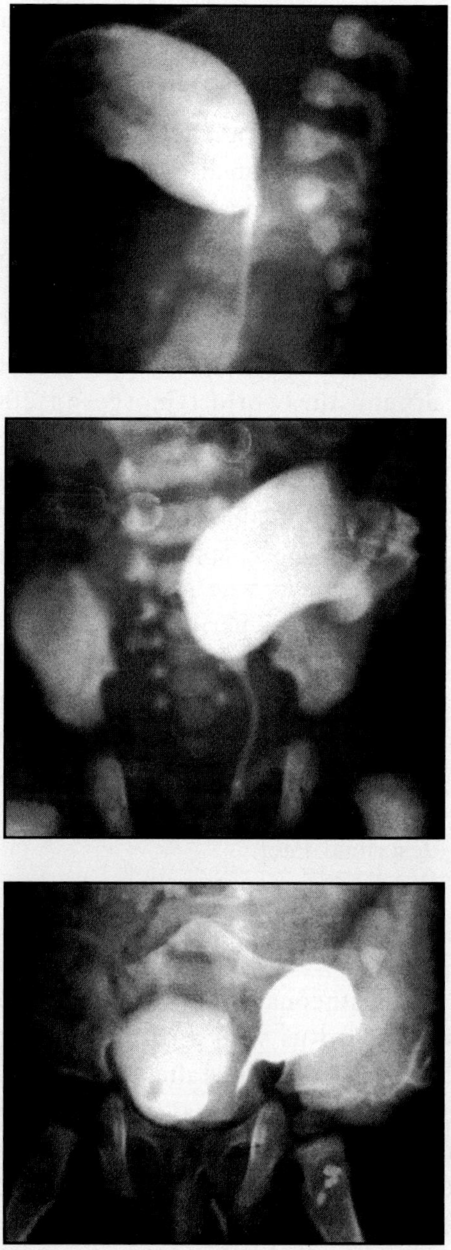

Figs. 8.11-13 Xray - distal cologram showing long fistula.

EXTRAPERITONEAL RECONSTRUCTIONS

1. Sacroperineal (SPR)

For a period of 14 years, from 1970 to 1984, SPR was the sheet anchor of our surgery for ARMs with the bowel ending between the 4th sacral vertebra and the I line. With minor modifications of the original Stephens operation, we could give countless children the gift of fecal continence. However, after Pena demonstrated that a midline incision in the perineum was harmless if the divided muscles were carefully repaired at the end of the procedure, the operation proposed by Pena and named Posterior Sagittal Ano-RectoPlasty (PSARP) has become the standard method of repairing major ARMs in most centers including our own. It has almost completely replaced SPR, almost, because surgeons in three important centers in India namely Chennai, Vellore and Calicut still perform SPR with some personal modifications.

2. Posterior sagittal (PSARP)

We changed over to PSARP, for the following reasons.

(i) The prime reason was that the most important step in SPR was performed blindly. The pullthrough was done with only a mental picture of the levator muscle as a guide. With PSARP all the structures of the region are exposed and the pullthrough is done under direct vision. Thus, the steps of PSARP can be clearly demonstrated to others.

(ii) In PSARP, most fistulas can be clearly defined and closed accurately. This is not so with SPR.

(iii) Bowel ending between the third and the fourth sacral vertebras could not have been exposed by SPR but can be mobilized to reach the perineum by PSARP; thus the need for intraperitoneal procedures is diminished.

(iv) Ectatic bowel encountered in the course of SPR posed an insoluble problem; it can easily be tapered during the course of PSARP.

(v) Finally, the sagittal splitting of the coccyx and lower sacrum necessary for PSARP is far less damaging than the wide transverse separation of coccyx and sacrum required for SPR. This will be discussed in Chapter 15.

(vi) We were initially worried about the fact that we did not possess a muscle stimulator.The stimulator became available in 1989; after we assessed its value in delineating the function of the different fibers, we reserved its use for teaching and for revisional surgery.

Our technique, in a boy with a colostomy (Figs. 8.14-21).

(a) Position

The spreadeagled position is eminently suited for this operation; in the absence of a stimulator, the surgeon should face the midline and not operate from one or other side.

(b) Preliminaries

Before the patient is turned prone, a flatus tube is passed down the distal colon and the bowel gently irrigated with dilute povidine iodine. The flatus tube is left in, and a cystourethroscopy is performed to confirm the presence and site of the fistula and the appearances of the ureteric orifices. After the patient is turned over and draped, a bougie is passed into the urethra.

(c) Incision

An inverted Y incision is made centered at the normal anal site; there is a short anterior V flap and a long sagittal stem reaching up to the lower sacrum. After the skin is incised, the knife is discarded in favor of a needletip cautery. Cautery is used both for cutting and for hemostasis throughout the operation. The parasagittal fibers of the external sphincter coursing from the coccyx to the normal anal site are exposed. At the normal anal site the vertical fibers of the sphincter can be identified. The anterior and posterior limits of these fibers are marked by fine stay sutures.

(d) Exposure

The parasagittal fibers with their covering fascia are incised strictly in the midline and then the posterior half of the vertical fibers are incised; this exposes the levator ani. Posterosuperiorly, the diaphragm fibers can be split in the midline down to the area where it fuses with the external sphincter. A self-retaining retractor is now placed in the wound and an excellent exposure is obtained. **The lower part of the striated muscle complex including the levator sling is left intact.**

(e) The rectum

This is covered with a layer of endopelvic fascia; it may reach as low as the sling fibers of the levator; on the other hand, it may end just in front of the lower sacrum. In the latter situation, the flatus tube introduced earlier is helpful; an assistant manipulating the tube from above can push the rectal pouch down into the wound. After the endopelvic fascia is incised, the rectum is picked up with stay sutures and the flatus tube removed. Identification and mobilization of the rectal pouch is easy if the urethral bougie is passed into it through the fistula. The rectum is mobilized posteriorly and laterally in the plane between the endopelvic fascia and the longitudinal smooth muscle. Care must be taken to remain close to the bowel wall and avoid damage to the pelvic nerves that course on either side to reach the urogenital organs in front. The middle rectal vessels need to be coagulated and divided, and then the bowel can be lifted up.

(f) The rectourethral separation

This is the most difficult part of the operation, irrespective of the level of the terminal bowel. The rectum that reaches a lower level is generally more intimately adherent to the urethra than one that ends higher up. The separation is carried out from within the lumen of the bowel. Its posterior wall is incised in the midline as low as possible and then its anterior wall is examined. After the fistula is found, a circumferential incision is made around it and the mucosa is mobilized above and lateral to the fistula. The urethral bougie helps in the smooth progress of this dissection. The bougie can be manipulated into the bladder or through the fistula into the rectum and this helps to define the structures. Further laterally, the full thickness of the bowel wall is incised on either side and these incisions meet the original incision made in the midline posteriorly. It is our endeavor to expose neither vas deferens nor seminal vesicle during the separation of a relatively lowly placed rectum with a RBUF. Some RBUFs are placed very low, in front of the sling fibers of the levator ani-deep

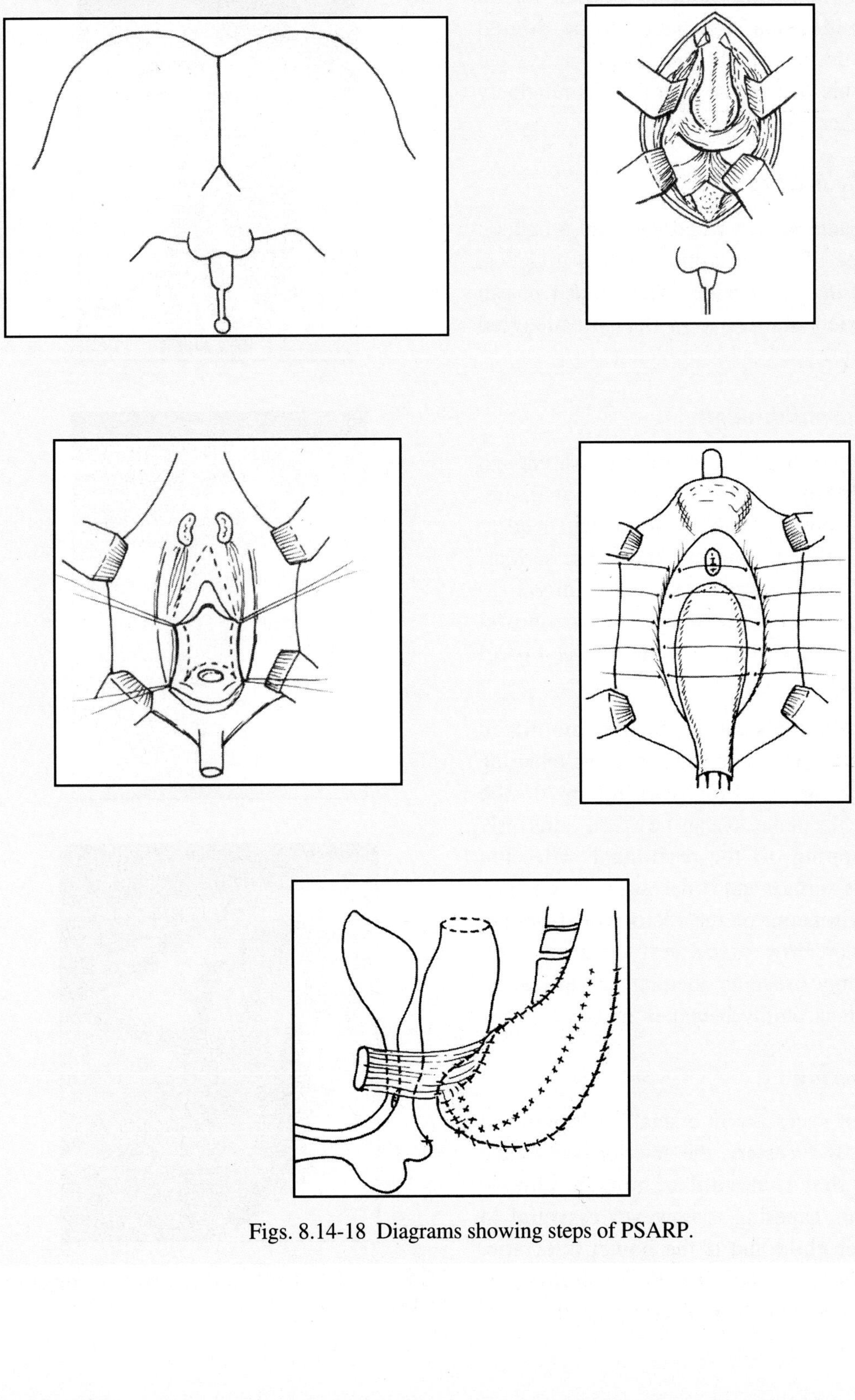

Figs. 8.14-18 Diagrams showing steps of PSARP.

external sphincter complex, which we do not divide; this area needs to be dilated before the rectourethral separation is carried out. This part of the operation is relatively easy when there is a RPUF.

(g) The urethra

The bougie is then withdrawn and a balloon catheter of a size appropriate for age is slipped into the bladder. This maneuver can be carried out easily in the spreadeagled position.

(h) The pullthrough

The rectum has to be mobilized just enough to enable it to reach the normal anal site. While excessive mobilization may lead to loss of afferent impulses and, more serious, loss of blood supply, inadequate mobilization will lead to tension at the skin-bowel suture line and retraction of the bowel upwards.

(i) The rectum can be further mobilized posteriorly by the division of some tethering vessels and a wider opening up of the retrorectal plane. It can be freed anteriorly by stripping off the peritoneal reflection from its surface and if necessary by opening the peritoneum of the rectovesical pouch. However, low placement of a sigmoid colostomy prevents adequate mobilization and a laparotomy becomes mandatory.

(j) Tapering

This not necessary in a small well-prepared infant. If necessary, the anterior wall of the bowel that is devoid of muscle can be plicated. Tapering is however essential in an older child and if the bowel is ectatic. Whether this should be done anteriorly or posteriorly should be decided on the spot.

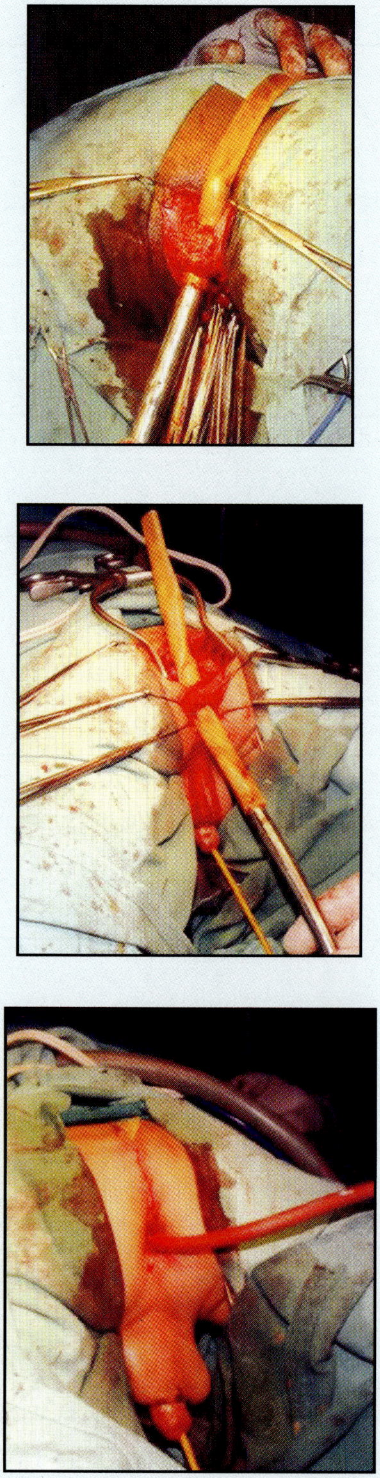

Figs. 8.19-21 Photographs showing steps of PSARP.

Generally posterior tapering is preferred because it allows the suture line on the bowel to remain far away from the urethral sutures; it also allows the region of the internal sphincter to be used as neoanus. However, if the anterior wall has been extensively denuded of muscle, anterior tapering is preferred and the incision on the posterior wall is closed. Tapering is carried out by excising an inferiorly based wedge and by repairing the defect with two rows of sutures. It is occasionally necessary to combine a posterior tapering with an anterior plication. After tapering, the bowel should accommodate a No.10 Hegar's dilator in an infant and a No.12 in an older child. Sutures, if any, on the anterior wall of the bowel stop 1 cm. short of the lower margin to provide space for the V flap of skin.

(k) Closure

The space between the urethra and the muscular sling that has been preserved is now dilated with a series of Hegar's dilators until there is sufficient space to accommodate the bowel. This is then pulled through and its terminal end placed in the trough formed by the undivided anterior fibers of the perpendicular part of the external sphincter. Repair is started from the posterosuperior end; the two segments of coccyx are approximated and then the diaphragm fibers of the levator are sutured. The external sphincter fibers and the divided posterior vertical fibers are then repaired behind the pulled through gut, taking bites of bowel muscle and striated muscle together. The anterior V flap of skin fits snugly into the gap in the anterior wall of the bowel. Then skin and mucosa are apposed and the wound is closed from behind the neoanus to the posterosuperior end of the incision by a continuous subcuticular suture. Our preferred suture material for the entire repair is polyglactin (vicryl).

(l) Postoperative care

The intravenous line is retained for 24 hours to give anantibacterial drugs and if necessary, a small transfusion of blood to ensure rapid healing. Normal feeds are resumed after 24 hours and then prophylactic antibiotcs are given orally. Dilatation of the neoanus is commenced with a soft pvc dilator after 3 days; the first Hegar's dilator is introduced after the wound is healed, round about the tenth day (Figs. 8.22-23).

Preservation of the sling fibers of the levator ani/external sphincter as described above has also been recommended by Smith (1987). In boys operated upon by me prior to 1987, the muscle complex was divided in its entirety as described by Pena (1982), and it was repaired around the tapered pulled through bowel. The only significant difference observed postoperatively between the two series is that dilatation of the new anorectum has been easier in the later series than in the earlier signifying that the scar tissue resulting from divided muscle is less pliant than that following stretching. Das and many of our other colleagues do not preserve the sling fibers and longterm results are no different.

The role of the internal anal sphincter has been a matter for debate ever since an internal sphincter anlage was found to surround the fistula between the bowel and the urogenital organs. Rintala and his group have tried to show by clinical and manometric studies that anorectal function is better if this sphincter is preserved and brought

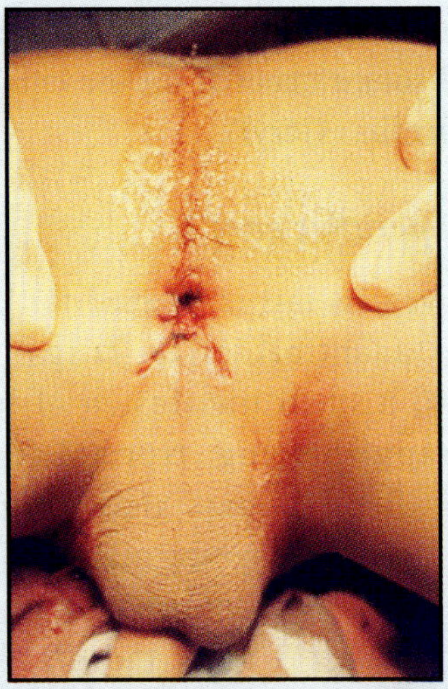

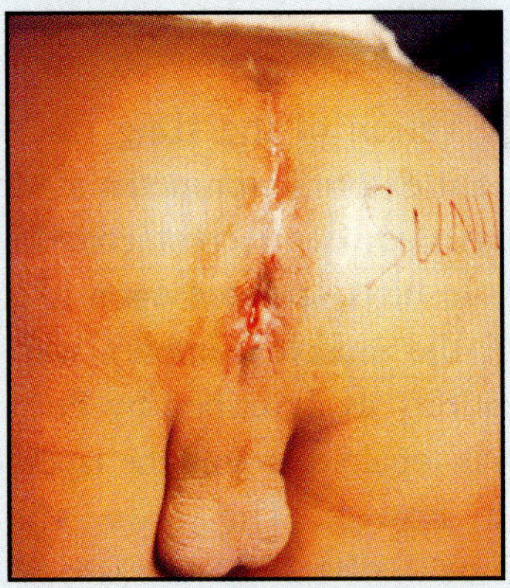

Figs. 8.22-23 Photographs after PSARP.

down to the normal anal site during the PSARP (Rintala, 1990, Husberg *et al* 1992, Rintala and Lindahl, 1995). Gangopadhyay and his group (2001) have also studied the fistula region and consider that the constipation that results from its preservation is preferable to the incontinence that may follow its destruction.

In our opinion, preservation of the fistula region is possible if this is low and the bowel shaped like a sledge. If the fistula is high and the bowel is retort shaped the fistula cannot be preserved with safety. Moreover, the bowel and the urethra often share a common wall without any intervening smooth muscle and there is in fact no sphincter. We have been able to preserve the internal sphincter in only a few cases; its value is still to be proved.

Surgeons who do not use the spread-eagled position start the operation by introducing a balloon catheter into the urethra while the patient is supine; the balloon is inflated if the catheter enters the bladder. If it does not enter the bladder it either lies in the urethra or enters the rectum. It has to be directed into the bladder when the fistula is exposed and then the balloon can be inflated.

When Gopal performs PSARP on a neonate without a colostomy, she mobilizes the meconium filled terminal bowel completely before opening it and divides the fistula. She opens and empties the bowel only after it has been firmly fixed at the normal anal site.

Prior to 1987 we performed suprapubic cystostomy whenever a large urethral fistula was encountered and maintained it for 10 days. Now we retain the urethral balloon catheter for about 5 to 7 days if we can get one into the bladder.

Until recently we had never had a problem introducing a balloon catheter of appropriate size. We now have 4 patients with RPUF on whom this was not possible because of a **narrow urethra** (Chatterjee *et al* 2003). All of them came after a neonatal colostomy.

In 2, the penis was deformed and flaccid and urinary obstruction was present from birth. One had a patent urachus and passed urine through the urachus, external urethral meatus and the distal limb of the colostomy. Investigations revealed that both kidneys were mildly dsyplastic. A catheter mounted on a stylet could be passed into the bladder for a voiding cystourethrogram (VCU). The contrast showed the narrow urethra (Fig. 8.24) and entered the urachus and the rectum. PSARP was done with a narrow catheter in the urethra; the rectourethral fistula was closed and suprapubic cystostomy was done. Subsequently, periodic urethral dilatations were done, the suprapubic tube was removed and the colostomy closed. At a second VCU reflux was seen into the right seminal vesicle and the right ureter and kidney. Episodes of urinary tract infection continued in spite of urethral dilatations. On cystoscopy a greatly dilated orifice of the right ejaculatory duct was seen. Fig. 8.25 shows the anatomy. The suprapubic tube was reinserted and removed 6 months later when micturition became normal. Episodes of urinary infection ceased and residual urine disappeared after the first year of life. However periodic urethral dilatations were advised. He lives far away and appointments are not maintained. He is now 7 years old and still suffers from bouts of urinary infection if he misses dates for dilatation.

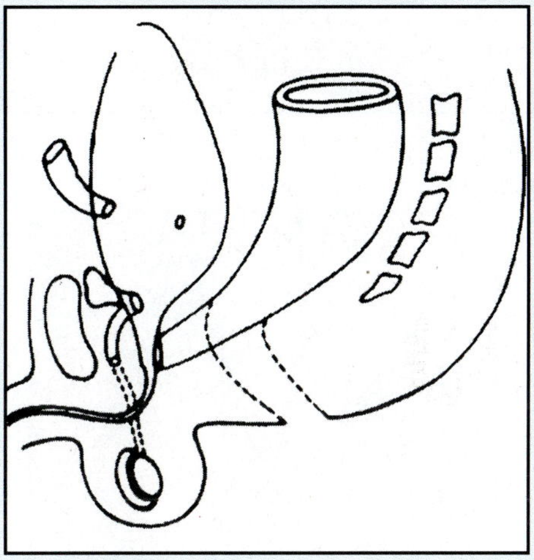

Fig. 8.25 Diagram showing urethral fistula & narrow urethra.

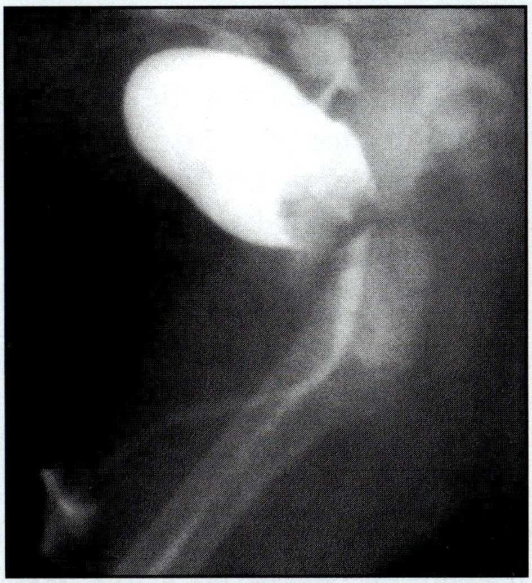

Fig. 8.24 Xray - urethrogram showing narrow urethra.

The other came at the age of 8 months because of obstructive uropathy and recurrent episodes of urinary infection follow-ing PSARP; this operation had been done with a narrow catheter in the urethra. He had a congenital urethral fistula in the midpenile region without hypospadias (Figs. 8.26-27).

Bilateral massive hydroureteronephrosis was seen on USG (Fig. 8.28) bilateral grade five reflux on VCU (Fig. 8. 29) and a duplex system on the left side on DTPA scan (Fig. 8.30). Fig. 8.31 shows the anatomy. Suprapubic cystostomy was done and he was put on a course of urethral dilatations. Subsequently his colostomy was closed and the suprapubic tube removed but episodes

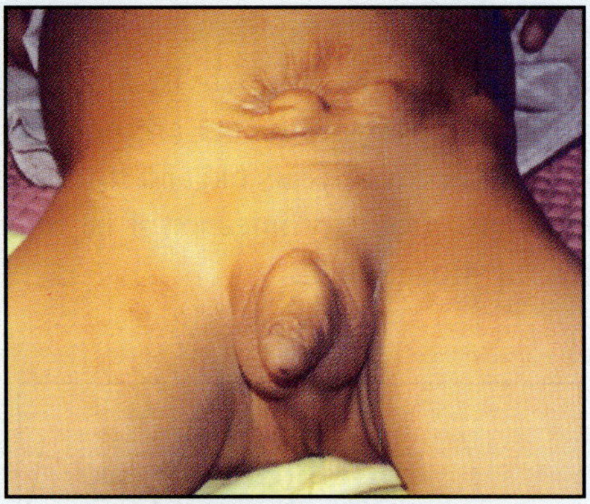

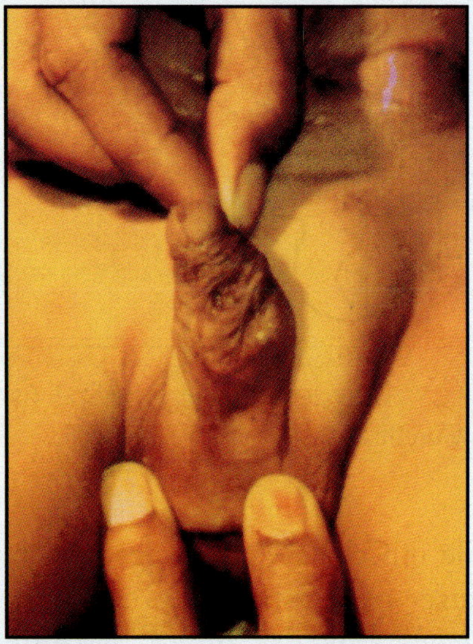

Figs. 8.26-27 Photographs of flaccid penis with narrow urethra.

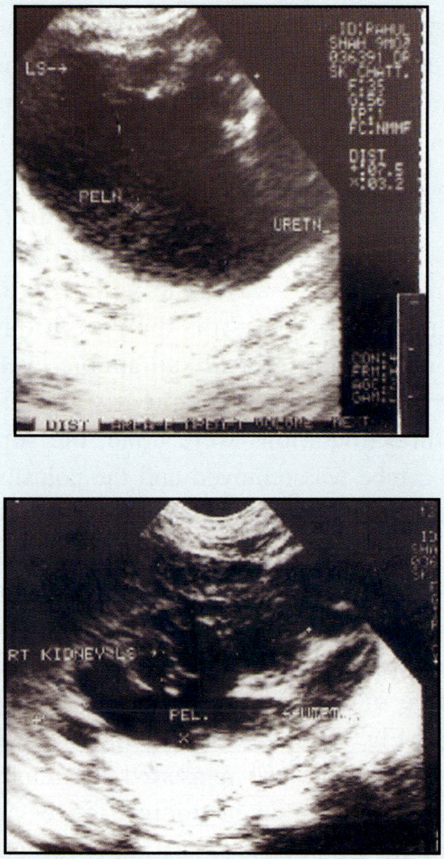

Fig. 8.28 USG showing bilateral hydronephrosis.

of urinary infection persisted and bilateral ureteroneocystostomies were done. In spite of regular urethral dilatations the bladder would not empty properly and he was put on clean intermittent catheterization; when this failed vesicostomy was done. This was closed after he improved. He was then put on a course of 6 monthly urethral dilatations. Subsequently the urethral fistula was repaired. However episodes of urinary infection continued. These ceased after the dilated nonfunctioning lower moiety of the left kidney was removed. He now passes urine well but has occasional mild urinary infec-tion specially when he is constipated. He is now 7 years old.

The third patient was treated by Banerjee. He had a midpenile hypospadias and a partially truncated sacrum. The narrow urethra was detected during PSARP. The urethral fistula was disconnected from the rectum and brought out on the perineum as an endurethrostomy (Fig. 8.32). After the colostomy was closed, the narrow urethra between the hypospadiac orifice and the bulbar fistula was laid open and partially

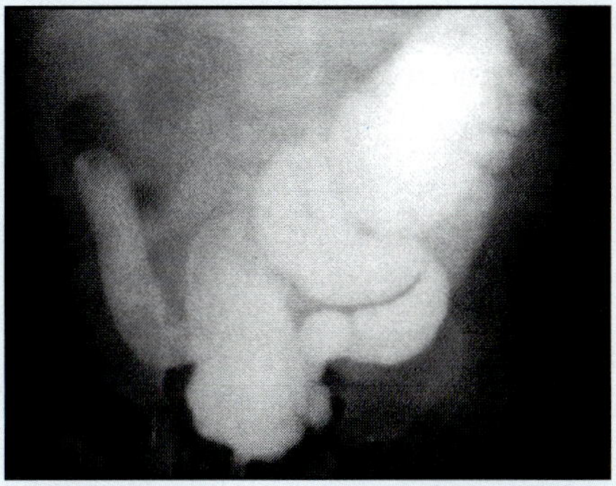

Fig. 8.29 Xray VCU of same baby showing bilateral massive reflux.

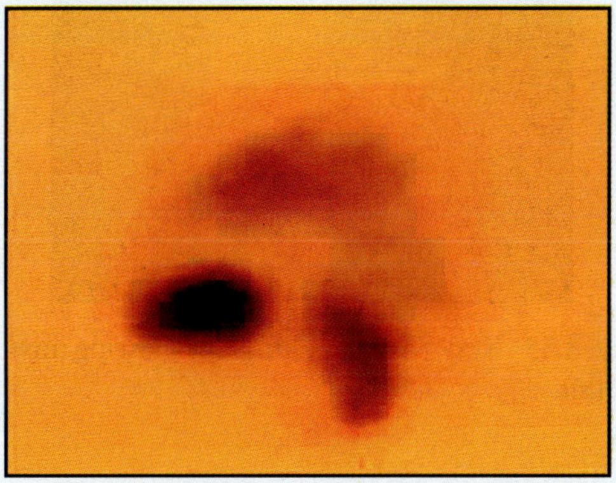

Fig. 8.30 DTPA scan of same baby showing duplex system L with bilateral hydronephrosis.

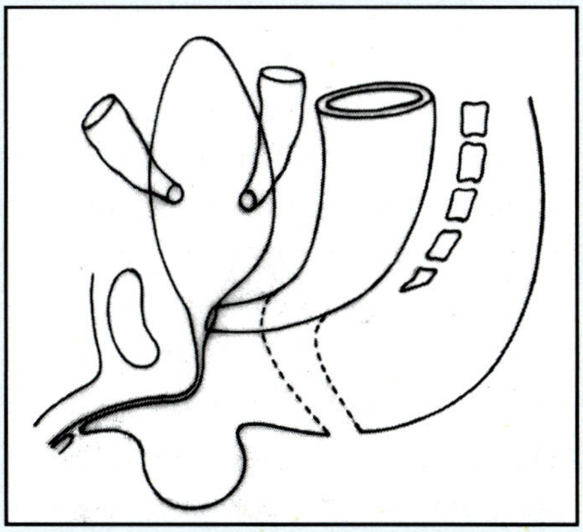

Fig. 8.31 Diagram of same baby .

closed with a skin tube. He is doing well.

The fourth patient was treated by Basak. A urethral catheter entered the rectum but would not enter the bladder during PSARP; hence suprapubic cystostomy was done. After a few postoperative urethral dilatations, micturition became normal and the suprapubic tube was removed.

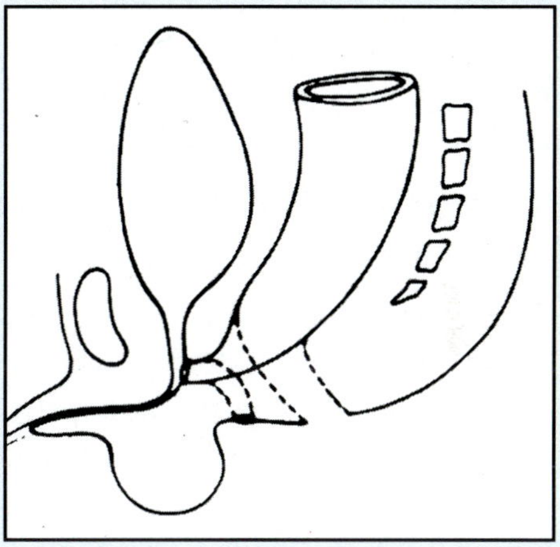

Fig. 8.32 Diagram of urethral fistula with narrow urethra treated by urethrostomy.

According to Pena (1988), 10% of patients cannot be reconstructed by PSARP, and need a laparotomy. We entirely agree. While it is generally possible to pick out this group on the basis of preoperative investigations and plan accordingly, the decision to stop and changeover to a laparotomy may have to be taken during the operation. This has rarely been necessary in my series, but Das opts for a laparotomy if there is the slightest tension in performing the pull-through extraperitoneally.

Whether postoperative anal dilatations are at all necessary is a question that has recently been raised by Kiely (2004). At present we dispense with dilatation on a neonate who does not have a colostomy but consider it essential if the patient has a colostomy.

We and Pena both feel that the operation is singularly free from complications. Nevertheless, **complications** have been described by Nakayama (1986), Gupta (2001) and many others. They can be divided into two groups, intestinal and urogenital.

Intestinal complications occurred in the following situations.

a) The patient did not have a fully defunctioning colostomy, oral feeds were started early in the postoperative period and feces leaked into the wound.
b) The terminal bowel had not been emptied fully of feces or meconium or injudiciously selected radio-opaque material.
c) Suturing either of the bowel or of the striated muscle wrap had been done under tension.
d) The tapering had been excessive.
e) There was ischemia of the pulled through bowel due to either excessive or inadequate mobilization,
f) Postoperative dilatations had been infrequent and inadequate or too vigorous
g) The colostomy had been closed before healing was complete.

The end result of all these mishaps is a fecal fistula, an annular or tubular stenosis or a presacral suppuration.

Urogenital complications included the following:

a) The fistula had been missed during the reconstruction. The high fistula associated with a low termination of the bowel is the one that is likely to be missed. We have recently closed a missed fistula by local revision; the fistula had fortunately been detected before the colostomy was closed (Fig. 8.33).

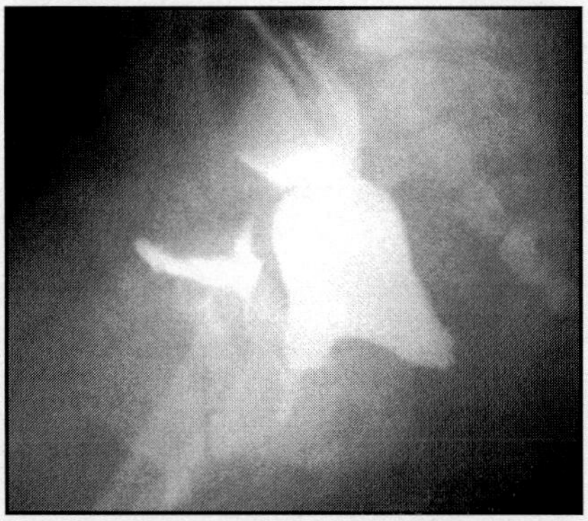

Fig. 8.33 Xray - cystourethrogram showing missed fistula.

b) The fistula had been identified and divided but the wound had broken down. A relatively low fistula is often associated with the bowel and the urethra sharing a common wall for some considerable distance. If these are not properly separated, there is tension at the suture lines and tissue necrosis. Suture lines also disrupt because of urinary leakage due to inefficient diversion of urine. It also results from fecal contamination if the bowel has not been snugly sutured and there is no defunctioning colostomy.
c) The urethra has been injured during the operation. Injuries are usually limited to the posterior wall of the bowel and occur while separating it from the bowel.

Fistulas persist only if the urethra is not repaired on the spot. Total transection of the urethra is more serious; I have done it once during revisional surgery and a third operation with both urinary and fecal diversion was necessary to effect a cure. A further problem will be discussed in Chapter 9.

d) The urethra has been injured by forcible postoperative dilatation of the anorectum, and revisional surgery was necessary to restore normal urinary flow

e) A ureter has been injured. An ectopic ureter is more vulnerable than a normal one; if not detected and repaired on the spot, major revisional surgery becomes inevitable.

f) Injuries to the vas deferenses and seminal vesicles do not manifest themselves till much later in life, but the seriousness of injuring both vas deferenses cannot be over emphasised.

g) Finally the presacral nerves coursing on either side of the midline are also vulnerable and injuries result in an acquired neurogenic bladder in childhood and more serious problems follow in adult life.

PSARP is the commonest major reconstruction that we have performed, not only for rectourethral fistulas, but also for agenesis without fistula, rectovaginal fistulas and some cloacal fistulas. We shall discuss the results together in Chapter 16.

3. *Anterior sagittal anorectoplasty (ASARP)*

This is done with the patient supine in the frog position; its merit lies in the fact that if the reconstruction cannot be accomplished extraperitoneally, the abdomen can be opened without turning the baby. Aluwihare has advocated this procedure for over a decade and manages to bring the rectum down through an undivided levator sling in most cases. without a laparotomy. Mollard (1989) has also described a modified version of his original operation in which he reconstructs the bowel without laparotomy. However his incision is not sagittal but more complicated; it has not caught on.

INTRAPERITONEAL RECONSTRUCTIONS

I. *Abdominoperineal anorectoplasty (APARP)*

The modern operation has evolved from the procedures practiced by Norris *et al* and Rhodes *et al* in the 1940s, by Swenson and Donnellan in the 1960s, by Mollard and his team in the 1970s and Laberge and his team in the 1980s. We perform this operation when the bowel ends above the level of the third sacral vertebra or when it is tethered by an incorrectly performed colostomy.

We use the FROG position, with a balloon catheter in the bladder. The abdomen is opened by a transverse suprapubic incision. After incising the peritoneum of the pelvic floor, the rectum is dissected free taking great care to avoid injury to the nerves coursing on either side. The rectum can be separated relatively easily from the urogenital organs in front. The fistula is isolated and divided after closing the urethral end with sutures. The bowel between the colostomy and the end of the rectum is then studied with reference to length, need to ligate and divide colonic vessels and need to taper. If the colostomy has been properly done and the colon is not malformed, there should be adequate bowel for the pull-

vessels should be above a major bifurcation so that an adequate collateral circulation is preserved. Tapering of course should be done along the antimesenteric surface.

If bowel distal to the colostomy is deemed insufficient, there are three options:

i) This bowel can be sacrificed and bowel proximal to the colostomy can be brought down to the perineum; if the proximal bowel is well prepared, the fecal stream need nor be diverted again and the patient managed postoperatively with intravenous medication. Alternatively, a concurrent transverse colostomy may be done.

ii) The colostomy can be closed and all available colon utilized for the pullhrough; a proximal diversion is essential.

iii) The colostomy can be translocated as described in Chapter 6.

While this is being done intraperitoneally, the perineal operator makes a horizontally disposed H incision. A midline incision is made between the base of the scrotum or the vulva to a little beyond the normal anal site. A transverse incision is then made at its upper end and another incision at its lower end; this is shorter and curves backwards as shown in Fig. 8.34.

At the posterior end, the anterior and posterior limits of the vertical fibers of the external sphincter are identified and marked with stay sutures. At the anterior end, the urethra and the surrounding levator sling are identified. All structures between these two landmarks are divided strictly in the midline. The space between the levator sling and the urogenital organs is opened up gradually by the perineal and the abdominal operators

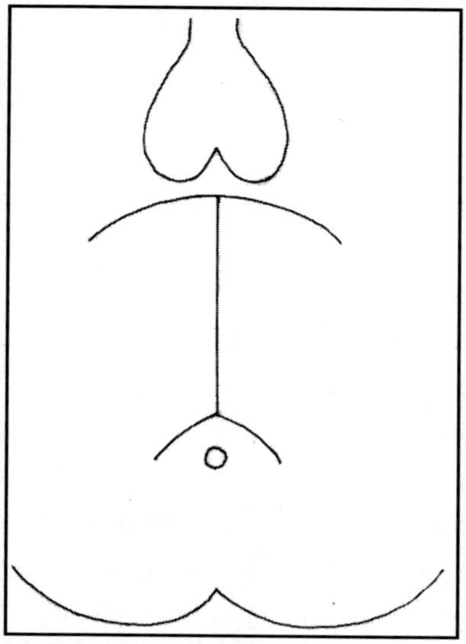

Fig. 8.34 Diagram of perineal incision for APARP.

through. The site of division of the colonic working together. A Penrose drain in gently inserted in this space; one end is in the peritoneum and the other in the perineal wound. A series of Hegar's dilators are passed through the Penrose drain to enlarge the space and allow pullthrough of the bowel from the abdomen to the perineum. When the space is considered adequate, the Penrose drain is removed and the bowel is pulled through. The perineal operator ensures that the mesocolic surface is posterior and brings the distal end of the bowel to the normal anal site. The bowel is fixed in place and the striated muscle complex is repaired around it. The flap of skin at the posterior end of the wound is tucked into the posterior surface of the bowel and the wound closed. By this time, the abdominal operator has closed the abdomen in layers.

The postoperative management is the same as for any major laparotomy with intravenous fluids, and gastrointestinal decompression for 3 to 4 days. Feeds can be started after this, except for patients whose colostomy has been discontinued; these patients will need a period of parenteral nutrition. The urethral catheter is removed after a week and dilatation of the neoanus

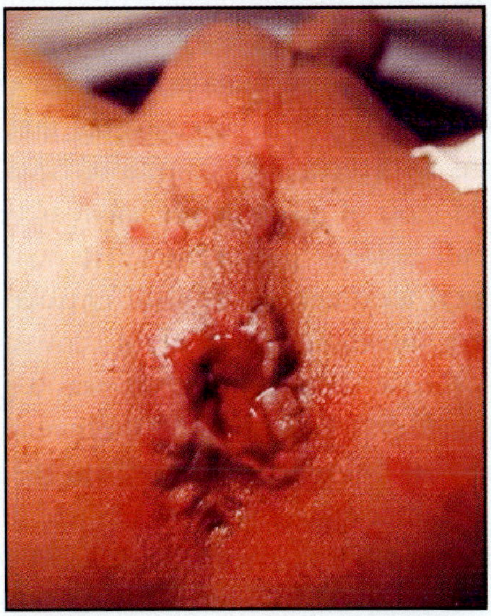

Fig. 8.35 Photograph after APARP

is started with soft instruments (Fig. 8.35).

2. *PSARP with laparotomy*

This is a more popular operation, performed by Das and most of our colleagues. It begins as a routine PSARP with the patient prone. However, when the presacral space is explored, the rectum either cannot be found or cannot be mobilized adequately. A rubber tube or an endotracheal tube of suitable caliber is then placed behind the urogenital organs and the striated muscles are repaired behind it. The posterior two-thirds of the wound is closed and a sterile dressing is applied. The patient is then turned over supine and placed in the FROG position.

The abdomen is opened by a transverse suprapubic incision and the fistula, the rectum and the sigmoid are dealt with as in APARP. The bowel is tapered to the size of the tube that had been previously inserted. The upper end of the tube is retrieved from the presacral space and terminal bowel is sutured to the tube with strong silk sutures.

The perineal operator then withdraws the tube, and with it, pulls through the bowel down to the normal anal site. The tube is then discarded and the terminal bowel takes its place. The striated muscle complex is repaired round it and the bowel muocsa is sutured to the skin margins. While this is being done, the abdominal operator closes the abdomen. Figs 8.36-37 show the procedure.

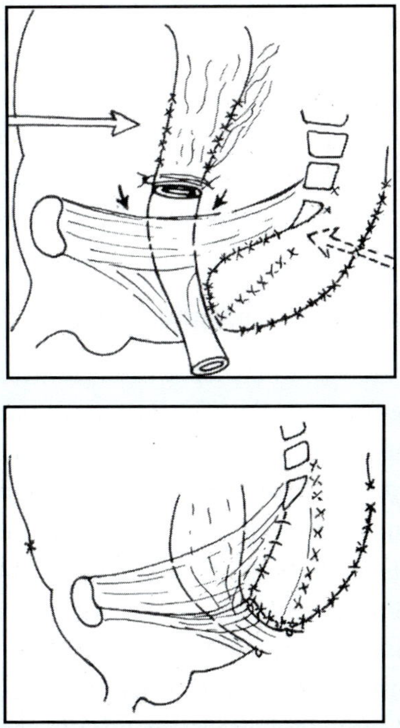

Figs. 8.36-37 Diagrams showing pullthrough, PSARP with Lap.

3. Laparoscopically assisted APARP

With the increasing popularity of Pediatric Laparoscopy, it was but inevitable that Laparoscopically assisted anorectoplasty would be widely practiced.

After Georgeson's description of Laparoscopically assisted pullthrough of the bowel for high anorectal malformations the operation has been performed in more and more centers all over the world. Laparoscopically assisted APARPs are being done in a number of centers in India notably Coimbatore (Raghupati *et al*, 2004) and Bangalore (Srimurti *et al* 2002). We have no firsthand experience of this operation and await longterm results. Nevertheless we believe that this will soon become the operation of choice for high lesions provided the anatomical landmarks are clearly identified and the pullthrough performed accurately. Whether this procedure should be done for lesions that are correctable extraperitoneally is a matter that is being hotly debated today. Personally we cannot justify an intraperitoneal procedure for a condition correctable by an extraperitoneal one.

Complications

Most of the complications mentioned in connection with PSARP also occur in patients requiring intraperitoneal procedures. In addition, they may have complications that may follow any intraperitoneal colonic operation, particularly small bowel obstruction. Prolapse of the neoanus is occasionally seen in patients submitted to APARP, It has once required correction by mobilizing the bowel through a circumferential incision and closing the wound snugly with a row of sutures.

The options regarding colostomy and postoperative management are the same as after APARP.

A major revision was necessary for a fistula missed during APARP elsewhere. Colostomy at birth had been followed by APARP with discontinuance of colostomy for a boy with a high lesion at the age of 16 months. After the operation, he passed stools normally through the neoanus, but this was mixed with urine. In course of time, he passed most of his urine per anum and only a small amount per urethra. He had had medical treatment to control episodes of urinary infection and numerous investigations. These showed that there was a good right kidney, a small poorly functioning left kidney with grade V reflux into the left ureter and considerable residual urine in the bladder. He was referred to us in 1994 when he was 18 years old with a diagnosis of missed rectourethral fistula. A huge megarectum with a rectourethral fistula was seen on Barium enema. Endoscopy revealed a large fistula between the bowel and the prostatic urethra, and a large left ureteric orifice with no efflux. Consent for surgery was obtained in 1995 and we performed a revisional PSARP. The fistula was closed, the bowel distal to this was discarded and the proximal bowel tapered to size. It was then brought out through the striated muscle complex and the muscles repaired. The muscle stimulator was of immense help. Concurrent colostomy was done. Normal micturition was restored as soon as the urethral catheter was removed and normal defecation was resumed as soon as the colostomy was closed. However attacks of urinary infection continued, and when the family finally agreed to further surgery a left sided ureteroneocystostomy was done in 1999. All problems then ceased and he now leads a normal life.

The special problem of high lesions is the diameter of the stem of the striated muscle funnel. A long narrow funnel calls for a great deal of bowel tapering, and this may compromise the blood supply of the bowel.

TWO : AGENESIS WITH VAGINAL FISTULA

This is the female counterpart of agenesis with urethral fistula in the males. It is, in our series, relatively rare; we have seen only 16 neonates and 6 older patients with this lesion. It is also very rare in Pena's series. Pena's group (Rosen *et al*, 2002) has suggested that its incidence was relatively greater in earlier series because of misdiagnosis. The opening of the bowel in the vestibule was either missed and rectovestibular fistulas were labeled as rectovaginal fistulas or an abnormal urogenital sinus was missed and the commoner but more problematic cloacal anomaly was labeled as a rectovaginal fistula. It is possible that there has been a real shift with time. On the other hand, rectovaginal fistulas have occasionally been labeled as rectovestibular and the correct diagnosis reached only at operation.

According to the Wingspread List, if the terminal bowel is above the P-C line and the fistula opens into the upper vagina, it is a high lesion, ANORECTAL AGENESIS WITH HIGH VAGINAL FISTULA. If the bowel terminates between the P-C line and the I line and the fistula opens into the lower vagina, it is an intermediate lesion, ANAL AGENESIS WITH LOW VAGINAL FISTULA. In all cases the urethra is normal (Figs. 8.38-39).

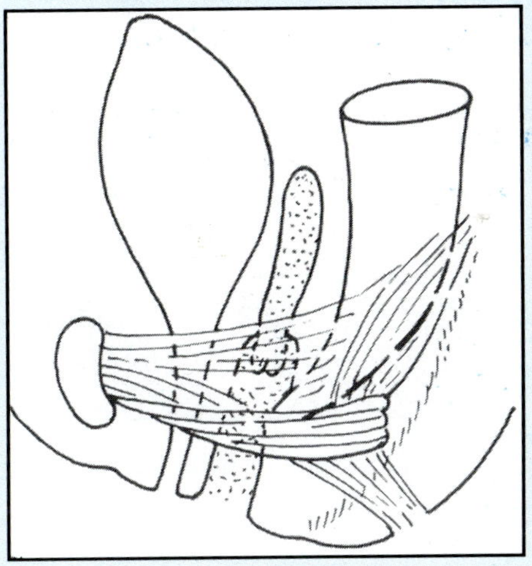

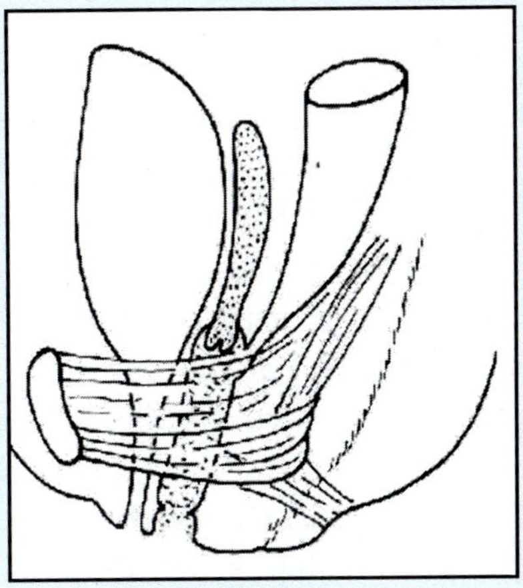

Figs. 8.38-39 Diagrams of rectovaginal fistula : intermediate, high.

The clinical features depend on the level and size of the fistula. If it is very small there will be features of intestinal obstruction (Fig. 8.40). If it is very large meconium is passed through the vagina. A low fistula can be seen after opening up the vaginal orifice by retraching the labia minora. A catheter inserted through the vagina has more chance

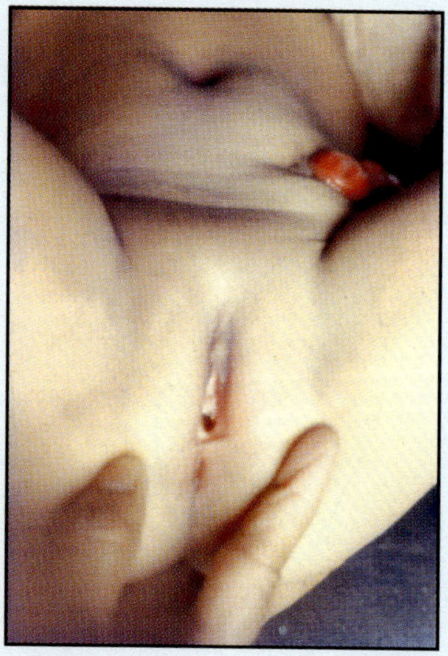

Fig. 8.40 Photograph of baby with rectovaginal fistula.

of reaching the retum if the fistula is low and large; the bowel can be decompressed through such a catheter. Sometimes the fustula is so large that there are intially no obstructive features and the patients are not presented in the neonatal period. Two of our patients presented at the age of 4 years without any previous treatment and one came at 6 years after having had a few vaginal washouts under anesthesia. Our last patient came at the age of 19 years long after the onset of menarche. She was fully continent and had no treatment whatever. Her mother brought her because she was about to be married. Das has a similar patient who was 23 when first seen. Gangopadhyaya's group (2004) has just encountered a patient with an undetected rectovaginal fistula; the condition was detected only after she delivered a stillborn baby. Fortunately, the family agreed to reconstructive surgery.

The standard method of delineating the anatomy of the anomaly is to inject radio-opaque dye through a vaginal catheter, and take a PA and lateral Xray; the dye generally reaches the rectum (Fig. 8.41). If it does not, vaginoscopy can be carried out and a catheter can be introduced into the fistula through the endoscope under direct vision; the bowel can then be decompressed and contrast Xray carried out. These examinations will reveal associated uterovaginal malformations, notably duplex systems and hydrocolpos. USG and MRI can also reveal Uterovaginal malformations.

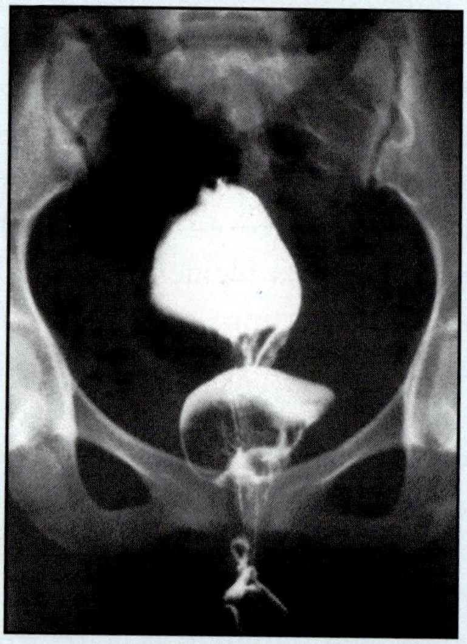

Fig. 8.41 Xray with contrast delineates vagina & rectum.

We have examined at autopsy a neonate who died with unrelieved intestinal obstruction due to Rectovaginal fistula. The bowel remained above the pelvic diaphragm and the fistula passed through the levator sling to reach the vagina.

Management in the Neonate

The standard treatment is **colostomy.** However, we had earlier performed PAT without colostomy on an otherwise healthy neonate with a low fistula large enough to allow complete decompression of the bowel through it. The operation was similar to what we did for a vestibular fistula except that the circumferential incision around the fistula had to be enlarged a few mm on either side to separate the bowel from the vagina. The bowel was treated as described earlier; the posterior vaginal wall repaired in two layers and the wound closed as before. Also, the operations available for male neonates with urethral fistula, namely ASARP, PSARP, APARP and Laparoscopically assisted APARP all have their advocates. Aluwihare in 1990 described the management of 10 neonates with high vaginal fistula by primary perineal rectovaginoanoplasty, a procedure we now name ASARVP.

Management in the Postneonatal Period

We perform **PSARVP;** it resembles the PSARP described for a boy, with minor modifications.

a) The endoscopic examination includes a vaginoscopy; a balloon catheter is placed in the bladder. In the spreadeagled position, the vagina is identified by a bougie introduced into it during the course of dissection.
b) The incision described for boys may suffice if the vagina is otherwise normal. However, if simultaneous reconstruction of an abnormal vagina is needed either because it is duplex or abnormally dilated a wider anterior exposure is required. The sagittal incision is extended up to the posterior limit of the vaginal opening and the striated muscle complex divided in its entirety; this provides wide access to the posterior wall of the vagina (Fig. 8.42).
c) After the posterior wall of the vagina is repaired, the perineal body is reconstructed. Then the anorectoplasty is done as for boys and the wound closed.

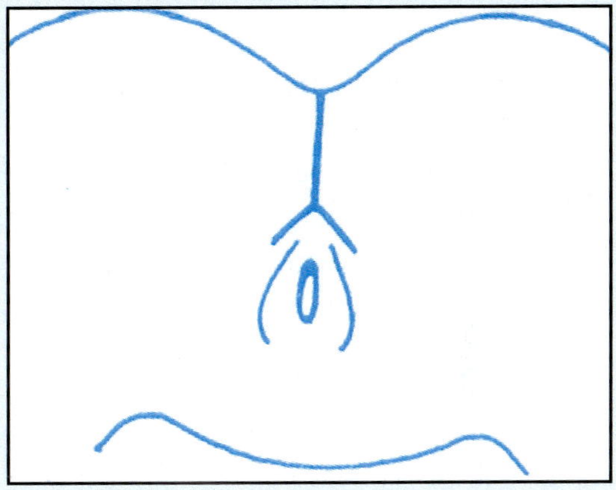

Fig. 8.42 Diagram to show incision for PSARVP.

The reconstruction may alternatively be done in the FROG position.

We also perform **PSARVP without a colostomy** in the healthy postneonate if the bowel can be completely decompressed. Our 19 year old patient had a hugely dilated rectum as well as a dilated vagina. Her large gut could be adequately prepared prior to reconstruction but because of the associated megarectum, a concurrent colostomy was performed.

The terminal bowel of patients with a high vaginal fistula cannot be reached extraperitoneally; it is then necessary to open the abdomen as in boys, by one of the methods already described. The fistula is closed and the bowel is brought down to the normal anal site. Das recently successfully reconstructed a 3 year old girl by **PSARVP with Laparotomy.**

Complications connected with the bowel resemble what has already been recorded for urethral fistulas. The additional problem concerns the state of the vagina; this may need revision (See Chapter 11).

Two patients required a major revision.

The first, born in 1974, had had a sigmoid colostomy at birth, a SPR at the age of 2 years and closure of the colostomy 3 months later. She did well for some time and then disappeared for 12 years. She was brought back after menarche. She had abdominal distension and constipation; she passed most of her stool through the vagina and only a small amount through a stenotic anus. The main reason for her return was dysmenorrhea. She was admitted and examined under anesthesia. After the rectum and distal colon was emptied, a large rectovaginal fistula was seen. On vaginoscopy, 2 vaginas were found; the right vagina was small and intact; the left was large and the bowel opened into it. The urinary organs were normal. She was prepared for revisional surgery and this was carried out. A hugely dilated rectum was disconnected from the vagina, tapered to size and brought down through the striated muscle complex to the normal site. The left vagina was trimmed to size and repaired. The distal half of the septum between the 2 vaginas was divided and a single vaginal opening created at the normal site. A concurrent transverse colostomy was done. Her postoperative course was uneventful. Dysmenorrhea disappeared and after the colostomy was closed, she began to pass stools normally. She married when she was 26 and was warned that cesarean section would be mandatory.

Obviously this girl could have been cured in infancy if we had learnt about the posterior sagittal approach in the 1970s.

The second born in 1982 had been reconstructed by PSARP in 1984 after a neonatal colostomy. She was one of the first patients submitted to this operation by us. There was wound infection; this responded to conservative treatment but flared up again after the colostomy was closed. There was osteitis of the sacrum and colostomy had to be done again to control the infection. A year later it was found that there was severe stenosis of the distal bowel and gross dilatation above. Basak carried out a revisional PSARP with laparotomy, tapering the megarectum to size. The colostomy was closed when healing was complete. She then recovered completely.

THREE : AGENESIS WITH VESICAL FISTULA

Rectovesical fistula is the name given to an invisible but manifest opening of the rectum into the urinary bladder. It is a **high** anomaly and should be named ANO-RECTAL AGENESIS WITH VESICAL FISTULA. The basic clinical features are the same as those of rectourethral fistula. In series reported prior to 1970 it was relatively common. A study of the records of the Children's Memorial Hospital, Chicago, of the period 1957-66 revealed that out of 250 cases of ARM, rectovesical fistula was diagnosed in 23 boys and 1 girl. It was deleted from the Wingspread list because of its rarity in subsequent series. This may be due to a real distal shift of the fistula with time. It may also be due to the fact that before the evolution of fiberoptic endoscopy and major extraperitoneal reconstructions, the precise relationship of the fistula to the vesicourethral junction was not always accurately determined and a fistula ending in the prostatic urethra was thought to end in the bladder (Fig. 8.43).

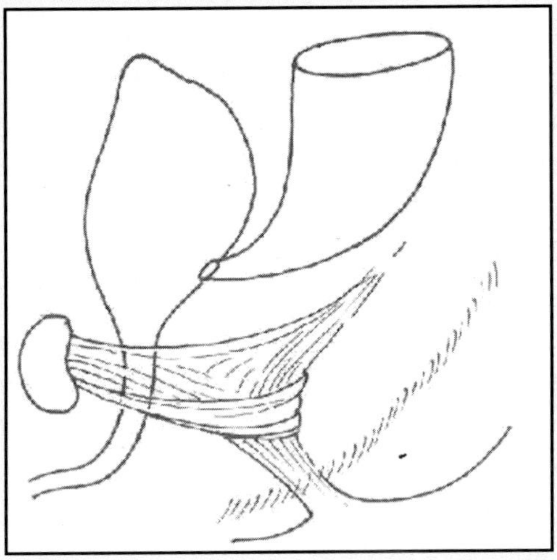

Fig. 8.43 Diagram of rectovesical fistula.

Rectovesical fistula is distinguished from rectourethral fistula by Xray after introducing contrast either through a urethral catheter in the neonate (VCU), or through the distal limb of a colostomy (Fig. 8.44).

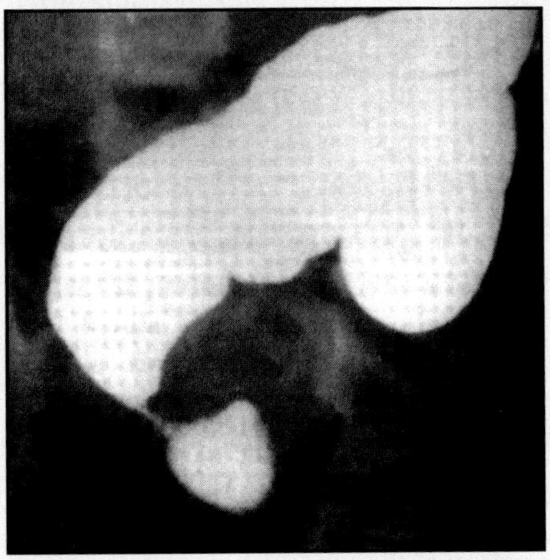

Fig. 8.44 Xray - distal cologram of above.

Today an additional imaging modality is MRI. The diagnosis is confirmed by endoscopy. The bowel generally opens in the trigone above the internal meatus, either in the midline or near the left ureteric opening.

The fundamental difference between rectovesical and rectourethral fistula lies in the incidence of associated malformations. Major malformations of the urinary tract are frequent accompaniments of rectovesical fistula. In 1972 and 1974, Magnus reported on 11 autopsy specimens and 5 patients, one of whom subsequently died at the age of 47 months. There were 12 males and 4 females in her series. Some patients labeled female by her would be considered intersex by us because their urethra and phallus were of the male type. About half of Magnus' cases had narrow urethras and all had major upper tract malformations. In many the musculature of the pelvic floor was inadequate.

There are 22 patients in our series, only 1 is a girl; 5 boys had **a narrow urethra** (Chatterjee *et al* 2001).

Details of a boy admitted the day after birth in 1979 are as follows. He was born without an anus and had not passed urine or stool since birth. His abdomen was greatly distended. Some urine emerged through an umbilical granuloma but a catheter could not be negotiated into the bladder. Intestinal and urinary obstruction were relieved by a right transverse colostomy and a suprapubic cystostomy. Subsequently urethrogram showed that the proximal urethra was occluded; distal cologram showed that the bowel ended with a fistula high up into the bladder base and USG failed to locate the kidneys. We decided to excise the urachus, perform a vesicostomy and send the baby home. He died soon after readmission at the age of 3 months with renal failure and septicemia. Autopsy revealed pyonephrosis of a solitary dysplastic kidney, both testes at the internal rings, high anorectal agenesis with a recto-vesical fistula, and ejaculatory ducts opening at the bladder base on either side of the rectal fistula (Fig. 8.45).

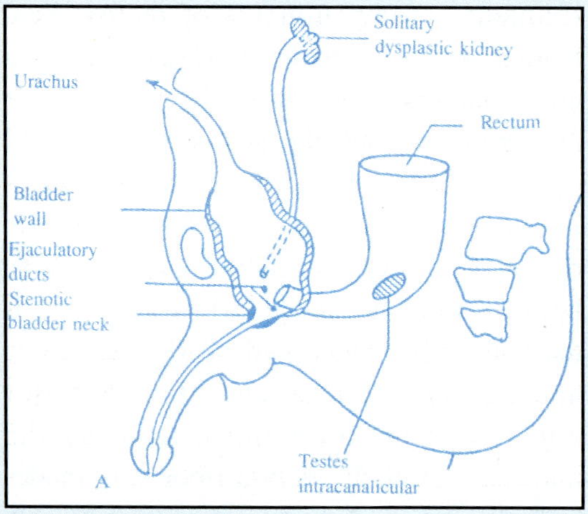

Fig. 8.45 Diagram of autopsy findings of baby with rectovesical fistula.

Management

A neonatal **colostomy** is mandatory. If there is bladder outlet obstruction, this should be relieved at the same time preferably by vesicostomy. USG followed by either an isotope renal scan or an intravenous urogram give details about renal function. The vesical fistula allows a free flow of urine into the bowel and hence hyperchloremic acidosis is likely. If there is massive vesico-ureteral reflux and ascending urinary infection vesicostomy may be needed even in the absence of bladder outlet obstruction.

Reconstructive surgery should only be performed after the urinary problems are stable. The alternatives are APARP, PSARP with Laparotomy and Laparoscopically assisted APARP.

We had earlier described a boy who was 3 months old when first seen in 1990. He was referred because of recurrent urinary infection and an inflammatory swelling of the right scrotum. He was born without an anus and had had a neonatal colostomy in the left lower quadrant. The colostomy had retracted and only one opening was seen. His urine contained plenty of pus cells and Pspyocyaneus was found on culture. VCU showed massive reflux into the right kidney and ureter, and displayed the right seminal vesicle; the contrast also passed into the bowel (Fig. 8.46). Distal cologram showed a very short length of bowel entering the bladder.

After the infection was controlled with antibiotics the colostomy was revised. Peroperative cystoscopy was planned but the instrument could not be passed into the bladder because of a narrow urethra. Intravenous urogram revealed bilateral hydronephroureter and considerable residual urine in the bladder (Fig. 8.47). After a course of urethral dilatation, the caliber of the urethra improved and cystourethroscopy could be done. There was an illdefined internal meatus and no verumontanum. Five orifices were seen, the bowel opening in the center, two dilated ureteric orifices on either side, and two dilated ejaculatory duct openings in the upper urethra (Fig. 8.48).

He was considered fit for reconstructive surgery when he was 8 months old. APARP was done with resection of bowel distal to the colostomy, repair of the bladder and suprapubic cystostomy. Both ureters and the right vas deferens and seminal vesicle were found to be greatly dilated; the left vas was

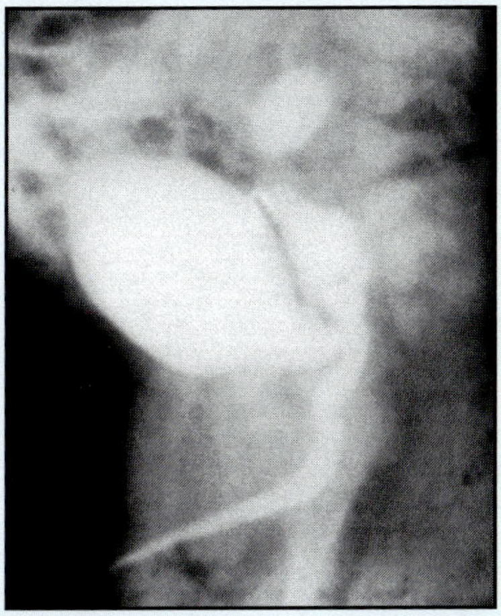

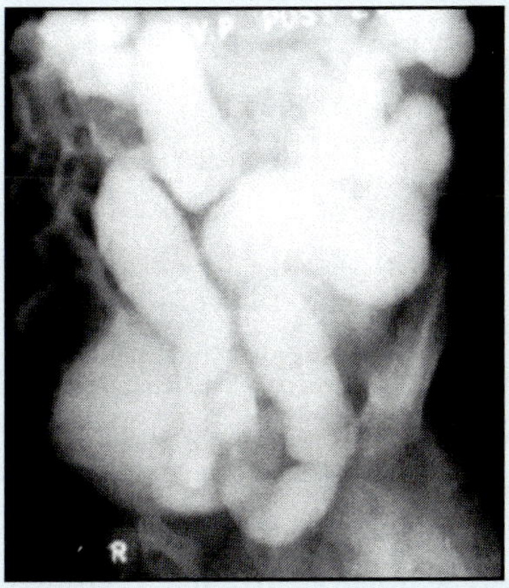

Figs. 8.46-47 Xray - cystourethrogram & IVU of baby with rectovesical fistula.

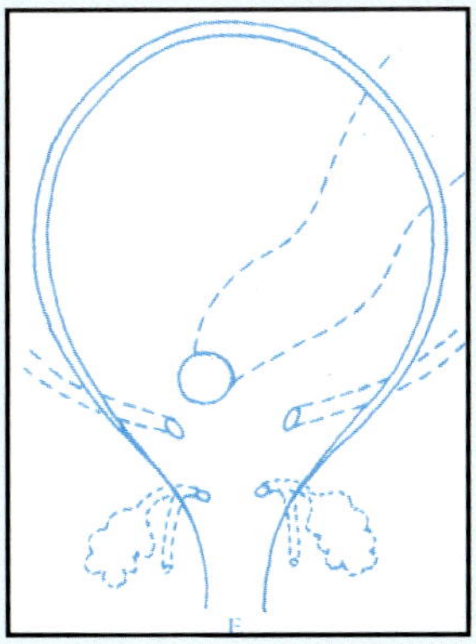

Fig. 8.48 Diagram - cystoscopic findings of same baby.

atrophic and led to a small intraabdominal testis; this was brought down to the scrotum. Recovery was uneventful but the testis atrophied.

The urethra was dilated periodically; after the suprapubic tube was removed he began to pass urine well, but the suprapubic fistula persisted for some time. He suffered from recurrent episodes of epididymitis, these only ceased after the right vas deferens was ligated and divided. He also suffered from recurrent episodes of urinary infection and bilateral grade 5 reflux was seen on VCU. Ureteroneocystostomies were done on both sides on two different days in 1992. Subsequent IVU showed improvement, but attacks of urinary infection continued. Urethral dilatations were necessary to maintain a good stream. A revisional anoplasty was done to control a bowel prolapse in September 1993, and the UNC had to be revised on the left side for recurrence of reflux in July 1994. Urethral dilatations were discontinued in 1996 and there has been no problem since. Investigations done in 1998 to show the status of the bowel and urinary tract revealed no abnormality other than mild hydroureteronephrosis. He was completely asymptomatic until his parents desired that we reconstruct the vas deferens leading down to a normal sized right testis. After this was done, he had an attack of epididymitis; this resolved with intravenous antibiotics. In 1998 Oguzkurt *et al* described 2 infants with ARM who had epididymo-orchitis due to reflux into the ejaculatory ducts.

Two boys treated more recently were more or less similar; both had colostomy soon after birth. In both a narrow urethra was identified during anorectoplasty and a balloon catheter could not be negotiated. Both had a PSARP with laparotomy. The first aged 7 years was operated by Basu with a narrow catheter in place. The second aged 2½ years was operated by Das. Das identified a stenosed segment of urethra; this was resected and an end-to-end anastomosis was done around an indwelling urethral catheter (Fig. 8.49). Suprapubic cystostomy was done in both cases after repair of the bladder fistula and the colon distal to the colostomy was brought down to the normal anal site. Subsequently their urethras were periodically dilated and both began to pass urine well. After colostomy closure, both began to pass stools well. They did not have any episode of urinary infection and no further investigations were done; however, after being lost to followup for some years, Das's patient came back with a recurrence of urethral narrowing and further surgery was necessary.

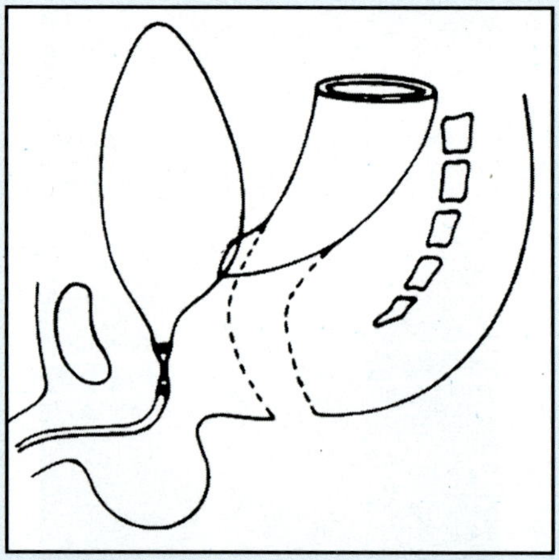

Fig. 8.49 Diagram of rectovesical fistula with narrow urethra.

We have done revisional surgery on one boy who had had APARP with discontinuance of colostomy elsewhere at the age of 7 months. He was totally incontinent and there was prolapse at the neoanus and perineal excoriation. Narrowing of the terminal bowel and a huge megarectum was seen on Barium enema. PSARP with concurrent colostomy was done; the rectum was tapered to size and brought down through the striated muscle complex to the normal anal site. Earlier it had been routed far anterior to the correct site. After discontinuance of colostomy, his continence has improved greatly but he still has some soiling when stools are loose. He is now 9.

In the other patients in the series, PSARP with laparotomy could be done without any untoward incident. They had a normal urethra; USG, VCU and isotope scan showed a normal urinary system with no vesicoureteric reflux and a normal verumontanum was seen on endoscopy. However in one boy, the left ureteric orifice was displaced laterally.

Rectovesical fistula in girls is a cloacal malformation and will be discussed in Chapter 11.

CHAPTER 9

NO MANIFEST OPENING

In this anomaly, the bowel terminates either blindly or with an opening that does not allow the passage of meconium to the exterior. Intestinal obstruction is therefore complete. According to the Wingspread List, when the bowel ends blindly above the P-C line, it is a **high** lesion and named ANORECTAL AGENESIS WITHOUT FISTULA; when it ends blindly between the P-C line and the I line, it is an **intermediate** lesion and named ANAL AGENESIS WITHOUT FISTULA. The Wingspread list omitted the condition wherein the bowel ends below the I line; this is a **low** lesion called COVERED ANUS COMPLETE (Figs. 9.1-3).

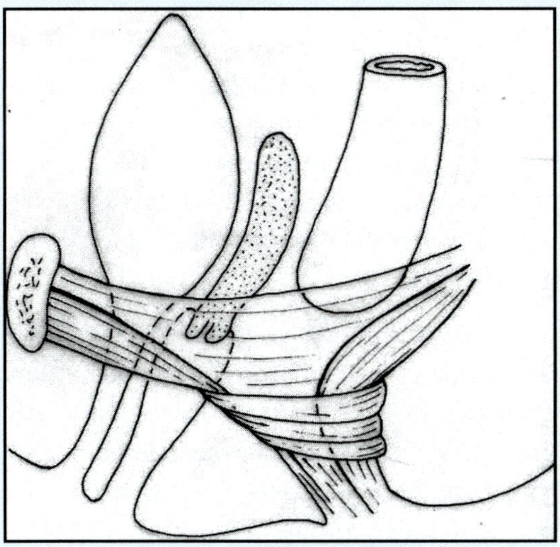

Fig. 9.1 Diagram showing high lesion.

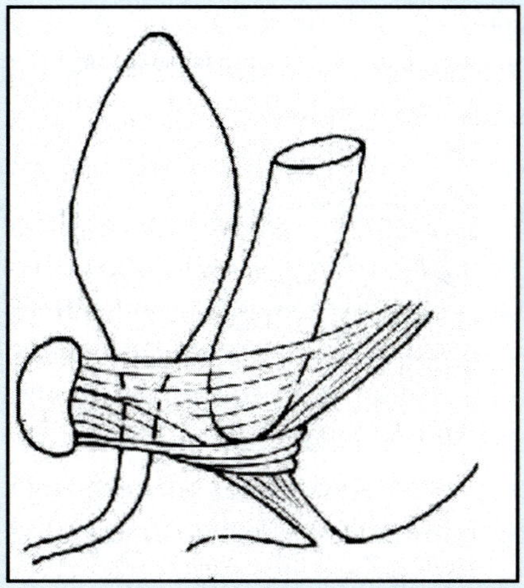

Fig. 9.2 Diagram showing intermediate lesion.

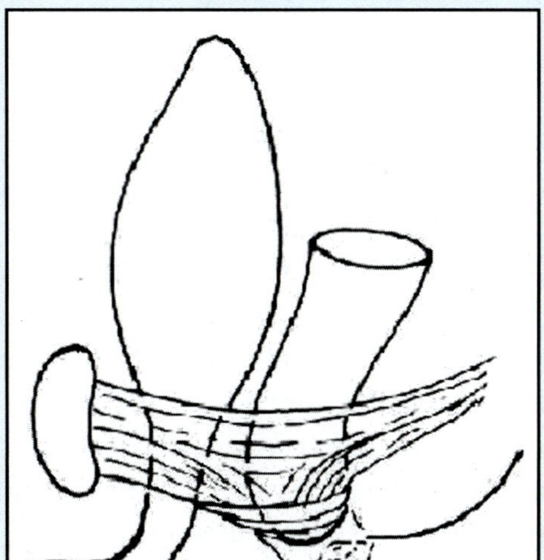

Fig. 9.3 Diagram showing low lesion.

The level of the terminal bowel can be determined by the methods already mentioned, namely USG, invertogram and MRI. Cystourethrography and endoscopy can reveal or exclude an occult fistula and urogenital anomalies.

In an earlier era we had examined at autopsy 13 males and 3 females with a blind ending bowel. It was above the P-C line in 7 males and 1 female; between the P-C line and I line in 3 males and below the I line in 3 males and 2 females. In 5, the terminal bowel nestled within the basket of striated muscle as described by Kiesewetter & Nixon in the following words. The blind pouch pushes its way down and through the puborectalis sling, carrying portions of the muscle around it to the point at which it reaches the perineum and perforates the anal plate'. In two specimens, the bowel was found emptied by a perineal incision that had gone through the fibers of the levator ani. In another, a lateral Xray was taken after the bottom of the pouch was smeared with barium paste; this showed that although the pouch ended above the levator, it was very low with reference to the pelvic skeleton. We had also examined a 4-day old boy who was born without an anus and died shortly after admission. He had been submitted to a perineal operation on the day after birth. He passed meconium through the opening thus made, but the next day a mass was seen to protrude through the wound, and he was brought to us. We found that there was a red fusiform mass at the anal site 10 cm. long. It was reducible; its surface appeared muscular; meconium emerged from its lumen and a finger could be passed into it (Fig. 9.4). Our explanation of the anatomy is shown diagrammatically (Fig. 9.5). The perineal operation divided the diaphragm fibres of the levator and opened the blind bowel; at the same time it opened up a plane of cleavage between the bowel and the levator. When the baby strained, the bowel having lost the support of the striated muscles was pushed out en masse.

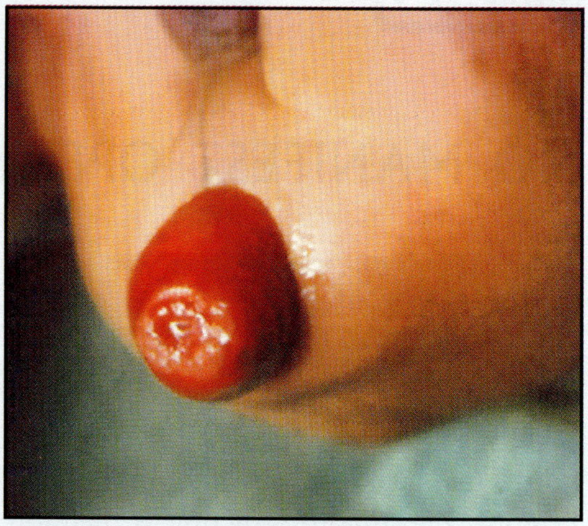

Fig. 9.4 Photograph of neonate with prolapse through an incision into the levator ani.

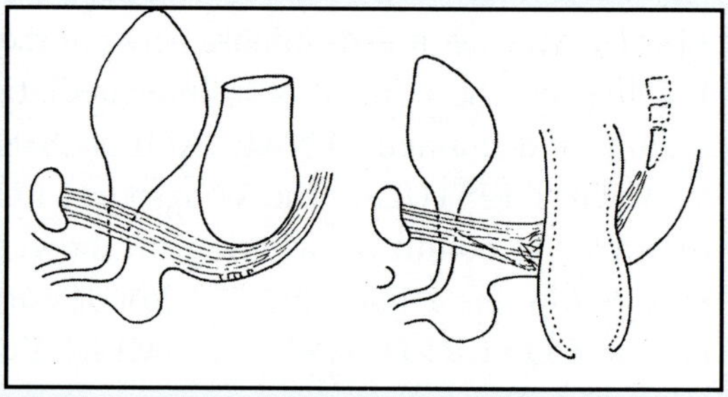

Fig. 9.5 Diagram of the above.

In Pena's series, a blind ending rectum is distinctly uncommon. It is much more common in the Japanese series; about one fifth of all high and intermediate anomalies ended without a fistula. In our series one third of these anomalies ended without a fistula. Moreover, we had 3 patients who had a demonstrable fistula in the neonatal period but this closed spontaneously by the time definitive surgery was performed. Martins *et al* (2003) have recently seen an obliterated rectourethral fistula during reconstructive surgery.

A number of surgeons, notably Ein (1997), Sharma (1995) and Gangopadhyaya (1997), have described patients with anorectal agenesis without a fistula and with associated more proximal atresias. These atresias were in the upper rectum or lower sigmoid All the patients had had a neonatal colostomy and the diagnosis was made either during PSARP or even later. MRI done on one occasion did not reveal the problem.

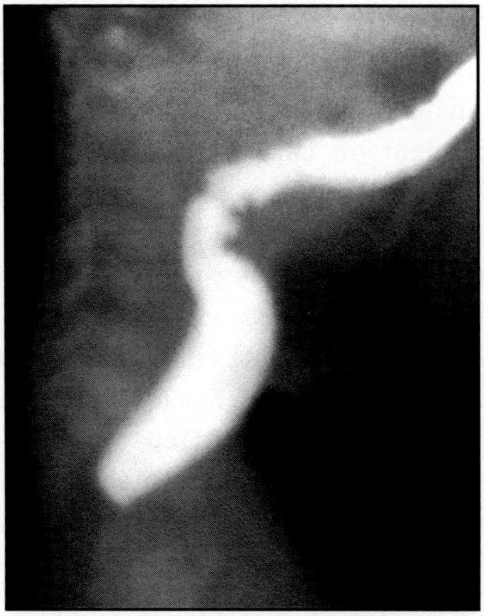

Fig. 9.6 Xray distal cologram.

Management

If the terminal bowel can be shown to be at or below the I line or within 1 cm. from the normal anal site, and a fistula can be excluded, the neonate should be submitted to **primary reconstruction** by a simple perineal procedure. The results have been excellent. The alternatives that are available for higher lesions are the same as for agenesis with urethral or vaginal fistula, namely **colostomy** or **primary reconstruction** by ASARP, PSARP or APARP. We have done ASARP once on a neonate with an intermediate lesion.

Postcolostomy reconstruction is carried out after a distal cologram (Fig. 9.6). The operations are the same as those described for agenesis with urethral, vaginal or vesical fistula but with some subtle differences. The absence of a fistula does not make the dissection any easier because the bowel adheres as intimately to the urogenital organs as in patients with a fistula. An area of muscular thickening that is often difficult to identify represents the internal sphincter. The surgeon who believes that a fistula should invariably be found in the course of a PSARP, has done neither an accurate distal cologram nor an endoscopy and is unable to pass a catheter into the bladder is in for trouble. Sarin in 2002 described a high anomaly in which the urethra was mistaken for fistula and was transected and the bladder was mistaken for rectum and was brought down to the surface. The mistake was detected when a suprapubic catheter failed to drain any urine and urine leaked continuously from the anoplasty site. A laparotomy was then performed and corrective steps were taken.

We have performed revisional surgery on 12 patients with ARM without a fistula either because of associated urogenital anomalies or because of poor postre construction anorectal function. Three of them had been initially reconstructed by us and have been followed up to adult life.

The first, born in 1972 had a SAPR for a high anomaly in 1974. This left him with accumulated feces with soiling and he was dependent on care by a doting grandmother. He had a truncated sacrum (see Chapter 15) and suffered from episodes of urinary infection. Investigations revealed that he had a dysplastic right kidney with VUR; on endoscopy the right ureter was seen to open into the prostatic urethra. The family agreed to revisional PSARP for a massive megarectum when he was 21; after this he was much less therapy dependent and kept clean. However consent for surgery for the urological problem was withheld for another 9 years. Finally right nephroureterectomy was done with relief; there was a duplex system with gross pyelonephrosis (Fig. 9.7).

The second born in 1978 had a SPR in 1979. He also had penoscrotal hypospadias with severe chordee and multiple hemivertebra. Investigations revealed that he had bilateral VUR with duplex systems on both sides. On endoscopy, four orifices were seen in the prostatic urethra and none in the bladder. Urine emerged from the two central orifices; the two lateral orifices were almost certainly the openings of the ejaculatory ducts. The hypospadias was repaired in stages between 1980 and 1984. He continued to suffer from ocasional attacks of urinary infection and had an attack of leftsided epididymitis resulting in a scrotal sinus. He generally remained clean with minimum dependence on therapy till he was 19. His main disability was scoliosis. Since episodes of urinary infection continued, the family agreed to a repeat endoscopy, On this occasion, three orifices were seen in the prostatic urethra two were cannulated and retrograde pyelograms were taken; there were duplex systems on both sides (Fig. 9.8). Apparently, the opening of the left ejaculatory duct was obliterated. Surgery was advised but consent was not forthcoming.

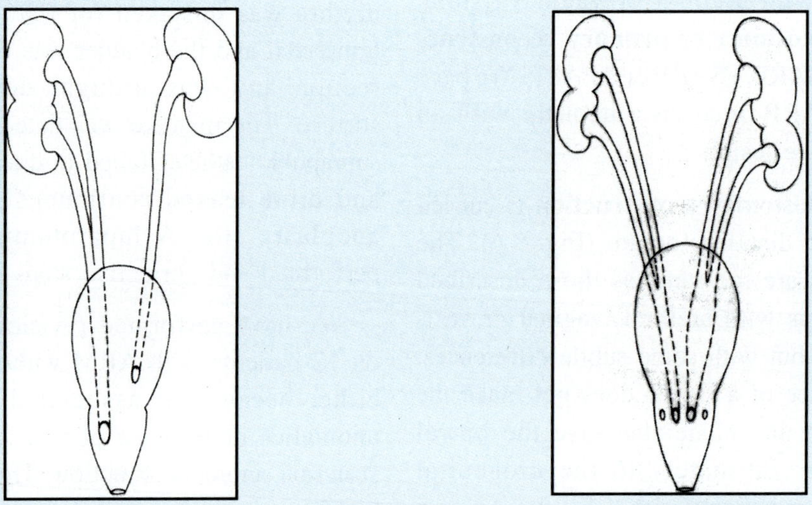

Figs. 9.7-8 Diagrams showing malformed urinary tracts in patients with blind ARM.

Subsequently bowel problems increased and there were episodes of rectal bleeding. A massive diverticulum on the anterior wall of the pulled through bowel was found; the family agreed to surgery only when he was 24. A revisional PSARP was done. The diverticulum was resected and bowel proximal to the diverticulum was brought down to the normal anal site. Concurrent colostomy was done; after this was closed he began to pass stools normally. He has again been strongly advised early ureteroneocystostomies.

The third patient born in 1992 had developed intractable constipation after an apparently routine PSARP done when he was 2½ years old. He had earlier had ureteroneocystostomy elsewhere for unilateral VUR. He had a large megarectum above an area of narrowing at the level of the third sacral vertebra; Banerjee performed a laparotomy and refashioned the bowel with relief when he was 12.

The remaining 9 patients had been reconstructed elsewhere either by perineal, abdominoperineal or posterior sagittal operations. Two had truncated sacrums (see Chapter 15). The bowel had either been pulled through an incorrect site with resulting incontinence (Fig. 9.9) or they developed stenosis and proximal megarectum. We performed a revisional PSARP on 8 and they all did well after revision.

The ninth one did not give permission for a reconstruction. He had first come to us at the age of 17. He had had an abdominoperineal pullthrough that left him with a tubular stenosis and then had multiple perineal operations during childhood. He came to us with a funnel shaped anal canal. Barium enema revealed an enormously distended sigmoid colon (Fig. 9.10).

We performed a laparotomy, the huge distal bowel was delivered out of the pelvis, tapered and left as an end colostomy; the rectal stump was closed. We had planned to carry out the reconstruction 6 months later. However, he disappeared and returned after 11 years, married and happy with his colostomy. He asked for treatment only because he was unable to father a child! He had a persistent fistula between the seminal vesicles and the rectum and seminal fluid would escape per anum after intercourse. He would not agree to a major revision.

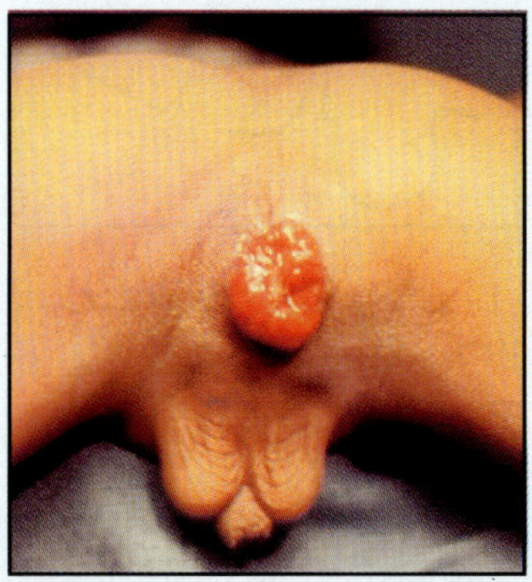

Fig. 9.9 Photograph of incorrect pullthrough.

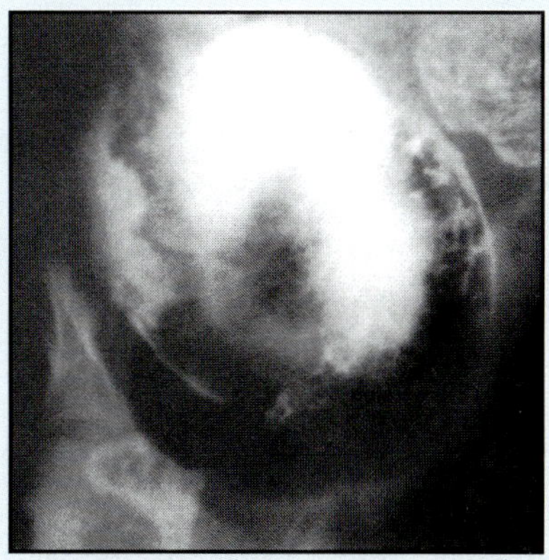

Fig. 9.10 Xray Barium enema - huge megarectum and megasigmoid.

CHAPTER 10

TWO MANIFEST ABNORMAL OPENINGS

In this malformation, the bowel opens through two abnormal openings in the perineum. It constitutes the first variety of **H FISTULA**.

In an article entitled 'H-type anorectal malformations' Rintala *et al* in 1996 described seven patients with the bowel ending with two abnormal openings. In the following year in an article entitled 'Perineal Canal', Wakhlu *et al* described six patients with two manifest abnormal openings.

IN BOYS

There were 5 boys in the series reported by Rintala *et al*; two had cardiac anomalies; a rectovesical and an anoperineal fistula were revealed at autopsy. One had an anobulbar and an anoperineal fistula and was repaired by a low operation. The fourth had had a cutback for an anoperineal fistula and the passage of urine from the anus led to the diagnosis of a urethral fistula later in infancy. The fifth had a fistula between the midurethra and a scrotal ectopic anal opening; this was diagnosed during delayed repair after a neonatal colostomy. Wakhlu *et al* had 4 cases. One died; he had a anourethral fistula and anterior ectopic anus; and also prunebelly syndrome. Three did well, of these 1 had anoperineal fistula and anal stenosis and 2 had anoperineal fistula and anterior ectopic anus.

We have 4 cases. Three came in a moribund state with intestinal and urinary obstruction. One came at three days; autopsy revealed the two fistulas one between the rectum and the prostatic urethra and the other between the rectum and the perineum at the penoscrotal junction. The urethra distal to the fistula was narrow (Fig. 10.1). The other two came at 3 and 4 months respectively; both had rectourethral fistula, anorectal stenosis and narrow urethra.

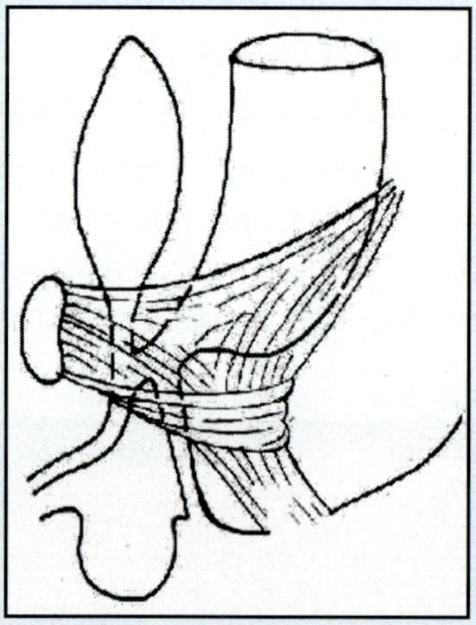

Fig. 10.1 Diagram – very narrow rectourethral and rectoperineal fistulas.

The fourth patient did well; he merits a detailed discussion. He came in 1972 at the age of 2 months; he was thought to have anal stenosis at birth and was submitted to cutback and dilatation elsewhere. After he was taken home the parents found that he passed urine through the neoanus. Xray with contrast led to the diagnosis of anal canal stenosis with rectobulbar urethral fistula (Fig. 10.2). He also had mutliple hemivertebra. SPR was carried out without a colostomy; the fistula was disconnected and bowel of normal caliber was brought out in the perineum; the initial result was very satisfactory. He was lost to followup for some years and reappeared at the age of 13 with recurrence of his urinary fistula. He passed approximately equal amounts of urine through the urethra and the neoanus, and occasionally feces and flatus through the urethra. He also had persistent soiling with fecal retention and multiple hemivertebra had resulted in severe scoliosis.

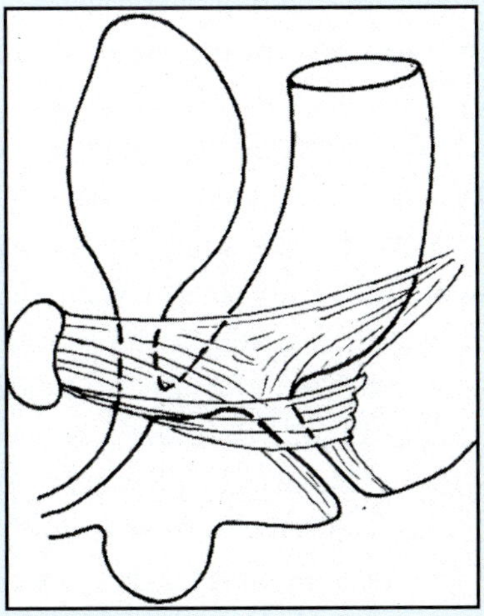

Fig. 10.2 Diagram – rectourethral fistula and anorectal stenosis.

Revisional surgery was advised but consent was initially withheld. In 1987, the family agreed to surgery to close the fistula but would not give consent to colostomy. The rectourethral fistula was isolated and closed by ASARP. Then the anterior half of the bowel was mobilized so as to bring the bowel above the fistula to the anal verge. The greatly dilated anorectum was not tapered. Suprapubic cystostomy was carried out. Healing was uneventful. The fistula closed but continence did not improve.

Finally, consent for concurrent colostomy was obtained and a revisional PSARP was done; the huge megarectum was tapered to size. Healing was uneventful and after closure of the colostomy continence has been excellent.

IN GIRLS

Wakhlu *et al* had two cases, both had an anterior ectopic anus and a vestibular fistula. Rintala *et al* also had 2 cases; one had a vulvar and a high vaginal fistula, and the other had a perineal and a low vaginal fistula. Bianchini in 2001 reported a single case of a girl with a very large rectovaginal fistula with a stenotic anal canal.

We have 5 cases.

The first presented in 1966, at the age of seven months. She passed stools through an opening on the anterior perineum since birth; after a period of constipation at the age of 5 months she began to pass stools through the vagina also. On examination, two openings of the bowel were seen, one in the vestibule and the other on the perineum, 1.5 cm. behind the vestibule. A probe could be easily passed from one to the other (Fig. 10.3).

The second presented in 1977, at the age of 5 years, with chronic intestinal obstruction. She passed stools through the vagina

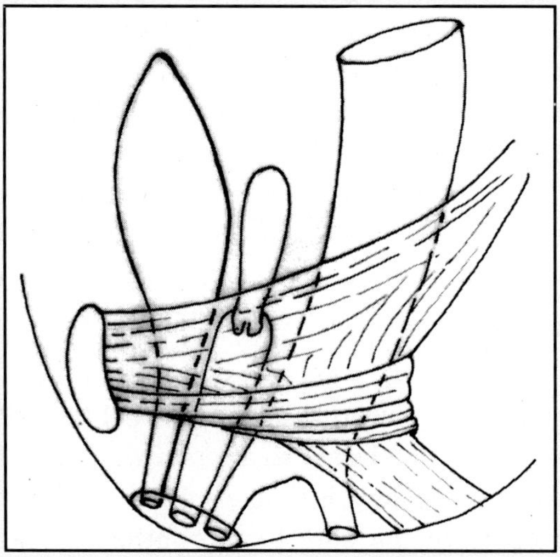

Fig. 10.3 Diagram showing vestibular and perineal fistulas.

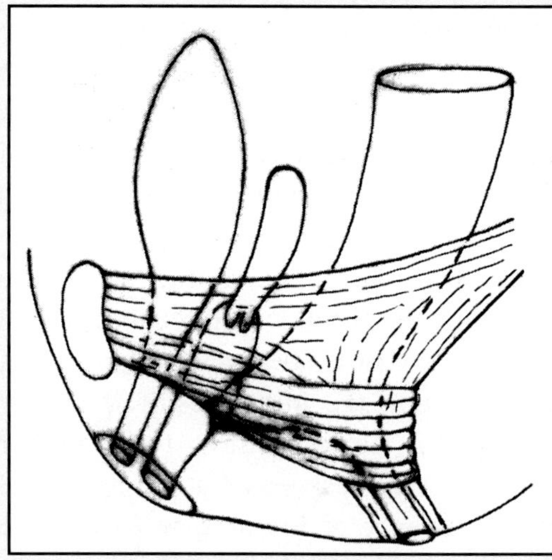

Fig. 10.4 Diagram showing vaginal and perineal fistulas.

as well as through a stenotic opening at the normal anal site. A cutback had been done in infancy to relieve obstruction. Xray with contrast showed a hugely dilated rectum with two narrow tracts leading down from it, one into the vagina and another on to the perineum (Fig. 10.4).

The third presented in 1989, at the age of two weeks, with abdominal distension and the passage of small amounts of feces through an opening in the vestibule; this had been dilated periodically elsewhere to relieve distension. On examination of the perineum, two openings were seen, one in the vestibule and another in the lower vagina. Xray after instillation of contrast revealed the two tracts and dilated bowel above.

In these patients, obstruction was initially relieved by laxatives, suppositories and washouts. They were then submitted to an almost identical operation. With a balloon catheter in the urethra, a circumferential incision was made around the anterior fistula. The anterior tract was dissected off the posterior wall of the vagina till dilated bowel above the levator was reached. Then through another circumferential incision made around the second fistula, the posterior tract was dissected free, and was drawn up to the anterior wound. The space between the vagina and levator sling was dilated, and the bowel drawn down through this. An incision was then made at the normal anal site as for the usual type of vestibular fistula. A tunnel was developed between the fibers of the external sphincter-striated muscle mass and the bowel drawn down through this into the normal anal site. It was fixed in place and the vaginal wound was closed. There was uneventful recovery in all.

The fourth, seen recently had a vestibular and a perineal fistula; she was successfully repaired by a sagittal exposure (ASARP). This is the operation we recommend at present.

Colostomy was not done in any of these cases.

The last case came to Basak with intestinal obstruction. She was 3 months old and had passed small quantities of stool through a small perineal opening and also through the vagina. The perineal opening could not be dilated and colostomy was done. Subsequently the bowel was reconstructed by SARP and the colostomy was closed.

When I studied the records of the Children's Memorial Hospital, Chicago in 1967, I found that out of 95 females with ARM, one had a double opening. This infant had no anus and was found to have a fistula at the fourchette. At operation by Potts in 1958, a second fistula was seen 1 cm. above this, and there was great difficulty in separating the rectum from the vagina. There was, moreover, a double vagina with a ridge going across just above the rectovaginal fistula. Potts concluded his description of the operation with these words: 'In the repair of rectovaginal fistula this was one of the most unsatisfactory operations because of the uncontrollable conditions which were the most difficult we have ever experienced'. Nevertheless, this patient when examined by me at the age of 8½ years was in an excellent state.

CHAPTER 11

ANY OF THE PRECEDING ANOMALIES WITH A UROGENITAL SINUS ANOMALY, NAMELY CLOACA

The word 'Cloaca' appears in the Wingspread List but the lesion is not elaborated in it. Cloaca still eludes a universally acceptable definition. We shall consider cloacal malformations to be those with coexisting anorectal and urogenital sinus malformations in females. The vast majority of girls with a cloacal malformation have a manifest invisible opening of the bowel in the urethrovaginal canal. Nevertheless, patients with a cloacal malformation may also have other anatomical features; these will be described later.

Till the mid 1970s, global experience on the subject was limited to small series reported by Gough (1959), Santulli *et al* (1965), Snyder *et al* (1966), Stephens & Smith (1968), Palken *et al* (1972) and Raffensperger *et al* (1973), there were also a few isolated case reports. Gough collected 18 cases, of whom 11 died; Snyder collected 7 cases, of whom 4 died; Palken collected 10 cases, of whom 1 died, 2 had permanent fecal diversion, 2 had permanent urinary diversion and 1 was treated elsewhere. Out of Raffensperger's 15 cases, 3 died and 7 continued to have major urological problems. This prompted him to offer one neonate the benefit of a one-stage total correction without a colostomy. On the other hand, Stephens and Smith had only three survivors who were all continent. They strongly advocated delaying the urethrovaginal separation. According to them, 'after an appropriate anorectal reconstruction, the patient should be observed until girl becomes woman. If continence of urine is satisfactory, no further reconstructive procedure is necessary. The urogenital sinus may continue to explicate, bringing the urethral and vaginal orifices closer to the exterior and may undergo considerable expansion at the time of puberty'.

The challenge of the cloaca was taken up in earnest by Hendren. A series of articles by him between 1977 and 1995 resulted in a radical change in approach. By 1987, Hendren had established the following.

1. The prime aim of management is a continent normally functioning urinary tract thus emphasizing the incidence of major associated anomalies and complications likely to be encountered in the urinary tracts of these patients
2. A defunctioning colostomy should be performed as early in life as possible, to eliminate intestinal obstruction and

to prevent the entry of bowel contents into the urogenital organs.

3. The precise arrangement of structures of all three systems should be clearly established before undertaking reconstructive operations.
4. The reconstruction should be a total correction of all three systems and should be delayed until the baby is fit for such an operation.

The other major contributor to our knowledge about cloaca is Pena. Between 1982 and 1989, Pena showed that many cloacas could be reconstructed at one sitting by an extraperitoneal extension of PSARP, which he named Posterior Sagittal Ano-Recto-Vagino-Urethro-Plasty (PSARVUP). He also showed that those cloacas that could not be dealt with extraperitoneally could be reconstructed by continuing the operation with a laparotomy. Until 1989 he had done this on 7 of his 54 patients. In 1997 he reported on a total of 177 patients, 139 underwent a primary repair and 38 required a secondary repair. In Pena's words, PSARVUP is a 'rather sophisticated operation; it requires a great deal of patience, a meticulous technique and finesse'. Urethrovaginal separation resulted in urethrovaginal fistulas in 7 to 11%, vaginal strictures in 10% and acquired vaginal atresia in 2%. Hence in 1997 he proposed what he considered 'an easier way to repair cloacas', namely Total Urogenital Mobilization (TUM). In this procedure, the common channel is widely opened up and mobilized as a whole by entering the space between the pubis and the urogenital organs. Traction is exerted on the margins of the urethra and vagina and avascular fibrous ligaments holding them up are divided so that the vaginal and urethral orifices reach the perineum. They are then sutured in place. A near normal appearance was restored in the 8 patients with a common channel less than 3cm. Three patients had a longer common channel and required urethrovaginal separation and an additional procedure. Hamza *et al* and Krstic *et al* both reported successes with TUM in 2001.

In 1992 Hendren reported on 105 patients; 4 died without surgery and 1 was lost to followup; 43 were treated after 1982; 12 were reconstructed by PSARVUP, 24 by PSARVUP with laparotomy and 7 by APARP. He altered the position of his patient several times during the course of an operation that often lasted 16 to 20 hours. Such an operation owes its success to an elaborate system of monitoring, replacement of fluid sometimes at the rate of 25 ml/kg/hour and ventilatory support for several days postoperatively. In the course of the discussion that followed one of his presentations in 1986, Hendren was asked 'if an individual surgeon does not have the stamina, expertise or renal capacity for a 16 hour operation, how should he or she handle the patient?' His reply has unfortunately not been published.

However, it is to this question that surgeons in the developing world interested in cloacal anomalies must address themselves. It is unlikely that expertise available in Boston will be available to all of them for some time to come and hence, alternative strategies have to be devised.

Patients with cloacal anomalies are presented to a surgeon either because they have a single opening in the perineum or because they have intestinal obstruction. In the developed world, most of them reach a surgeon soon after birth. In the developing world, some come in the neonatal period, others reach months or years after birth with chronic or acute-on-chronic intestinal obstruction or features of obstructive uropathy. In 1990, my gynecological colleague Sen Gupta reported details about a 24-year old girl who was brought to him by her husband some time after marriage because of unsatisfactory intercourse. Apparently she had been micturating and defecating through a single opening all her life without much distress!

The common variety of Cloaca with a manifest abnormal opening is divided into 2 groups depending on the level at which bowel of normal or greater caliber ends.

If the bowel ends at or below the third sacral vertebra it is an intermediate anomaly; if it ends above the third sacral vertebra it is a high anomaly. The anomaly was considered intermediate in 66 patients and high in 14 patients; the level of the lesion could not be determined in 5.

INTERMEDIATE ANOMALIES

In this condition, there is a rounded perineum without an anus and a small vestibule with a single opening; both urine and meconium emerge freely through this and the baby is rarely obstructed at birth (Fig. 11.1).

The single vestibular orifice can be opened up under sedation to reveal the urethral and rectal orifices. A catheter can be passed into the rectum; it can be utilized to decompress the bowel and instill radio-opaque dye. A catheter can also be passed into the urethra and radio-opaque dye can be instilled through it. Xray reveals bowel of normal or greater caliber below the third sacral vertebra, and a fistula opening into the posterior wall of the lower third of the vagina. The urethra is relatively long and usually meets the vagina anteriorly at about the same level as the rectum. The common channel is less than 3 cm. long (Fig. 11.2). The status of the urinary system is assessed by routine examination of blood and urine and USG. Major obstructive uropathies are relatively uncommon with this type of malformation. However, if USG reveals such an anomaly, other imaging procedures are mandatory.

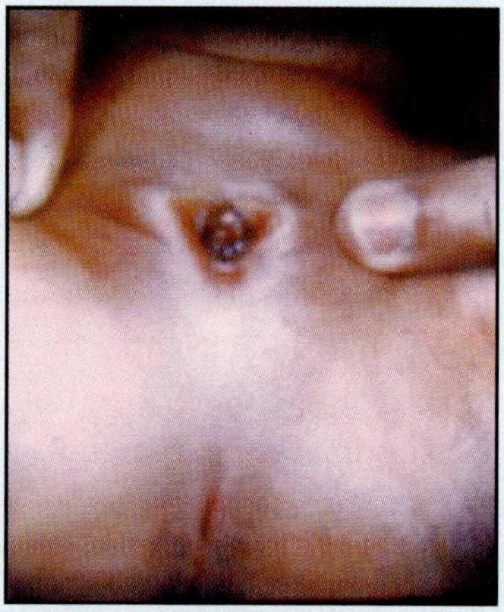

Fig. 11.1 Photograph of intermediate anomaly.

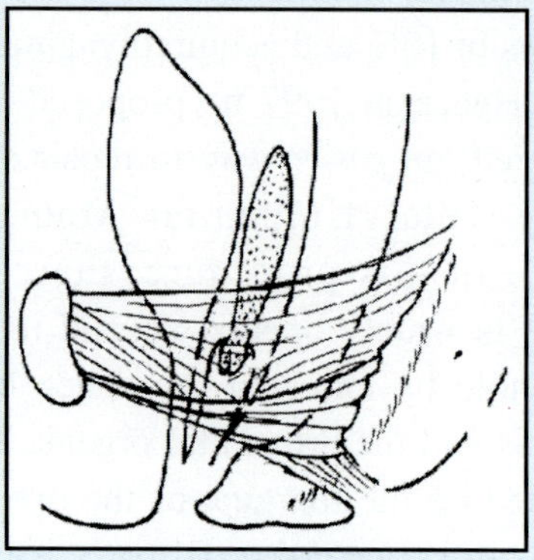

Fig. 11.2 Diagram of above.

Earlier we had studied 28 patients, 18 of whom had reached us as neonates. We have subsequently studied 38 patients, 11 of whom reached us as neonates.

Management

We now perform a **colostomy** on all patients. It is necessary to ensure that there is a free flow of urine in the period between the colostomy and the reconstruction.

The reconstruction, named **PSARVUP** is done at about the age of 4 months provided the baby is healthy and weighs about 6 kg. We agree with Pena that this operation should only be performed in centers where necessary finesse for carrying this out is available. At present we do not consider TUM to be an easier way to repair cloacas.

The operation begins only after the anatomy has been clearly defined by pre-operative distal cologram and cloacogram and peroperative endoscopy.

The operation begins as a PSARP for vaginal fistula with a balloon catheter in the common channel. The incision reaches anteriorly up to the posterior margin of the single orifice and the striated muscle complex is divided completely (Figs. 11.3-8). The rectovaginal separation is carried out as already described for recto bulbar urethral separation and the anorectum is kept

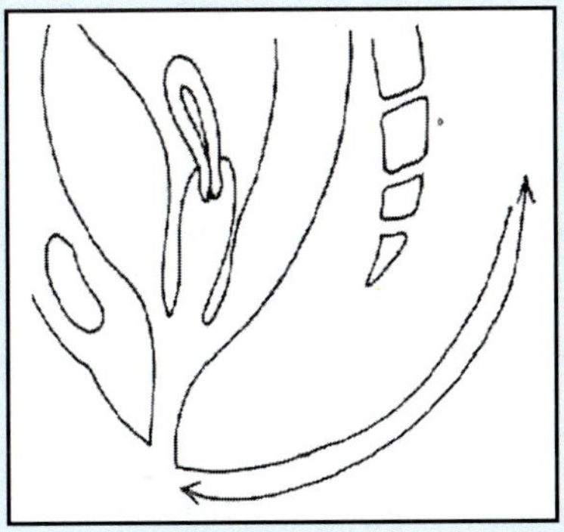

Fig. 11.3 Diagrams of operation PSARVUP – incision.

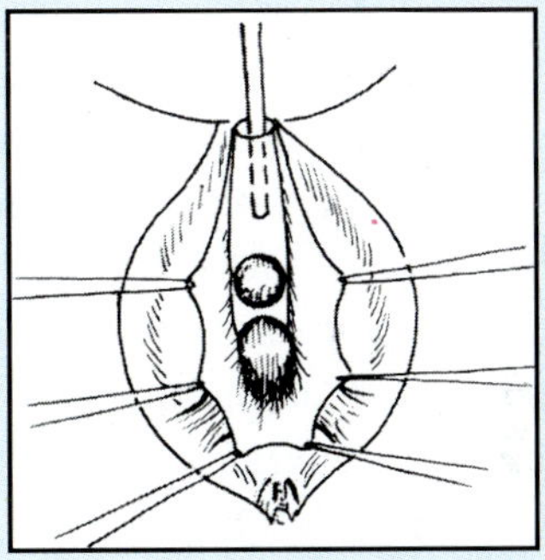

Fig. 11.5 PSARVUP - view of perineum showing incisions.

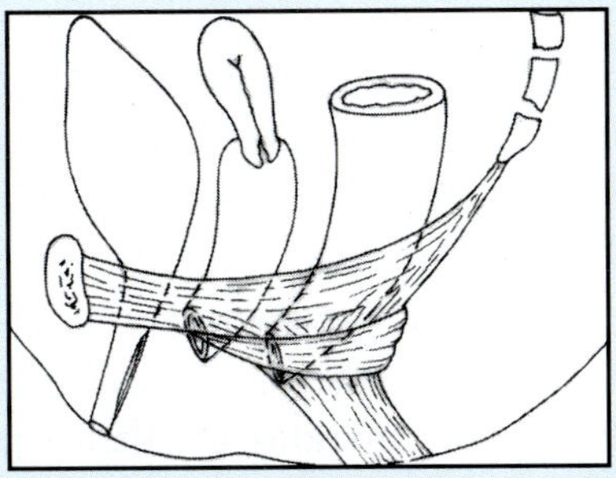

Fig. 11.4 PSARVUP - sagittal view after separation of bowel & vagina.

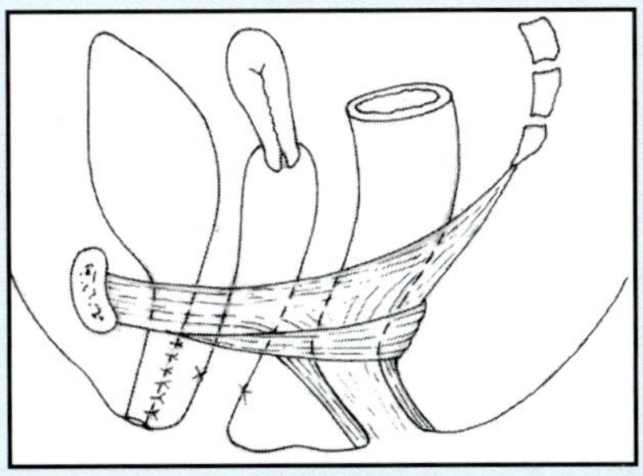

11.6 PSARVUP - sagittal view after reconstruction.

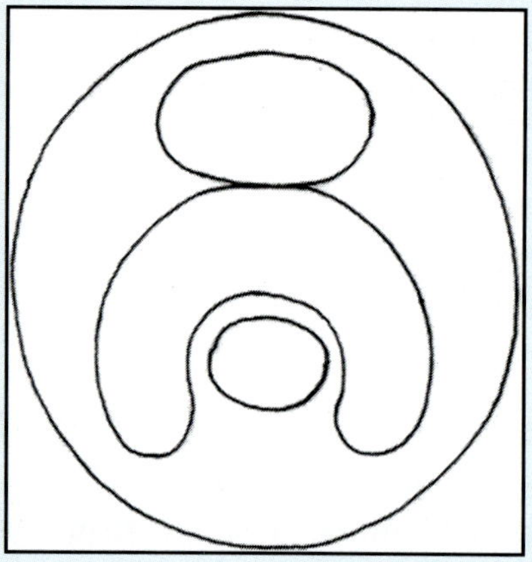

Fig. 11.7 PSARVUP – showing relation of vagina to urethra.

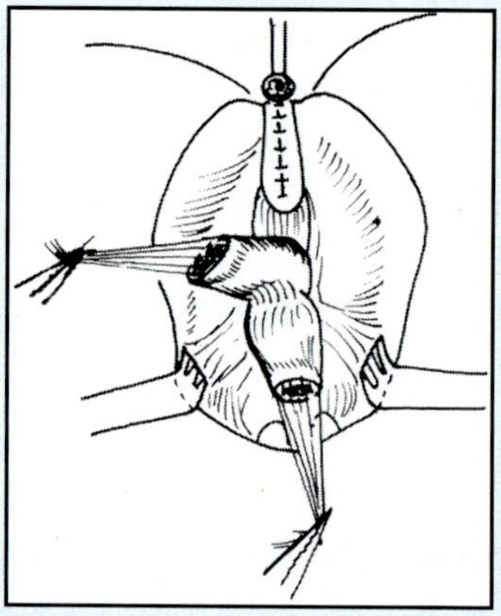

Fig. 11.8 PSARVUP – view of perineum showing repair.

ready for pullthrough. The posterior and lateral walls of the vagina are then mobilized so that these reach the surface.

Attention is then directed to the anterior wall of the vagina and the urethra. We strive to use the common channel as urethra; a midline vertical incision on the posterior wall of the vagina above the confluence gives a good exposure of the anterior wall of the vagina. This is picked up with stay sutures above the confluence. A transverse incision is then made on the epithelium of the vagina and a plane is developed between the posterior wall of the urethra and the anterior wall of the vagina. Gradually the vagina is lifted off the posterior wall of the urethra. This separation is difficult because the structures are inelastic and the vagina wraps the back and sides of the urethra and bladder neck in a semicircular fashion. When the separation is complete the balloon catheter is passed into the bladder and the posterior wall of the urethra is repaired over the catheter.

We now turn our attention to the vagina. If it is capacious and its posterior wall has reached the surface, the anterior wall can be separated from the bladder base up to the peritoneal reflection and brought down; if necessary the peritoneum can be opened to facilitate mobilization. If it does not reach the surface, lateral skin flaps can be developed and turned in. If there is hydrocolpos, the posterior half of the dilated vagina can be brought down on an anteroinferior pedicle distally and the vagina repaired by a row of sutures in the midline posteriorly. Pena has named this maneuver a dome flap; (Figs. 11.9-10); we have found it very effective.

The repair is started from the front. The urethral rent is closed and the perineal muscles are apposed between the urethra and the vagina. Simultaneous dissection on both surfaces of the vagina may devitalize the vagina anteriorly. In order to prevent contact between the sutured posterior urethra and the devitalized vagina, it may be necessary to rotate the vagina through 90°. The vaginal margins are then sutured to the skin on either side. The perineal body is then reconstructed behind the vagina. The anorectum is then pulled through to the

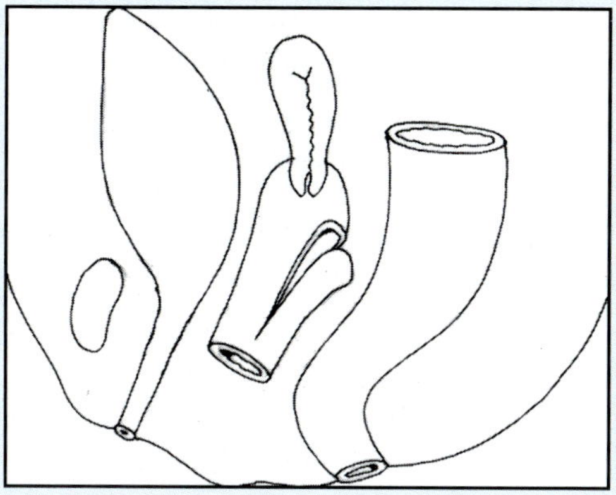

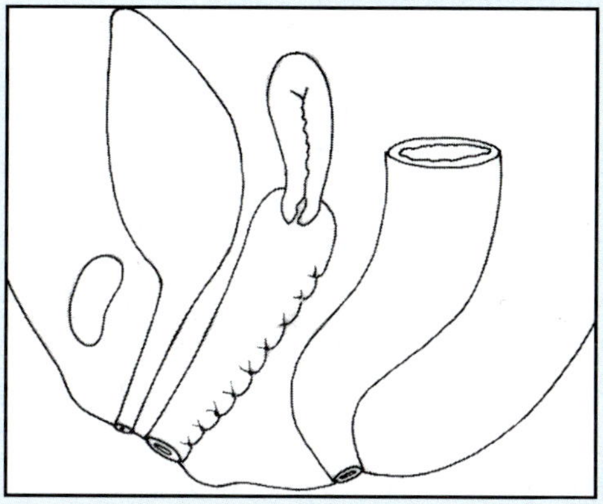

Figs. 11.9-10 Diagrams to show construction of dome flap for vagina.

normal anal site through the levator sling and between the vertical fibers of the external sphincter. The levator ani and the posterior half of the striated muscle mass are repaired behind the bowel; the anterior half is repaired in front of it. The neoanus is then sutured to the skin margins on either side. The remaining part of the wound is closed by apposition of the skin margins in the midline.

Alternative Procedures

In an earlier era we had staged the repair, carrying out the anorectal reconstruction first and postponing the urethrovaginal separation for another day. Prior to 1984, we had done postcolostomy SPR on 4 girls between the ages of 6 and 12 months with success. Concerned at the high dropout rate after colostomy, we had done primary SPR without colostomy on three neonates and on five older girls who were only mildly obstructed and whose large bowel could be completely decompressed by laxatives and washouts. While 6 patients regained normal bowel function, two neonates died and the procedure was abandoned. After 1984, we did postcolostomy PSARP on two babies when they were about 3 months old and weighed about 5 kg. The operative technique was the same as that described for anorectal agenesis with vaginal fistula. When healing was complete, the colostomy was closed and normal defecation was restored.

Disconnecting the bowel from the urethrovaginal canal eliminated a safety valve against the ravages of urinary obstruction. This could be controlled by periodic dilatation of the common channel during the time interval between the anorectal reconstruction and the urethrovaginal separation.

Until 1988, we carried out the urethrovaginal separation before the child began school, between the ages of 3 to 4 years. By then, the perineum had grown and there was space between the neoanus and the posterior margin of the urethrovaginal opening. Also there was some explication and enlargement of the urogenital sinus, as described by Stephens and Smith (1968). We recommend this plan even now for surgeons who for one reason or another did not think that one stage correction was justified; we shall therefore describe our technique.

Urethrovaginal separation for staged procedure

With the patient in the spreadeagled or the frog position, a posterior V flap of skin is raised with its apex at the posterior margin of the common channel. Its posterior wall is then mobilized by extending the incision laterally from the tip of the V along the mucocutaneous junction on both sides.

A sagittal incision is made on the posterior wall of the common channel extending to the vagina to accommodate the V flap. This flap is then sutured in place with interrupted sutures, thus widening the vagina posteriorly; if there is hydrocolpos a dome flap can be used.

Two stay sutures are placed on the upper margin of the urethrovaginal fistula.The epithelium is incised transversely between these, and the posterior wall of the urethra and the anterior wall of the vagina are separated as already described. When the separation is complete, the distal urethra reaches the surface; a balloon catheter is left in to drain the bladder. The anterior wall of the vagina may reach the surface directly or may do so only after tapering, namely after excision of redundant epithelium and suturing in the midline.

Two transverse V flaps of skin are then raised on either side. The perineal muscles are apposed in the midline to fill up the gap between the vagina and urethra and the skin flaps are then suitably sutured

An alternative procedure recommended by Das is to use a sagittal incision between the posterior margin of the vagina and the anterior margin of the neoanus. If the space available is insufficient, the anterior wall of the anorectum can be divided in the midline, and repaired after the urethrovaginal reconstruction is completed.

Results

Two patients of an earlier era on whom anorectal reconstruction and discontinuance of colostomy were successfully completed were found at followup to have a reasonable explication of the vagina and were left alone. Out of the three who had secondary urethrovaginoplasty only one has reported regularly. She is now twenty four and happily married. The others have been lost to followup.

So far, 26 patients have been operated by PSARVUP. There was one death following colostomy closure and one required a laparotomy for a secondary hydrocolpos in a duplex system; this was producing obstructive uropathy and recurrent urinary tract infection. There has been a few minor urethrovaginal leaks. All other patients are doing well (Fig. 11.11). They have normal urinary continence and initial constipation and soiling disappeared with passage of time.

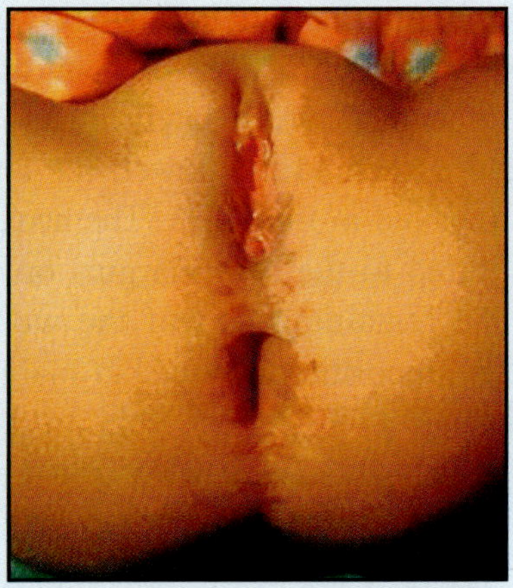

Fig. 11.11 Photograph after PSARVUP.

HIGH ANOMALIES

In the high lesion there is a relatively flat perineum without an anus and a relatively small vestibule with a single opening (Fig. 11.12). Urine is voided through this opening; the amount of meconium passed through it depends on the size of the fistula. If the fistula is very narrow, no meconium is passed and obstruction is complete. On the other hand, if the fistula is large, there may be a free flow of meconium and the baby may survive for many weeks without surgery.

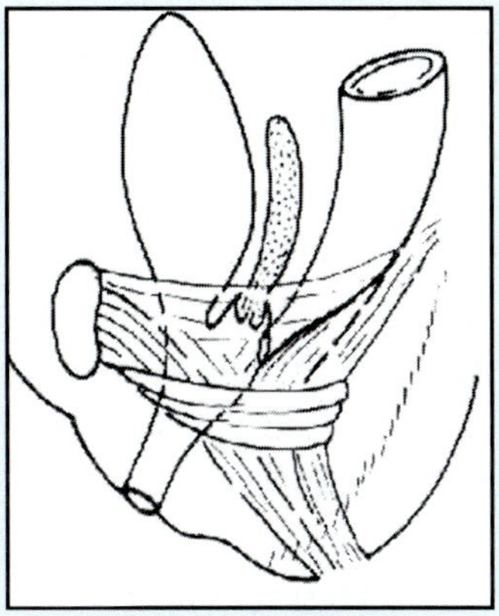

Fig. 11.13 Diagram of high anomalies.

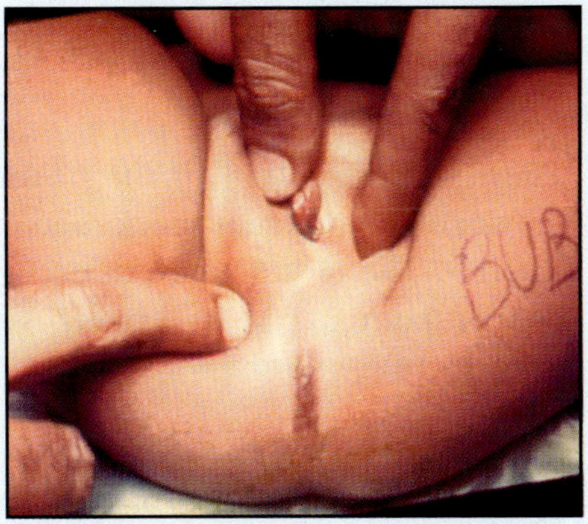

Fig. 11.12 Photograph of high anomaly.

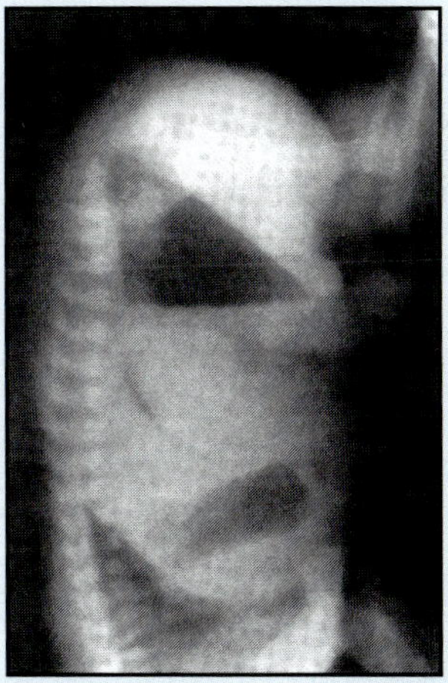

Fig. 11.14 Xray – invertogram showing gas in bowel and vagina.

In this anomaly, the common channel is longer than 3 cm. and the openings of the urethra and rectum into it can only be seen with the help of an endoscope (Fig. 11.13). In the obstructed neonate, an invertogram shows bowel at or above the P-C line and gas in the bladder (Fig. 11.14). Contrast fluid instilled into the common channel is unlikely to enter the bowel unless there is a very large fistula. The structure of the urinary tract is outlined by USG and this may be followed up by MRI scan. If a catheter can be passed into the bladder, a VCU can be done (Fig. 11.15).

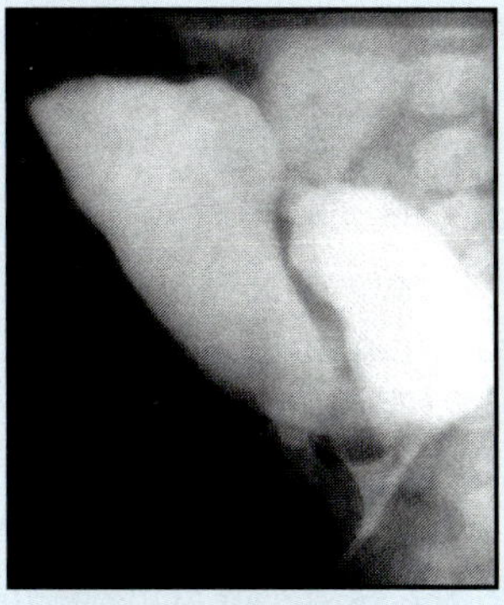

Fig. 11.15 Xray – cloacogram showing dye in vagina and bladder, reflux into ureter.

We have 14 cases. Autopsies had been carried out on two who came in an earlier era. In one there was a unicornuate uterovaginal system; the rectum opened into the upper end and the urethra into the lower end. In the other there was a massive hydrocolpos with the rectum entering posterosuperiorly and the urethra anteriorly. Both had bilateral dysplastic kidneys.

Management

The management is beset with many problems.

A neonatal colostomy is of course mandatory; a concurrent endoscopic assessment can be carried out if weight is satisfactory and the abdomen is not greatly distended; otherwise this is postponed till the day of reconstruction.

With an endoscope in the common channel, the presence or absence of meconium or feces in it can be detected and the shape and size of the channel can be determined. After the instrument enters the vagina, the cervix uteri can be seen at the dome. The urethral orifice is seen on the anterior wall and the instrument can be passed through it into the bladder for a routine cystourethroscopy. Usually the bladder and the internal meatus are normal; the length of urethra between the vesicourethral junction and the urethrovaginal junction is short. A catheter can be introduced through the endoscope into the bladder and a VCU carried out to record the anatomy and demonstrate or exclude vesicoureteric reflux. After this, attention is directed to the posterior wall of the vagina. The rectal opening is often difficult to identify, but with patience a catheter can be introduced to decompress the bowel and instil radio-opaque fluid.

Endoscopy and Xray studies can establish that the rectum in these babies opens into the upper two thirds of the posterior wall of the vagina, and bowel of normal or greater caliber lies above the third sacral vertebra. The rectum and urethra generally meet the vagina at about the same level.

A postcolostomy distal cologram is followed by a detailed study of urinary structure and function, either with radioisotope scans or intravenous urography.

The urological status of these patients is disturbed by two factors:

1. There is obstruction of the channel between the bladder neck and the exterior. The obstruction can occur at one or both of the following sites (Fig. 11.16).

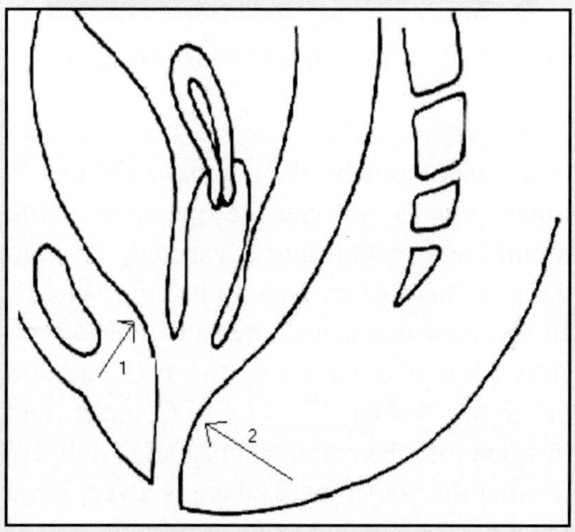

Fig. 11.16 Diagram showing obstruction to urinaryflow 1) at bladder outlet and 2) at urogenital sinus.

a) Between the bladder neck and urethrovaginal canal. This produces the classical features of bladder outlet obstruction with bilateral hydroureteronephrosis.

b) Between the urethrovaginal junction and the exterior. Stenosis of the common channel produces three problems.

i) A large rectocloacal fistula allows urine to escape into the bowel. Absorption of the urinary constituents by the bowel mucosa gives rise to hyperchloremic acidosis; its intensity depends on the size of the fistula, the extent of the outlet obstruction and above all, the length of bowel between the fistula and the colostomy. It is therefore more severe if the colostomy is transverse and not sigmoid. The fistula also protects the upper urinary tracts; this protective action is lost when the bowel is reconstructed without disturbing the urethrovaginal connection.

ii) If the rectocloacal fistula is small, urine flows freely into the vagina from the urethra. The vagina distends with urine and **Urocolpos** results with consequent upper tract dilatation seen on USG and VCU.

iii) When both fistulas are large, the vagina distends with both urine and bowel contents; the condition is named **Pneumourocolpos** (Fig. 11.17). Intestinal gas is seen in the vagina on a neonatal erect Xray.

2. There are associated malformations. These include VUR, obstructive hydroureteronephrosis, an absent or dysplastic kidney and duplex pelviureteric systems. Reflux in a baby with a cloaca permits bowel organisms to enter the pelvicalyceal system and cause pyelonephritis and pyonephrosis.

The data collected allows a decision to be taken as to whether or not to intervene in the urinary tract. Hendren in 1986 advised periodic dilatation of either the urogenital sinus or the urethra or a small cutback to enlarge the orifice. In his subsequent study in 1992 he found that 27 patients came with a prior urinary diversion. Pena in 1989 also found it necessary to perform various forms of urinary diversion.

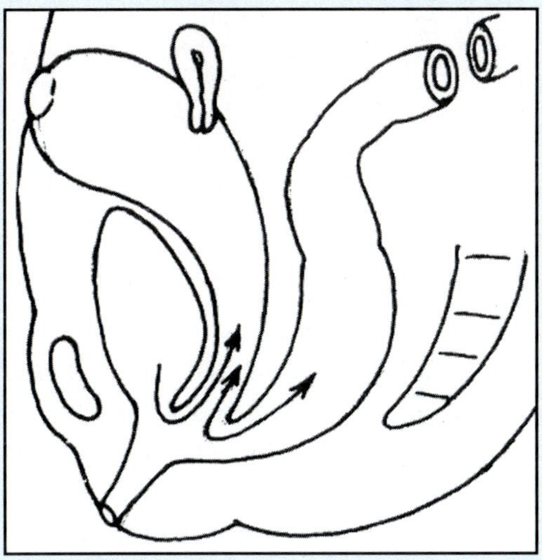

Fig. 11.17 Diagram of pneumourocolpos with vaginostomy, showing flow of urine.

We perform a vaginostomy if there is a very large urocolpos. In all other situations we proceed to vesicostomy (Fig. 11.18) if periodic dilatations fail to keep the urinary tract in good shape. This protects the upper tracts, prevents hyperchloremic acidosis, gives time to decide on the form of reconstruction, does not interfere with the method of reconstruction and can be closed when no longer required. However, ureterostomy may have to be done if a supravesical diversion is thought necessary.

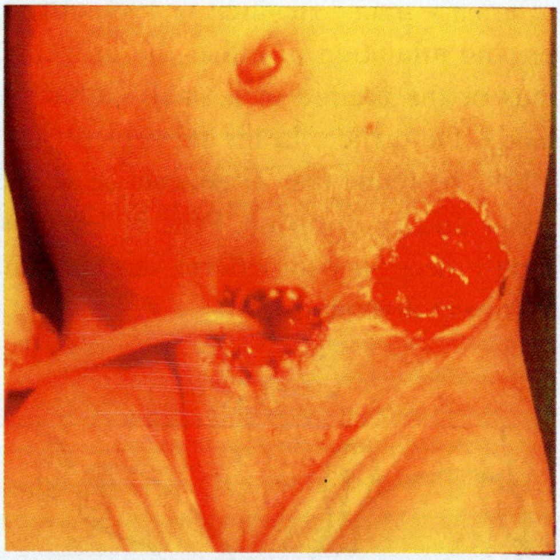

Fig. 11.18 Photograph of vesicostomy and colostomy.

Earlier, we believed that the repair of this anomaly should be staged, even if there were no major associated problems. We would carry out the anorectal reconstruction at about the age of 4 months and leave the urethrovaginal separation till the age of 4 years. Prior to 1984, APARP was done for all high lesions; subsequently we explored the malformation by the posterior sagittal route. If the rectum ended at the third sacral vertebra we found that we could detach it more easily from the posterior vaginal wall than the rectum that opened lower down and shared a common wall. If the rectum was not found, the patient was turned over for laparotomy.

The urethrovaginal separation was done after an endoscopic examination; this helped to decide whether to separate by the perineal route only or to carry out an abdominoperineal procedure. After separation, the entire common channel became the new urethra, and the vagina had to be brought to the surface by other means.

Today we feel that onestage correction can justifiably be performed in a center of excellence by a combined abdomino-perineal procedure, either PSARVUP with laparotomy or APARVUP with or without laparoscopy.

Results

We had earlier studied 8 patients with a high anomaly. Five had died; one after an abdominoperineal reconstruction, 2 soon after colostomy and 2 after going home with a colostomy. The last patient had a massive urocolpos and bladder outlet obstruction but the parents would not agree to any form of urinary diversion.

There were only 3 survivors. The first had a Mollard type of abdominoperineal reconstruction in 1983 and a perineal urethrovaginal separation in 1989. She was doing well when last seen. The second born in 1966 came to us at the age of one year with intestinal obstruction and severe urinary tract infection. She was born with a single opening in the vestibule and had had a perineal operation elsewhere to relieve intestinal obstruction; this opening closed. A colostomy was done and investigations revealed a high cloacal malformation. We performed a Swenson Donnellan type of APARP and closed the colostomy. She was lost to followup for some years and was brought back after menarche with incontinence and prolapse. Perineal revisional surgery and urethrova-ginal separation was carried out; she again disappeared and came to see us when she was 18. She had no urinary problems but had vaginal stenosis and fecal retention and soiling. More revisions were carried out but she was not satisfied and one day she ran away from home never to return!

We have a complete followup of the third patient, first seen in 1967 when she was a year old. She had a neonatal left lower quadrant colostomy and suffered from recurrent bouts of urinary infection and mild azotemia. She passed urine through a small opening between the labia. Contrast Xray revealed that the rectum ended high up into a massive hydrocolpos. There was a septate vagina and a grade 4 reflux up the left ureter. Poorly functioning kidneys and bilateral hydroureteronephrosis were seen on intra-venous urography. At endoscopy, a high urethrovaginal connection, hydrocolpos, bladder trabeculations and wide ureteric orifices with poor efflux were seen.

At the age of 14 months, a Swenson-Donnellan type of APARP together with a suprapubic cystostomy was done. Consent for a more permanent urinary diversion was not given. The colostomy was closed at the age of 20 months and she began to defecate normally. However she continued to suffer from recurrent episodes of urinary infection, retention of urine and dribbling. She responded to antibacterial drugs and periodic dilatations.

When she was 5 years old, the cloacal channel was enlarged by Y-V plasty. This relieved the obstructive uropathy but she did not achieve urinary continence. An intravenous urogram done a year later showed remarkable improvement. She was then lost to followup and was brought back after menarche with severe dysmenorrhea and scanty menstrual discharge. Examination under anesthesia at the age of 15 years revealed a tight stenosis of the urethrovaginal canal above the site of the previous Y-V plasty, with retention of urine and menstrual fluid above the stenosis. The collection was evacuated after dilatation, and she was relieved for some time. Periodic dilatations were continued until finally consent for major surgery was obtained.

In collaboration with a gynecological colleague an abdominoperineal reconstruction was done in 1982. We found that she had two normal looking uteruses at the superolateral angles of a huge hydrohematocolpos. After this was emptied of its contents, the urethral opening was found in the anterior wall. The capacious vagina continued below the urethrovaginal junction as a stenotic tube. We performed an abdominoperineal urethrovaginoplasty; the tubular stenosis was resected, the vagina was tapered to size and brought down to the perineum. Though the urethrovaginal fistula remained, the hydrocolpos and obstruction to the flow of urine and menstrual fluid were eliminated.

Three years later, the urethrovaginal separation was carried out by the method described by Hendren and Mitchell (1982) (Figs. 11.19-21).

She was placed in the prone position. The urethrovaginal canal was opened by an oblique incision. A U-shaped incision on the anterior wall of the vagina enabled reconstruction of the urethra over an indwelling catheter. Then a buttock flap was raised and rotated into the lumen to fill up the defect created on the anterior vaginal

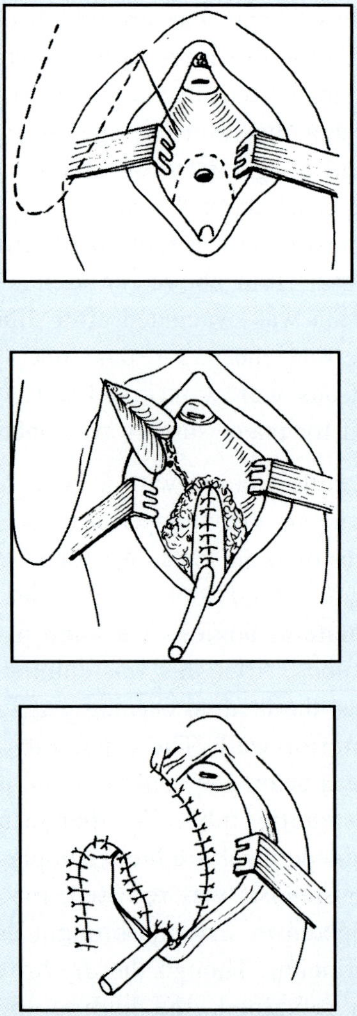

Figs. 11.19-21 Diagrams showing perineal vaginoplasty.

wall. The defect in the buttock was repaired by rearrangement of local tissue. When healing was complete, the urethral catheter was withdrawn and she could micturate normally for the first time in her life. Her subsequent urological status has been excellent. Hendren in 1998 reported his study of 40 cases operated with this technique.

Our patient belongs to the top socio-economic group of Indian society, has a happy home, had pursued postgraduate studies, is married but has not become a mother. Although she did not have the benefit of the treatment that has now evolved for the type of lesion she was born with she has done very well, thanks to parental support.

We have studied 6 new patients in the last two decades.

Three patients are available for followup. Two had had PSARVUP with laparotomy and are doing well. The third had an APARP for a high lesion 13 years ago. She had severe sacral truncation and urinary incontinence. She survives with good parental care and both fecal and urinary continence has improved with time; the parents have not given consent to urethrovaginal separation.

There were 2 deaths. One death was unfortunate She had survived a right upper quadrant colostomy and a vesicostomy and was put up for a onestage correction when she was 10 months old. Das performed a PSARVUP with laparotomy, and reconstructed the vagina with a segment of colon. Postoperative septicemia led to death. The second presented with a massive pneum-ourocolpos, an absent kidney on one side and hydroureteronephrosis on the other, and azotemia. Colostomy and vesicostomy were done but the parents would not agree to further surgery.

The last patient had been treated elsewhere. PSARVUP with laparotomy had been done, but since there was insufficient bowel distal to the colostomy this was resected and colon proximal to the colostomy brought down to the normal anal site. The wound unprotected by a colostomy had broken down and there was a continuous flow of urine and feces through it. The parents would not agree to a second colostomy.

UNUSUAL FORMS OF CLOACA

1. A Urogental Sinus with the bowel opening on the surface anterior to the normal anal site

This is considered by Hendren (1986) to be the least pronounced cloacal anomaly. There are two varieties.

(a) In one of them the bowel opens in the perineum behind the vestibule; its caliber may be normal or narrow (Fig. 11.22). Even if normal, it should be moved back to the normal anal site to provide space in the perineum to accommodate the vaginal orifice after the vagina is separated from the urethra. The only patient in our series came the day after birth with obstruction; this was relieved by a washout. There were ambiguous genitalia with one descended gonad. USG revealed a single ectopic kidney.and blood examination showed a high estrogen level. A successful PAT was done, but after some time renal failure supervened and the father did not wish to continue treatment.

(b) In the other one, the bowel opens in the vestibule just behind the common urethrovaginal opening. In the only patient in our series Basu performed a neonatal SARP and left the urethrovaginal canal alone for another day.

2. Atresia of the Vagina

The vagina may be atretic either at the outlet or higher up and the bowel may end as a urethral, vestibular or perineal fistula. (Fig. 11.23). Secretions retained in the vagina produce a variety of hydrocolpos known as **Mucocolpos** (Fig. 11.24). There may be a palpable hypogastric swelling and consequent obstructive uropathy. The diagnosis is confirmed by USG. It is generally managed during the course of the anorectoplasty using a dome flap; occasionally a vaginostomy is necessary.

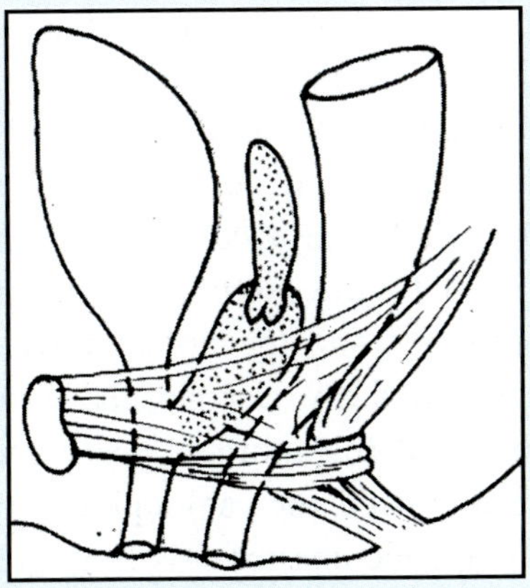

Fig. 11.22 Diagram of anoperineal fistula with urogenital sinus.

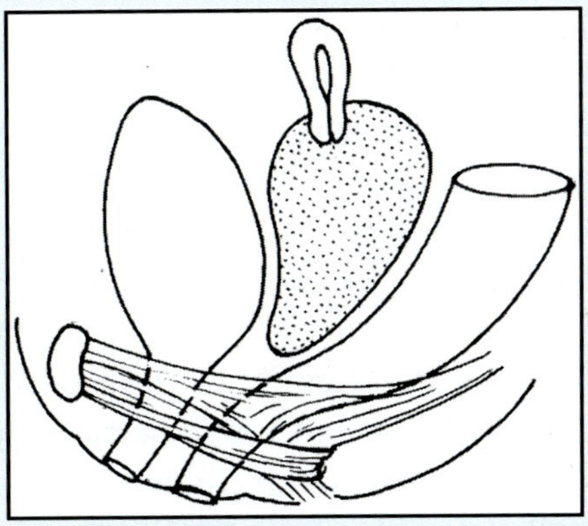

Fig. 11.23 Diagram of vaginal atresia and rectovestibular fistula.

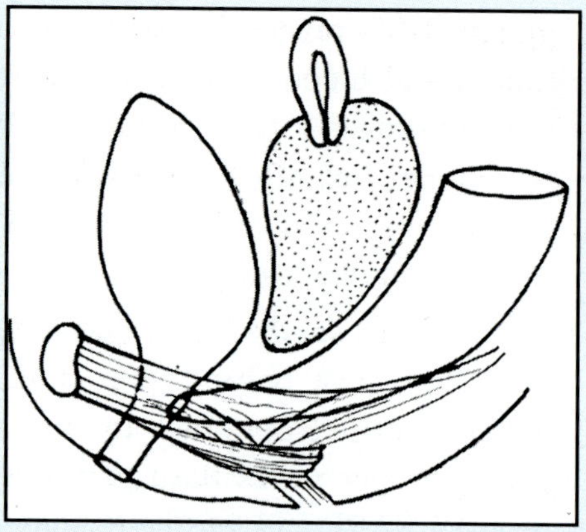

Fig. 11.24 Diagram of vaginal atresia and mucocolpos.

3. Agenesis of the Vagina

This condition has been reported by Cohn *et al* in 1956 and by Ein *et al* in 1971. In 1998 Levitt *et al* reported 8 cases. In 6 the uterus was also absent and a vaginoplasty was done with the terminal 8 cm of bowel; the bowel above this was brought to the normal anal site. In 2 there was a uterus and upper vagina. An end to end anastomosis was done between the upper vagina and the neovagina; one during closure of the colostomy and the other in the course of the main repair, completing the PSARVUP with a laparotomy. In 2002, Sarin reported 4 cases. Two presented with amenorrhea in adult life after a successful anorectoplasty in infancy and two were diagnosed during the anorectoplasty. The vagina was reconstructed in one patient with small bowel and in the other with sigmoid colon. In 2003, Deshpandey *et al* from Mumbai reported on an adult who presented with hematocolpos and a recto-vestibular fistula; she had vaginal atresia and a functioning uterus.

We have 2 patients. In one, the absence of the uterus and vagina was detected by USG before anorectoplasty was done (Fig. 11.25). The other presented at the age of 15 years with primary amenorrhea having had only a cutback in infancy. She had soiling but no obstruction. Laparoscopy revealed two rudimentary uteruses and tubes and two normal ovaries. Das reconstructed a vagina from an isolated segment of sigmoid colon.

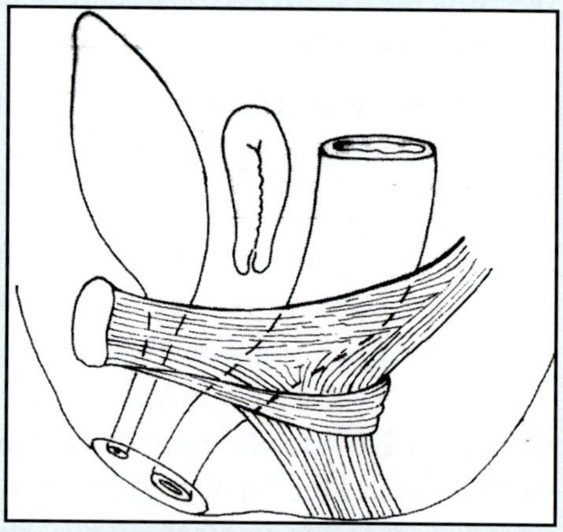

Fig. 11.25 Diagram of agenesis of vagina.

Intraperitoneal vaginal reconstruction

A loop of colon is brought down on a vascular pedicle. Colovaginoplasty was easy in the girl with a neonatal cutback because she did not have a colostomy at all. It is also relatively easy if the original colostomy is in the transverse colon. There are two options. First, the distal bowel immediately proximal to the fistula can be used for vaginoplasty and the bowel above it used for anorectoplasty. Second, the distal bowel can be used for anorectoplasty and bowel above this used for vaginoplasty; this calls for a colocolic anastomosis (Figs. 11.26-27). In spite of this, Das prefers the second option because the distalmost segment of bowel is the best replacement for the anorectum and the colocolic anastomosis is protected by the colostomy. After the bowel is pulled through into the perineum, the perineal operator does the colocutaneous anastomosis.

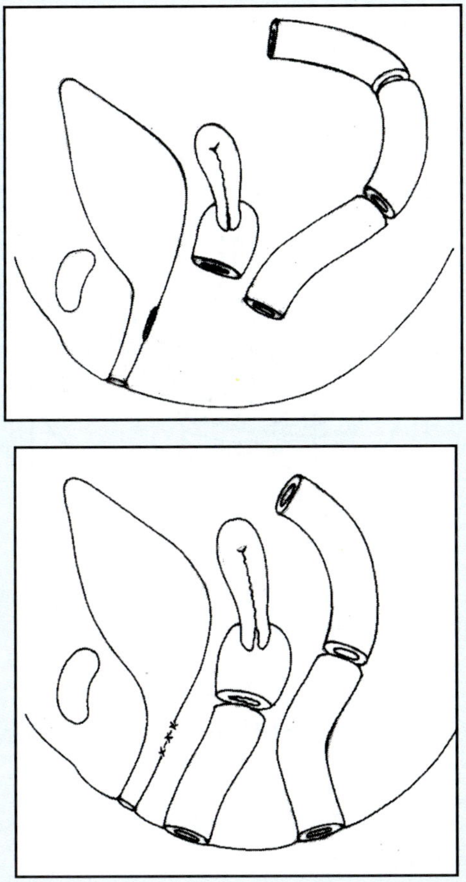

Figs. 11.26-27 Diagrams showing intraperitoneal colovaginoplasty.

If there is insufficient bowel distal to the original colostomy, there are again two options. First, the vaginoplasty may be done with colon after dismantling the colostomy and a more proximal colostomy can be done to protect both the anastomoses. Since it is difficult to identify and preserve the vascular arcades, Das prefers to use a loop of ileum. Ileovaginoplasty is a much simpler operation but excessive mucus secretion at the introitus may be troublesome. This, in Das's experience disappears in about 4 to 6 weeks.

If there is a adequate uterus and upper vagina, the operation is concluded by an intraperitoneal colo- or ileo-vaginoplasty.

4. Other Malformations of the Mullerian System

These include duplex systems with two separate uteruses and vaginas opening into a common channel (Figs. 11.28-29) or a bicornuate or septate uterovaginal canal.

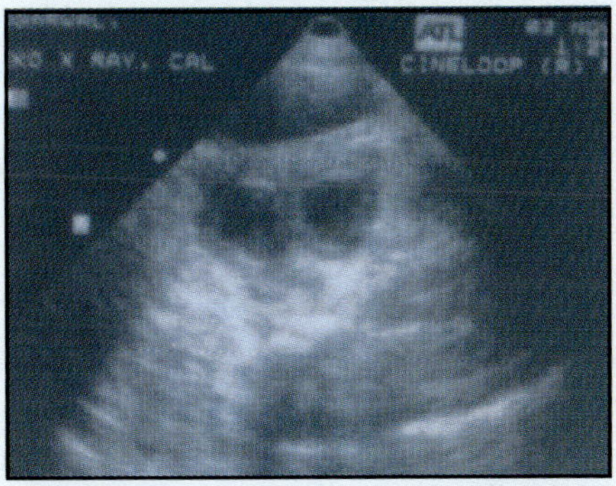

Fig. 11.28 USG showing double vagina.

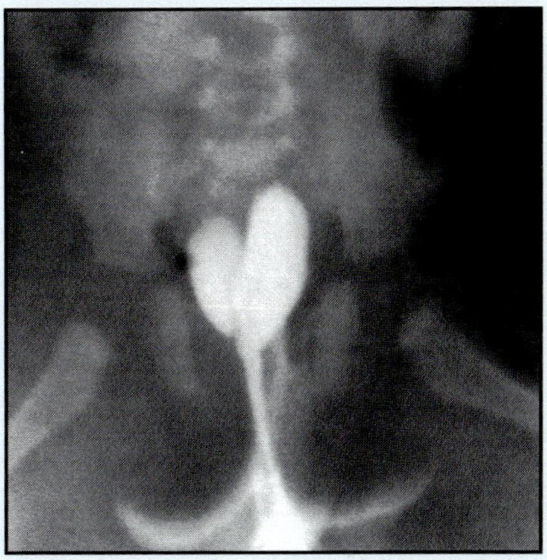

Fig. 11.29 X ray with contrast of the above.

Again, one system may be atrophic or hypoplastic. With a duplex system, the urethra may open into one vagina and the rectum into the other. For a patient with a duplex vagina and 2 separate uteruses, Pena has recommended a relatively simple vaginoplasty named 'vaginal switch'. One uterus can be sacrificed, the vaginal septum can be excised and the hemivagina now devoid of uterus can be rotated down to reach the perineum.

In 1998, Levitt *et al* reported their study on 22 girls who had reached puberty. In 7 there was no uterus and in 9 there was obstruction to the flow of menstrual fluid with consequent pain and intraabdominal mass and operative treatment was required. Only 6 girls had a normal genital system.

5. A Urogenital Sinus with the Bowel Opening into the Bladder

A rectovesical fistula in a girl is only possible if there is a duplex or a unicornuate uterovaginal system (Fig. 11.30). Stephens has described both. We have one patient who had a common urethrovaginal canal, a duplex system, a total colonic pouch and a colovesical fistula (see Chapter 14).

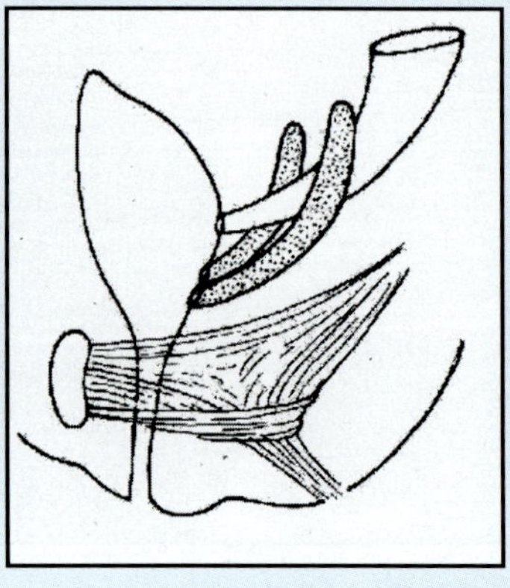

Fig. 11.30 Diagram of rectovesical fistula.

6. A Urogenital Sinus with the Bowel Ending Blindly

We have 2 patients. Urgent colostomy was necessary, subsequently one patient had PSARVUP; the other was lost to followup. (Fig. 11.31).

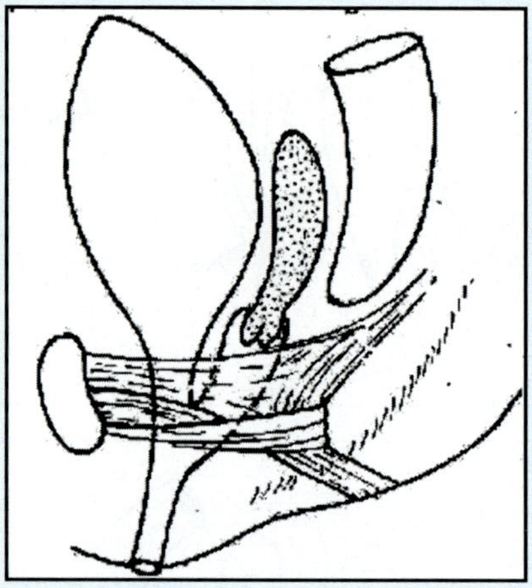

Fig. 11.31 Diagram of blind termination of bowel with urogenital sinus.

7. A Urogenital Sinus with a Colonic Pouch

There are 5 patients; these will be discussed in Chapter 14.

8. A Urogenital Sinus with an H Fistula

We have a single patient who presented in 1988, at the age of 2 years with microcephaly, mental retardation, protein-energy-malnutrition and chronic intestinal obstruction. She could neither talk nor walk. She had a most unusual perineum. There was a single opening between the labia through which both urine and feces emerged. In addition, there was a small opening far behind the normal anal site through which feces also emerged (Fig. 11.32). This opening had been dilated several times in the past to relieve obstruction.

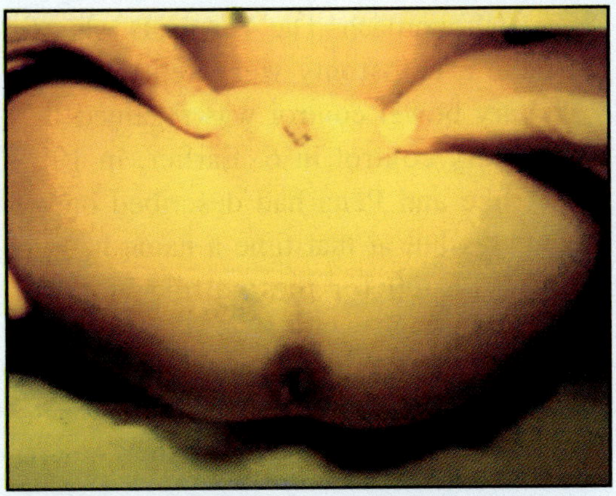

Fig. 11.32 Photograph showing urethral and cloacal fistula.

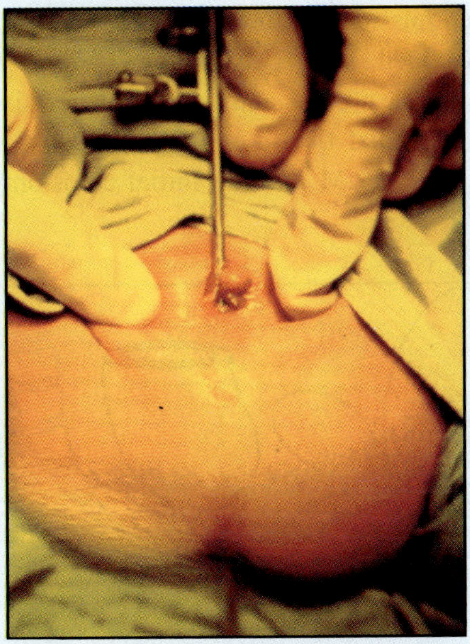

Fig. 11.33 Photograph with cystoscope in place.

Radio-opaque dye studies revealed a cloacal fistula and a posterior perineal fistula. On USG, no internal genitalia were seen; her karyotype was 46XX, 45X0. Endoscopy was next done; the proximal urethra, bladder and ureteric orifices were normal. The vagina could not be seen. The endoscope easily entered the bowel, and could be maneuvered out through the perineal fistula (Fig. 11.33).

It was obvious that this fistula could not be closed successfully without prior fecal diversion, and so a left lower quadrant colostomy was carried out. Her health and mental status improved greatly and she was accepted for reconstruction by PSARP. When the perineum was opened, the dilated rectum was found ending in two fistulous tracts. One led backwards to the perineal opening, and the other continued forwards to join the common urethrovaginal canal (Fig. 11.34). Both tracts were dissected free; the bowel was suitably tapered, and placed in the normal position; the muscles were then repaired. An indwelling urethral catheter and a suprapubic tube were inserted and the wound closed; the urethrovaginal separation was postponed (Fig. 11.35). The colostomy was closed three months later. In the course of this operation the pelvic organs were examined. There was no uterus or ovaries, only a streak gonad was found on the left side.

She came very irregularly for followup and continued to have retained feces and soiling. This improved with institutional treatment and Y-V vaginoplasty was carried out. She then disappeared for 7 years. When last seen she could walk and talk, and had good fecal continence but poor urinary continence. The repair could have been completed with a buttock flap urethroplasty, but permission for further surgery could not be obtained. Vaidya in 2003 reported a girl who had a normal anus, a urogenital sinus and a vaginal fistula and was successfully treated by TUM after an initial colostomy.

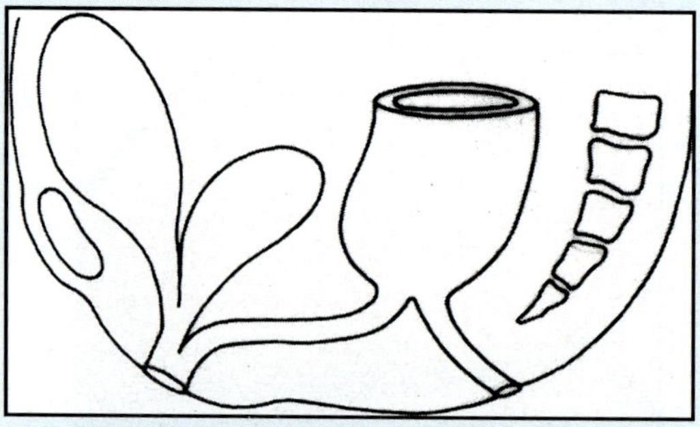

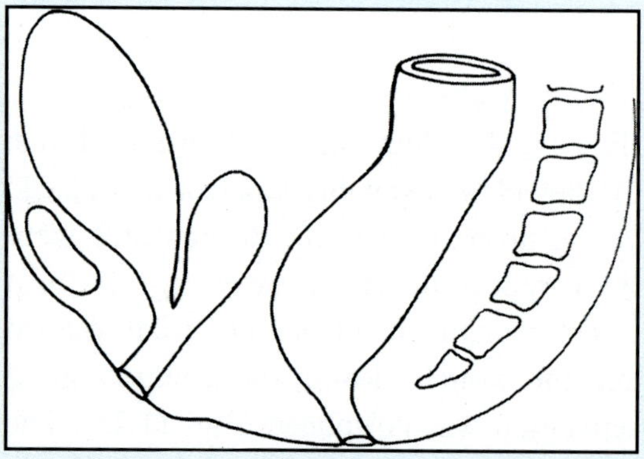

Figs. 11.34-35 Diagrams preoperative & postoperative.

9. Posterior Cloaca

In 1998, Pena described 9 patients who had a unique defect that he named Posterior Cloaca. The urogenital sinus opened on to the anterior rectal wall in 5 and immediately anterior to it in the remaining 4; 5 came with colostomy. In 8, there were associated urogenital defects like hydrocolpos, vesicoureteral reflux, hydronephrosis, absent kidney, uterovaginal septational disorders, rudimentary urethra opening at the tip of the phallus, bladder diverticulum and dysplastic sacrum. The rectum was either well located or minimally anteriorly mislocated. They were corrected by a posterior sagittal transrectal approach. The 4 patients who did not have a colostomy were kept on TPN. Voluntary bowel control was regained in 7 and urinary control in 6. Earlier, in 1991, Leditschke and Pena had described one of these cases but at that time a name had not been suggested for the malformation. In 2001, Krstic *et al* described the successful repair of 3 cases with transanorectal TUM.

In our opinion, girls with a urogenital sinus opening anterior to a normal anus cannot really be considered to have an ARM. Earlier we (Chatterjee *et al*, 1999) had described 2 such patients who had in addition clitoromegaly and a duplex urethra; the urethra bifurcated into a smaller male component opening at the tip of the phallus and a larger female component uniting with the vagina. In our opinion, this was a variety of nonadrenogenic female pseudo-hermaphroditism (NAFPH). However in the two patients with NAFPH reported by Dougherty and Spencer (1982) and by Sen Gupta (1992), the urogenital sinus did indeed open into the anal canal posteriorly.

We studied a patient with posterior cloaca in 1993. She presented at the age of 3½ years with a history of passage of urine and stool through a normally placed anus. There were episodes of fever, vomiting, abdominal distension and retention of stool and urine temporarily relieved in various hospitals by antibiotics and decompression. She had had some investigations but no surgical treatment.

When examined by us she was very ill. She was febrile and toxic; she had a greatly distended abdomen and a tense mass in the suprapubic region. There was a completely flat anterior perineum with a midline groove and without any vestibule or clitoris. The anus was normally placed and admitted a finger; copious hard feces was felt in a hugely dilated anorectum. When the finger was withdrawn, foul smelling purulent fluid emerged.

A plain erect Xray showed grossly distended loops of bowel, Barium enema showed huge megarectum and megasigmoid, and IV urogram showed bilateral hydroureteronephrosis with poor renal function. Her urine was loaded with pus cells and Klebs were isolated. Her hemoglobin was 10g/dl, and creatinine was 1mg/dl. USG confirmed bilateral hydroureteronephrosis but the internal genital organs could not be identified. Her karyotype was 46XX.

Examination under anesthesia was carried out after bowel decompression and antibiotics. An orifice was seen on the anterior wall of the bowel 3 cm from the anal verge. A catheter was introduced through it into the bladder and a cystourethrogram was taken; this excluded reflux. Endoscopy was then performed. The instrument passed through the bowel fistula into a distended inflamed vagina, and then through a second fistula into the bladder. There was gross cystitis and the ureteric orifices could not be identified. The bladder neck was normal and a short urethra opened into the common urethrovaginal passage. The anatomy is depicted in Fig. 11.36.

A left lower quadrant colostomy was carried out together with suprapubic cystostomy. The hydrocolpos was emptied through the urethra; two uteruses with ovaries were found in the course of the operation (Figs. 11.37-38).

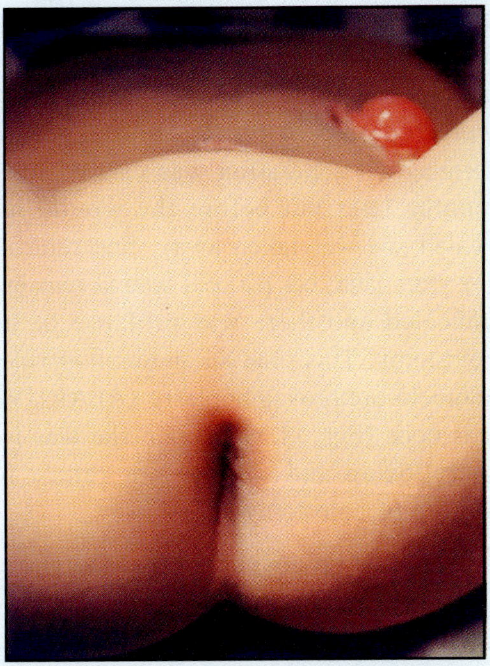

Fig. 11.36 Photograph of posterior cloaca showing perineum.

Three months later, ASARP was done. The common urethrovaginal canal was separated from the bowel and placed

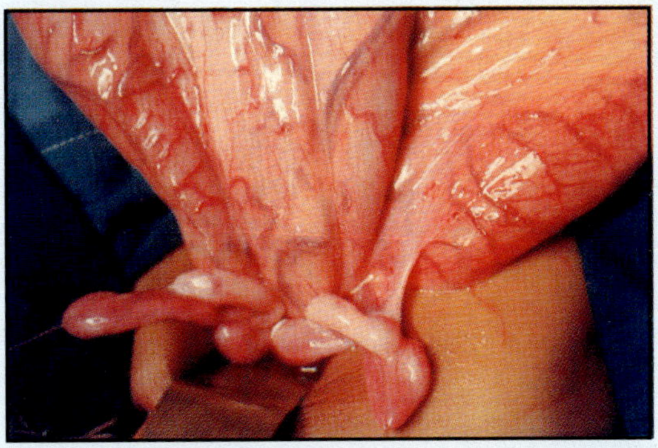

Fig. 11.37 Photograph of posterior cloaca showing pelvic organs at laparotomy.

behind the pubic arch as far anterior as possible The bowel was tapered by resecting an anterior V and the muscles and skin flaps were repaired in the midline. The urethrovaginal separation was carried out 2 months later but before the wound had healed she was taken away. She returned 1½ years later; her perineal wound remained unhealed and there was prolapse of her colostomy. This time an abdominoperineal anorecto-urethrovaginoplasty (APARUVP) was done (Fig. 11.39). Again she was lost to followup and she did not return for closure of colostomy.

We have no doubt now that the correct management for this condition should have been colostomy and vesicostomy followed by PSARVUP through a sagittal incision splitting the anorectum in the midline front and back A total urethrovaginal mobilization (TUM) could then have placed the urogenital organs in their correct location. The bowel could then have been repaired and the vesicostomy and colostomy discontinued at a suitable time.

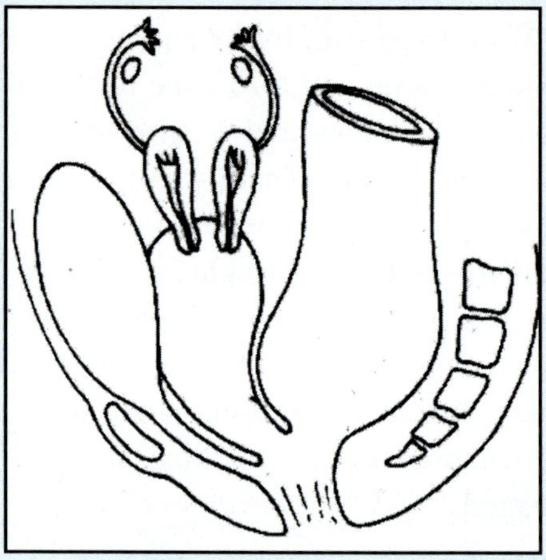

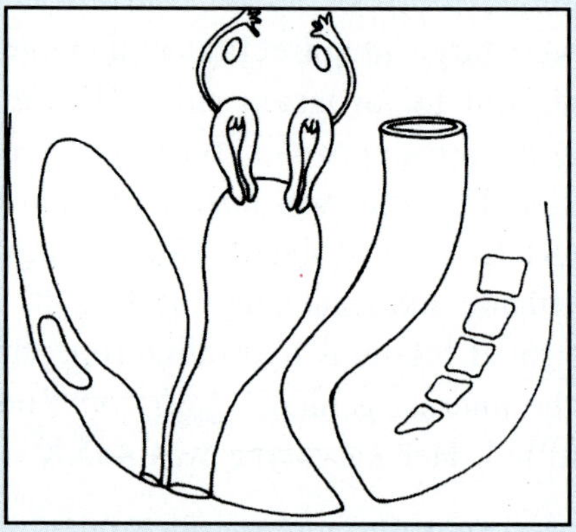

Figs. 11.38-39 Diagrams of posterior cloaca, preoperative & postoperative.

CHAPTER 12

A NORMAL ANUS WITH AN ABNORMAL ANORECTUM

RECTAL ATRESIA

This is the only true major 'supralevator' lesion. The infralevator region inamely the anal canal with the striated muscle complex around it is normal. The rectum ends blindly above the levator ani and is separated from the anal canal either by a septum or a short gap bridged by a fibrous band or by a long gap (Figs. 12.1-3).

In our series this lesion is very rare. We have only 9 babies, 5 boys and 4 girls. It is equally rare in most other series except in those emerging from southern India. Out of 1,024 children with anorectal malformation treated by Dorairajan in Madurai between 1962 and 1978, 147 or 14% had rectal atresia. However, in recent years, the incidence of rectal atresia in this region also appears to be falling significantly (Dorairajan 1988, 1989).

Because there is a normal anus, rectal atresia is rarely diagnosed before features of intestinal obstruction set in. A catheter introduced up the anus is obstructed within 1 to 3 cm. from the anus. When an invertogram is taken with a bougie in the anal canal, the gap between the gas filled rectum and the tip of the bougie indicates the gap between the two ends (Fig. 12.4). CT and MRI reveal the anatomy more clearly.

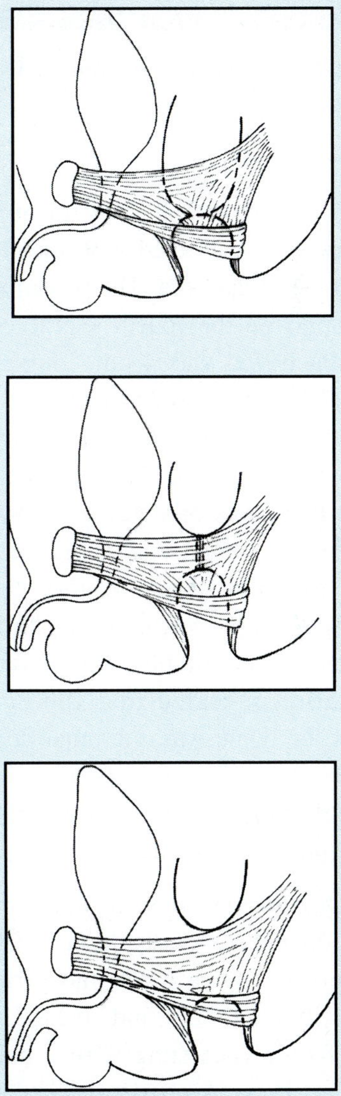

Figs. 12.1-3 Diagrams of rectal atresia - common wall; intervening band; long gap.

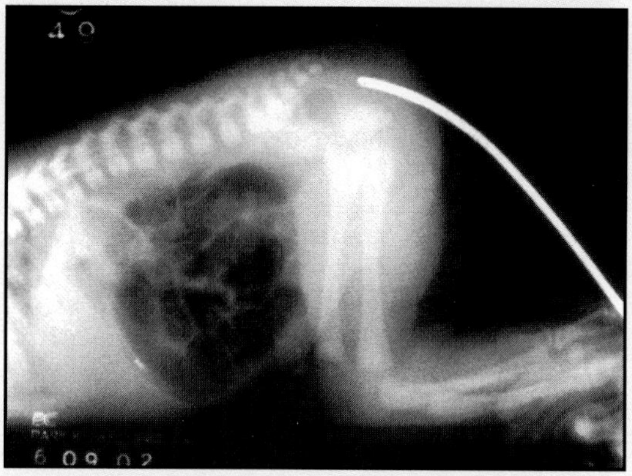

Fig. 12.4 Xray showing proximity of 2 ends.

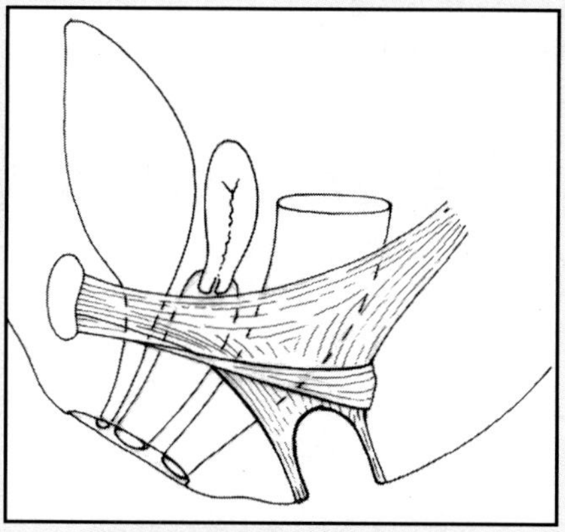

Fig. 12.5 Diagram of rectal atresia with vestibular fistula.

In the 1970s we studied at autopsy 2 male newborns who died with rectal atresia. The first was 4 days old. The proximal bowel ended opposite the fourth sacral vertebra. The distal bowel was 4 cm. long and was surrounded by the striated muscle complex; its upper end reached close to the lower end of the proximal bowel. The second case died because there was bilateral renal dysplasia. The proximal bowel ended high up at the level of the third sacral vertebra; the distal bowel was only 15 mm. long and ended below the pelvic diaphragm. Histological examination revealed that the epithelial lining at the dome was columnar and that it gradually changed to stratified squamous at the anal verge, this confirming the endodermal origin of the atretic region.

The proximal bowel of babies with Rectal Atresia do not generally have a fistula to the exterior but we have one girl with a rectovestibular fistula and one girl with a cloacal fistula coexisting with a blind anal canal (Fig. 12.5). A proximal rectal stenosis coexisting with rectal atresia has been reported from Varanasi in 2004.

Management

The standard treatment is **Colostomy.** However, if the 2 ends of the bowel can be shown to be adjacent to each other, it may be possible to perforate the septum by means of an adult cystourethroscope, and then to dilate the opening, thus allowing meconium to flow out. In a recent case, we could establish by a plain lateral Xray that the 2 ends were adjacent to each other. We carried out an end to end anastomosis through a limited PSARP that stopped 3 cm. short of the anal verge (Fig. 12.6). However the wound did not look healthy and a protective colostomy was done 48 hours later. Recovery was uneventful and after a course of anorectal dilatations, the colostomy was closed a month later and normal defecation took place.

Repair of Rectal atresia is generally done after neonatal colostomy. If the 2 segments of bowel are adjacent (Fig. 12.7), end to end anastomosis is done through a posterior sagittal incision that does not disturb the anus or the striated muscle complex. Alternatively, an adult cystourethoscope can be

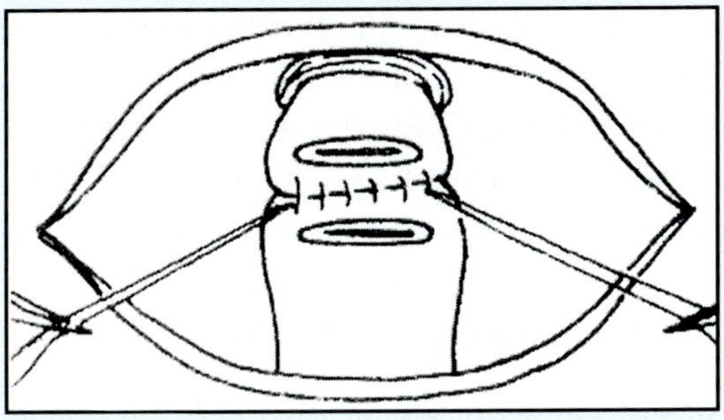

Fig. 12.6 Diagram to show end to end anastomosis.

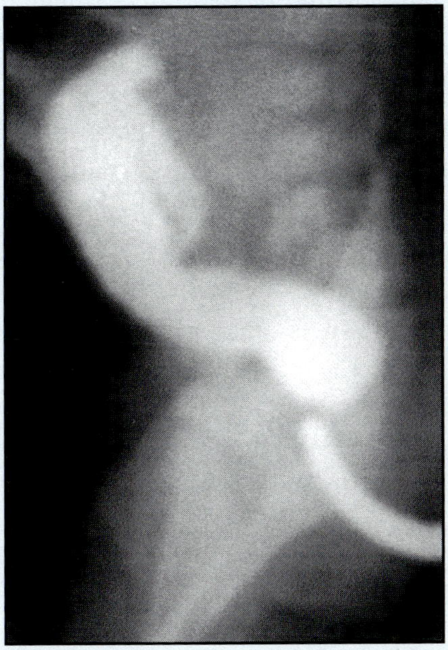

Fig. 12.7 Xray - distal cologram with bougie in anus.

used and transanal endoscopic fulguration of the adjacent walls of the bowel can be done after introducing a solution of methylene blue through the colostomy; this is followed by periodic dilatations (Borwankar, 1987). If there is a large gap between the 2 segments, an abdomino-perineal procedure as used for Hirsch-sprung's disease, is required (Halimul *et al*, 1981). The baby with the associated rectovestibular fistula could be corrected by a neonatal ASARP without colostomy. We have described in Chapter 3 the baby who had rectal atresia and associated Hirsch-sprung's disease.

RECTAL STENOSIS

This is a condition in which the rectum and anal canal are joined by a narrow piece of bowel of variable length (Fig. 12.8). We have 3 cases.

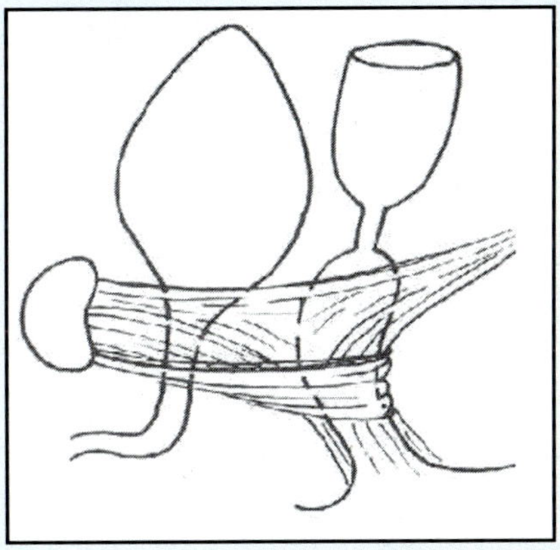

Fig. 12.8 Diagram of rectal stenosis.

The first was a 6-month old boy weighing 5 kg. referred in 1983 with a clinical diagnosis of Hirschsprung's Disease. He had intractible constipation, abdominal distension and vomiting. When we examined the anorectum digitally an unyielding annular narrowing was felt. A stiff flatus tube could be passed through it guided by the finger. A bowel wash was given through it and then contrast fluid was instilled; Xray confirmed the diagnosis of rectal stenosis at the level of the fourth sacral vertebra. (Fig. 12.9). We performed a twostage reconstruction. At the first operation, a left lower

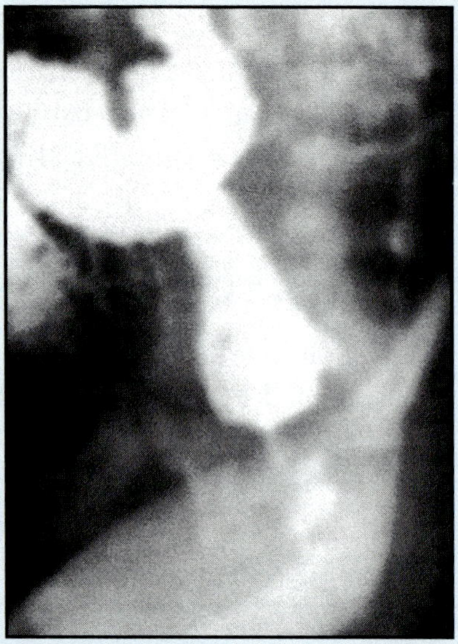

Fig. 12.9 Xray of rectal stenosis – distal cologram.

quadrant loop colostomy was carried out low down in the sigmoid colon. Two months later, the colostomy was dismantled, the bowel between the distal stoma and the stenosis was resected and the proximal colon was pulled through to the anus in the endorectal plane as in a Soave operation for Hirschsprung's Disease. There was uneventful recovery. Probably the result would have been equally satisfactory if we had carried out the reconstruction in the manner described for rectal atresia. The second case was 3 months old and came with severe rectal bleeding requiring blood transfusion. There was stenosis 3 cm. from the anal verge. He was relieved with dilatations and oral prednisolone and continues to remain well.

The third patient was more difficult. He reached us at the age of 11 years with a colostomy that had been done elsewhere when he was 9; until this age he was managed with periodic dilatations and washouts. His anal canal admitted a finger but there was a block above; the stenosis and the huge megarectum above was revealed by Barium enema. We performed PSARP after tapering the rectum to aize and closed the colostomy a few weeks later. After this he has had no problems.

CONGENITAL FUNNEL ANUS

In this condition the stenosis is lower down, that is, within the muscular cuff (Nixon 1984). The anus is normal but there is great resistance to the passage of a finger or an instrument at the anal canal. We have 3 cases.

In one girl who reached us at the age of 3 weeks with a hugely distended abdomen, attempted dilatation resulted in a false passage (Figs. 12.10-11). Xray with contrast showed that the dye had entered the peritoneum and urgent laparotomy and colostomy was done. The extent of the narrowing could not be determined at that time. A subsequent distal cologram showed bowel of normal caliber up to the anorectal junction. The stenosis could be fully dilated and the colostomy was closed. She has had no problems since.

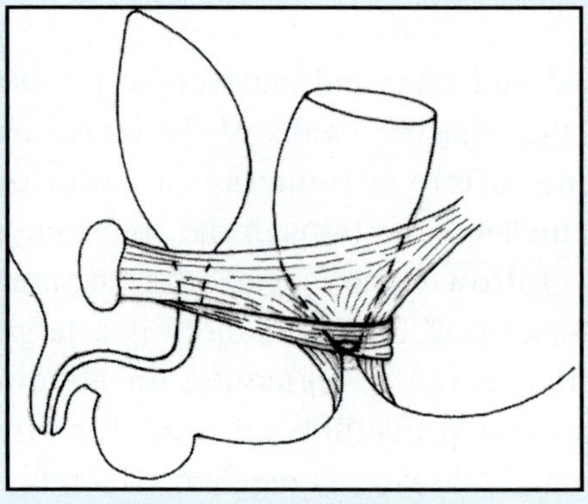

Fig. 12.10 Diagram of funnel anus.

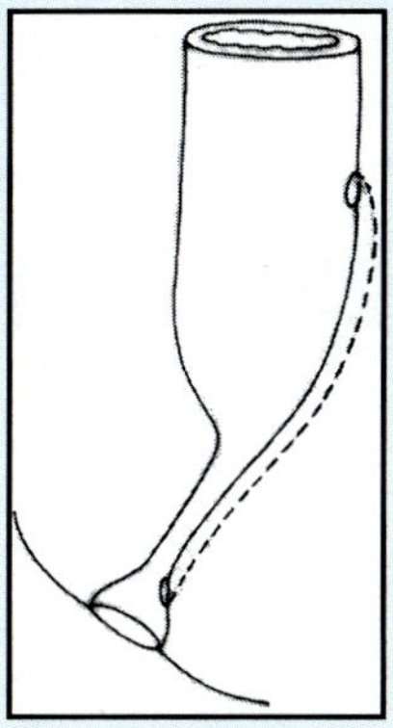

Fig. 12.11 Diagram of false passage after attempting to dilate funnel anus.

Another girl came when 6 weeks old with severe constipation. Barium enema showed a narrow anal canal with hugely dilated bowel above. An extended Y-V plasty was done and the bowel was emptied. After she went home she continued to have bouts of constipation and was unfortunately neglected. She was last seen when she was 8 years old. The anorectum easily allowed a finger to enter but the rectum would not empty without enemas or bowel washes. Revisional surgery was advised but consent was not forthcoming.

The third patient was a boy aged 3 years; he also came with massive megarectum. He was successfully treated by an extended Y-V plasty.

CHAPTER 13

A NORMAL ANUS AND ANORECTUM WITH A FISTULA

A normal anus and anorectum with a fistula is the second variety of **H FISTULA.**

IN BOYS

The fistula is generally invisible and connects to the urethra. The urethra may be otherwise normal or may be deformed.

An otherwise normal urethra and a fistula

Stephens and Donnellan described one case in 1977. Subsequently, in 1992, Hong *et al* from Montreal described two patients aged 4 and 5 years with recurrent attacks of urinary infection. The tract was visualized by voiding cystogram, sinogram and endoscopy. The tract was excised by an anterior perineal approach. In 1996, Rintala *et al* described a boy with a normal anus, a rectoprostatic urethral fistula and rectal stenosis above the fistula; the diagnosis was made after colostomy and the repair of rectal stenosis by PSARP. In 2002 Sharma *et al* describd a 3 year old boy who came with recurrent urinary tract infection and the passage of urine per anum. A fistula between the posterior urethra and the rectum was seen on VCU; this was closed by an anterior perineal approach

Earlier we had described two patients who had come in 1975 and in 1980; both were 3 years old. In both there was a history of passage of feces and flatus with urine since infancy, of episodes of strangury relieved after the passage of pellets of feces through the urethra, and of occasional passage of watery stools. There was normal urinary and fecal continence and no detectable clinical abnormality. The parents of the first patient did not agree to have any investigation or treatment. In the second, the fistula connecting the lower rectum to the bulbous urethra was demonstrated by contrast Xray and bouginage; the urinary system and the lower alimentary tract were normal (Figs. 13.1-2).

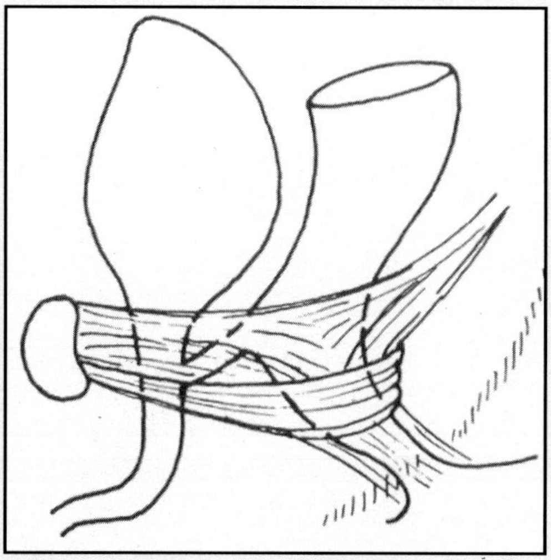

Fig. 13.1 Diagram of normal anus and urethra and rectourethral fistula.

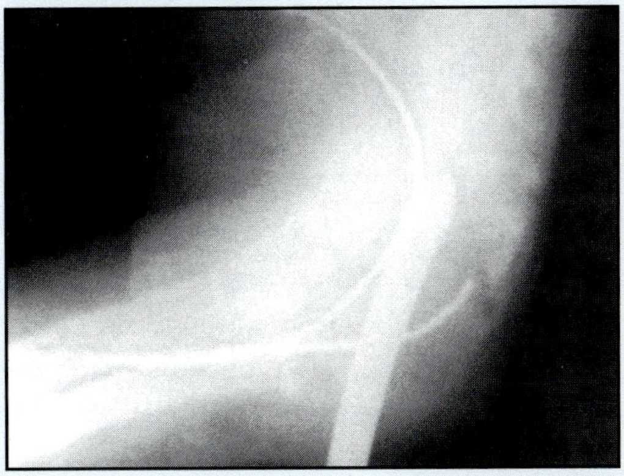

Fig. 13.2 Xray of above - two small bougies through the urethra, one entering bladder and the other entering rectum, and a large bougie through anus into rectum.

At operation the bulbous urethra was approached by a transverse perineal incision behind the scrotum.The fistula was disconnected and the urethra was closed. The fistula was then inverted into the anorectum and the rectal end closed from within the bowel. A suprapubic cystostomy was done. The postoperative course was uneventful, and normal micturition was restored after the suprapubic tube was withdrawn. Stools were passed normally from the third day. The anatomical characters of this fistula between the lower rectum and the bulbous urethra were the same as those of the common rectobulbar fistula with anal agenesis. Although this patient did well, we have no doubt that today a fistula such as this should be exposed and closed by a sagittal incision and that an indwelling urethral catheter would suffice.

A malformed urethra and a fistula

There were several reports of this anomaly in the 1970s by deVries and Friedland (1974), Stephens and Donnellan (1977), Belman (1977) and White *et al* (1978). Earlier we had described a single patient. He was 18 years old and had, ever since he could remember, passed most of his urine per anum and only a small amount per urethra. He had a small external urethral orifice through which urine would dribble in drops resembling tear drops on attempted micturation. A uniformly narrow anterior urethra was seen on a urethrogram, and neither catheter nor bougie could negotiate the phallic urethra even under anesthesia. However, a cystoscope could be passed through the anal canal and the rectoprostatic fistula into the bladder. The bladder and prostatic urethra were normal and the urethra bifurcated a little below the verumontanum into a wide posterior channel entering the rectum, and a narrow anterior channel passing along the course of a normally placed anterior urethra. This was confirmed by a voiding cystourethrogram, after contrast fluid was introduced into the bladder through the fistula (Figs. 13.3-4). The fistula was disconnected from the rectum and brought out on the perineum as an end-urethrostomy. Urethroplasty was carried out later.

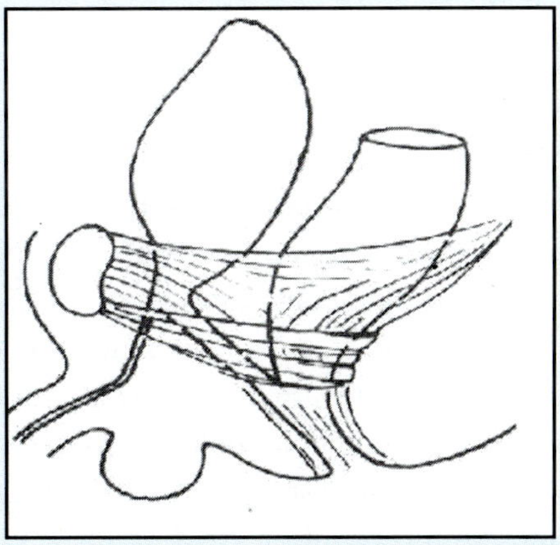

Fig. 13.3 Diagram of normal anus and narrow urethra and rectourethral fistula.

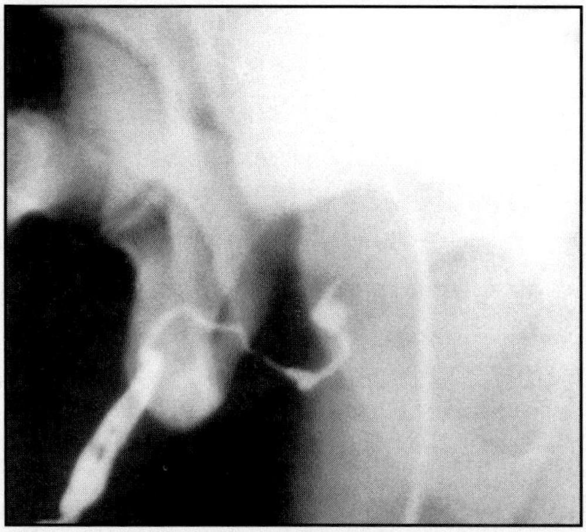

Fig. 13.4 Xray of above-voiding cystourethrogram with bladder filled per anum.

In the 1990s cases were seen worldwide and four different types of management were proposed. Senocak and Buyukpamukeu's patient was 3 years old; a colostomy was done and two years later a suprapubic cystostomy. Then a tubularized skin flap was made on the penis and perineum. One end was joined to the normal-sized glandular urethra and the other to the fistula after disconnecting it from the bowel. An indwelling urethral catheter was left in place. Rizalar *et al* performed a colostomy and suprapubic cystostomy on a patient aged 4 months and carried out dilatations for 6 months, they then excised the fistula and continued with dilatations. The patient described by Lal *et al* was 5 months old; the fistula was closed and the urethra repaired under colostomy cover and a suprapubic cystostomy. Finally, Al-Bassam *et al* treated a patient aged 5 years with a program named PADUA, namely Progressive Augmentation by Dilatation of the Urethra Anterior. The anterior urethra initially allowed only a No.4 stent; it could be dilated in 6 weeks to accommodate a No.14 stent. At that time, the fistula was closed and a balloon catheter was left in place for 10 days. Al-Bassam has credited Passerini-Ghazel for first proposing the PADUA technique.

We have treated two infants; in both we dissected the urethra from the anal canal, performed an end-urethrostomy and closed the anorectum in two layers. One was subsequently treated by a plastic surgeon; in the other we carried out the PADUA procedure (Chatterjee *et al* 2001). We dilated the anterior urethra from the external meatus to the bulbar urethra with a No.2 bougie; the segment between this and the junction between the two urethras was impassable. A urethrotomy was done over the tip of the bougie and a stent was placed in the anterior urethra; its proximal end was brought out on the perineum. After two weeks the anterior urethra was again dilated and a larger stent was left in place; three weeks later the anterior urethra became sufficiently wide to accommodate a No.12 catheter. We then tried to join the two ends of the urethra in the perineum. There was a wound breakdown and a stent was left in place for some time. Ultimately the wound healed after a period of diversion with a suprapubic cystostomy. He is now passing urine normally (Figs. 13.5-8), but has a diverticulum at the anastomotic site.

The urethroanorectal fistula associated with apenia bears a striking resemblance to the above lesion except that the phallus and phallic urethra are also missing. Our primary operation for apenia has been the same as described above; namely an end-perineal-urethrostomy. The subsequent management depends on the decision regarding sex of rearing and is beyond the scope of this presentation.

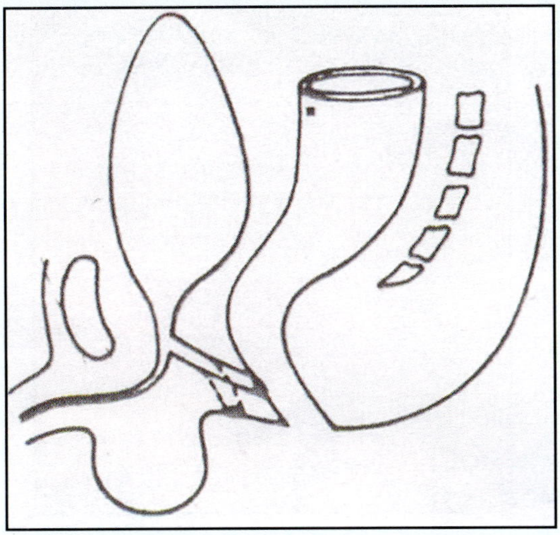

Fig. 13.5 Diagram of normal anus and very narrow urethra and fistula; dotted lines show planned end - urethrostomy.

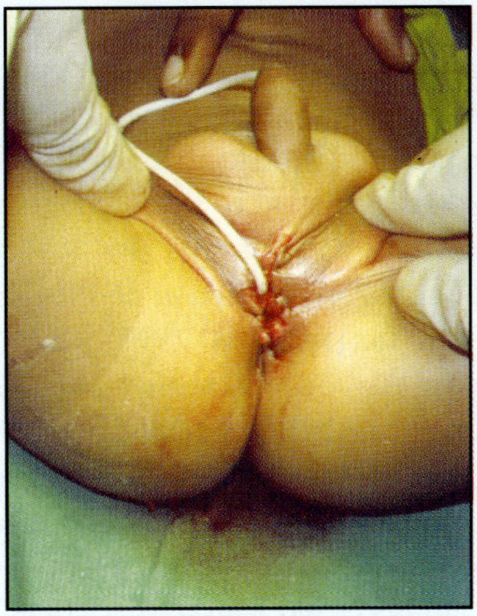

Fig. 13.7 Photograph with indwelling tube between tip of urethra and perineal urethrostomy.

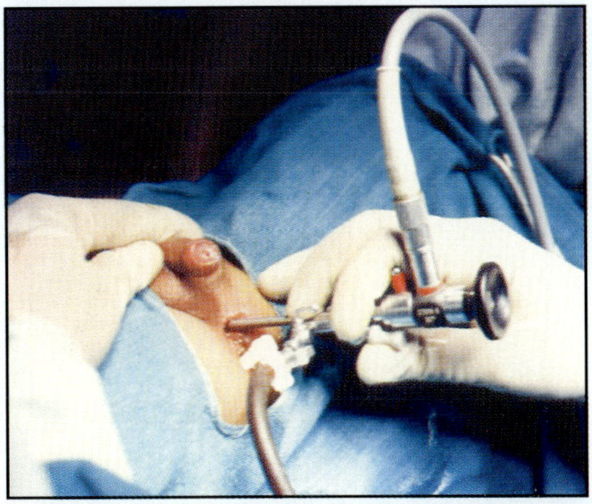

Fig. 13.6 Photograph of patient with cystoscope through the anus.

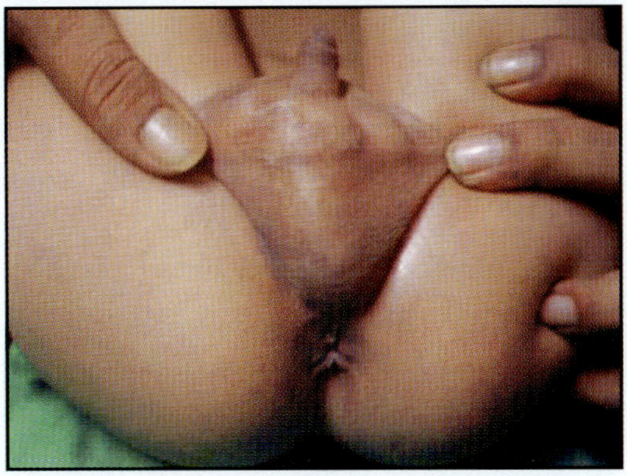

Fig. 13.8 Photograph of end result.

IN GIRLS

Vestibular Fistula coexisting with an otherwise Normal Anorectum

This is a relatively common anomaly. In 1969, we (Chatterjee and Talukdar) reported 7 patients with a condition we had named 'double termination of the alimentary tract'. In 6 of them, a normal anorectum coexisted with an anorectovestibular fistula. In 1980, we added 10 new cases and described the features that distinguished rectovestibular fistula, an intermediate anomaly from anovestibular fistula, a low anomaly. This malformation was first reported by Bryndorf and Madsen in 1959. It is rarely seen in Europe and America; however Rintala *et al* have reported on 12 girls in 1996. In 10 the fistula was low down and in 2 it connected the rectum to the vagina. It is fairly common in many Asian countries and relatively large series have been reported from Japan, China and Vietnam (Ito 1976, Ninh 1970, Sai 1975, Tsuchida *et al* 1984, Zhang 1984 and Tsugawa *et al* 1999). Cases have subsequently been reported from Egypt (Mahmoud, 1982), Pakistan (Mirza, 1997) and Qatar (Ismail, 1994). Our colleagues in India have reported a large number of cases, notably H Chatterjee, Narasinharao (1993), Wakhlu (1997) and Kulshrestha (1998). Out of the 10 congenital cases Kulshresta described, ten had low lesions and two intermediate lesions. Wakhlu's series is the largest with 58. In 2003, Arora described a 5 month old girl who passed stool through a normal anus and also through two openings, one on either side of the fourchette. 3.5 cm. from the anal verge. Brem *et al* in 1989 described this lesion in two girls of Asian origin living in USA.

We now have 52 patients with the low anomaly and nine with the intermediate one. These girls pass stools not only through the anus but also through an opening in the vestibule. This unusual phenomenon may begin at birth or days or weeks later; it may occur only during defecation or independently and may take place daily or only when stools are loose. The perineum has four openings. In addition to the three normal openings, there is one in the fossa navicularis either in the midline or on one or other side of it. Three of our patients presented with local inflammation and a fifth opening further laterally (Figs. 13.9-11). Occasionally, the abnormal opening is not obvious during the initial examination and is recognized only during an episode of

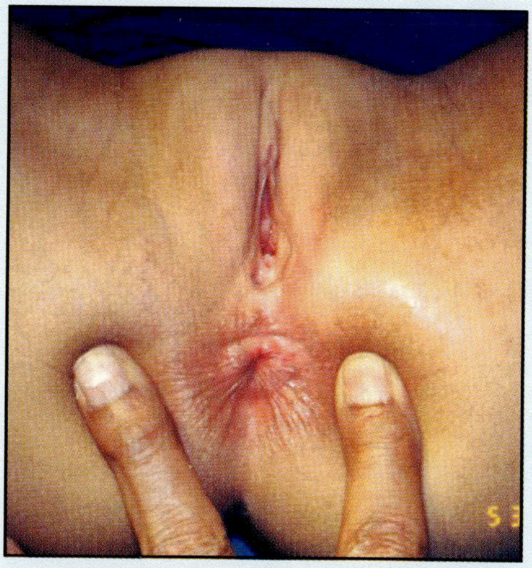

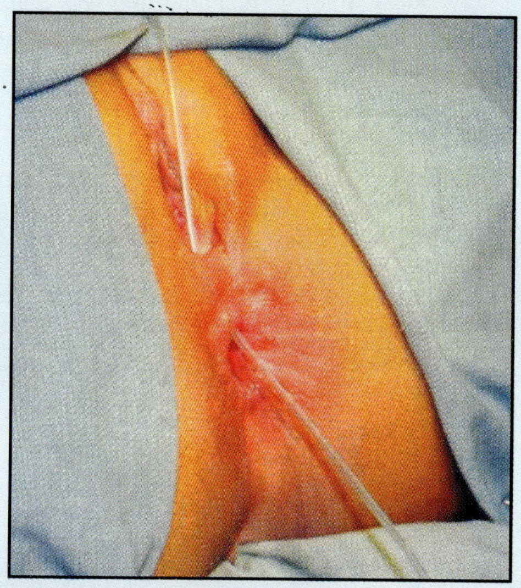

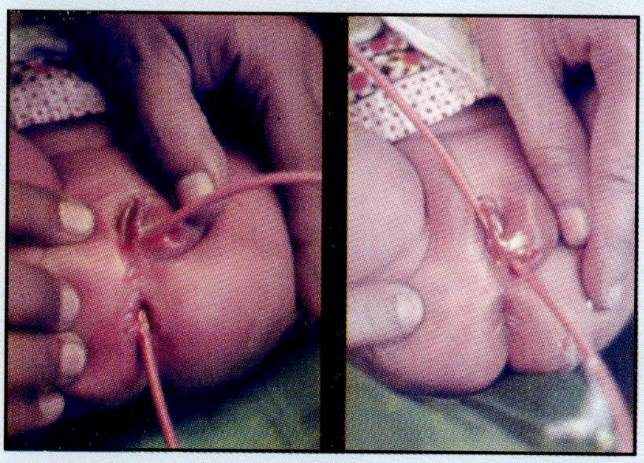

Figs. 13.9-11 Photographs of normal anus and Vestibular fistula.

diarrhea. Generally a probe can be passed through the vestibular opening into the anorectum. If not, the tract can be demonstrated by the method described by Tsuchida *et al.* Lateral radiographs are taken after introducing contrast fluid into the bowel through a balloon catheter with a perforation below and not above the balloon (Fig. 13.12).

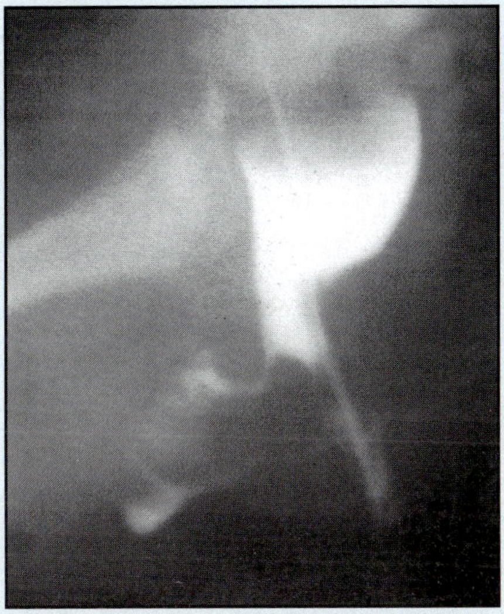

Fig. 13.12 Xray with contrast showing 2 channels.

The two varieties can usually be distinguished fairly easily. The anovestibular fistula lies subcutaneously between the fossa navicularis and the anterior wall of the anal canal at or superficial to the site of the anal valves. This conforms to Stephens and Smith's description of Perineal Canal in1971. The rectovestibular fistula, on the other hand, issues from the anterior wall of the rectum above the levator and then passes down along the posterior wall of the vagina to open at the fossa navicularis. Thus this fistula resembles the common rectovestibular fistula with anorectal agenesis. The rectaltal end is usually funnel-shaped and the vestibular end is narrow (Figs. 13.13-14). Undoubtedly there are shades of gray between the two groups.

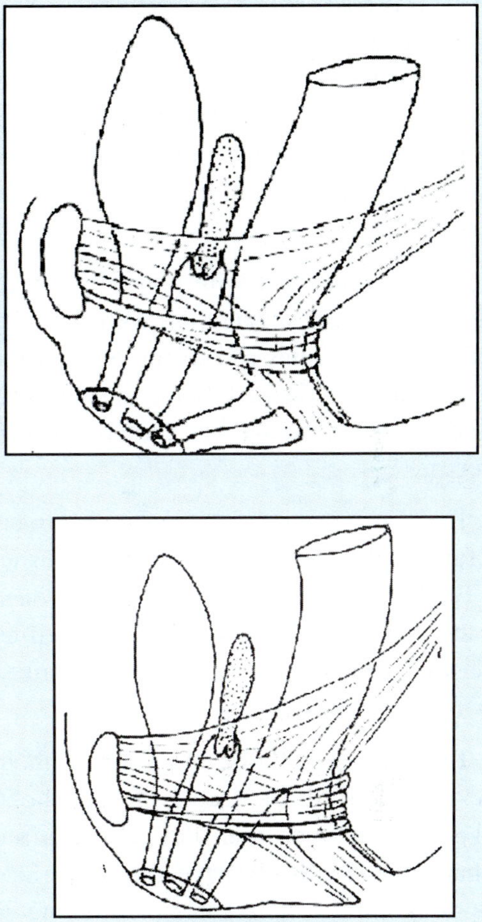

Figs. 13.13-14 Diagrams, low and intermediate types.

Management

The operation we perform at present for patients with a rectovestibular fistula and a normal anus is SARP without a colostomy. We had initially suggested a procedure we had named Vestibulorectal Pullthrough (VRPT), an operation resembling PAT. The fistula was dissected out from the vestibule, pulled through into the lumen of the anorectum and excised; the vestibule and the bowel were repaired and there was no incision on the perineum. A changeover to SARP was made after three recurrences; two have had a successful revision. We have found that SARP provides a better exposure, but Das is happy with VRPT. The relation of the fistula to the posterior wall of the vagina is crucial; separation may be easy or very difficult.

The two patients with abnormal openings due to local suppuration were initially treated by antibiotics and laying open of the second tract into the first. Some months later, the definitive operation was carried out with success.

The management of anovestibular tracts is far simpler. Spontaneous cure occurred in 10; 2 were cured by a simple laying open of the tract and the remaining four cured by excision of the tract in the manner described for rectovestibular tracts.

There has been an ongoing debate about the origin of these tracts. It has been suggested by some that they are acquired (Zhang, 1984). We believe that the tracts are congenital. Their anterior opening is either sagittal or parasagittal; it never extends more laterally. Although in a few patients feces appears at the vestibule for the first time during an episode of diarrhea or of constipation secondary to anal fissure and sphincter spasm, the fistula is manifest soon after birth in most patients, before any episode of suppuration has occurred. There are indeed clear evidences of suppuration in a number of patients. The congenital origin of the lesions cannot be excluded by this because it is well-known that secondary infection often supervenes on all types of congenital sinuses and fistulas, for example in the face and neck, and even in the cardiovascular system. We have histologically examined a number of excised tracts and have not found any evidence of inflammation (Figs. 13.15-16).

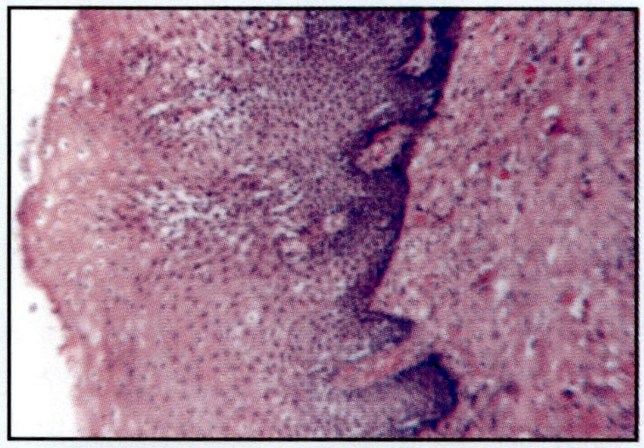

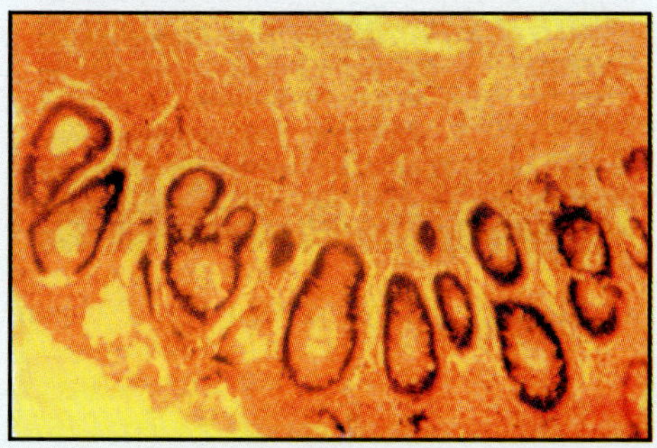

Figs. 13.15-16 Photomicrographs of vestibular fistula, showing normal epithelium and absence of inflammation.

Vaginal Fistula with an Otherwise Normal Anorectum

This is indeed rare; we have a single case. A 7-year old girl presented in 1989 with a history of chronic constipation and soiling since birth. She had mild abdominal distension; both the vestibule and anus appeared normal except for the presence of feces in the lower vagina. Under anesthesia, a huge fistula was demonstrated between the vagina and rectum. We disconnected the fistula and restored continence by ASARP after routine bowel preparation and a concurrent colostomy (Figs. 13.17-18).

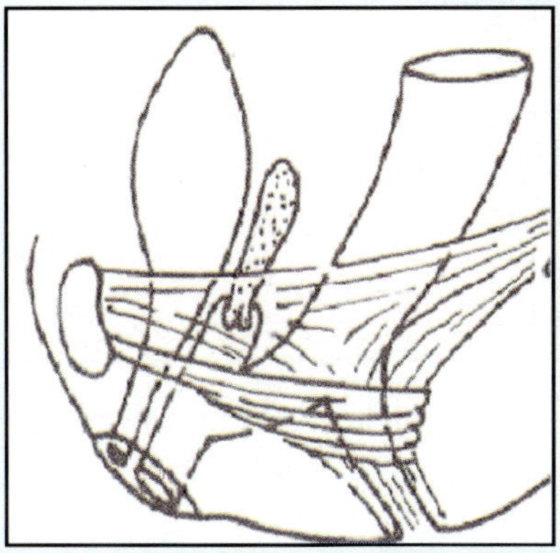

Fig. 13.17 Diagram of vaginal fistula and normal anus.

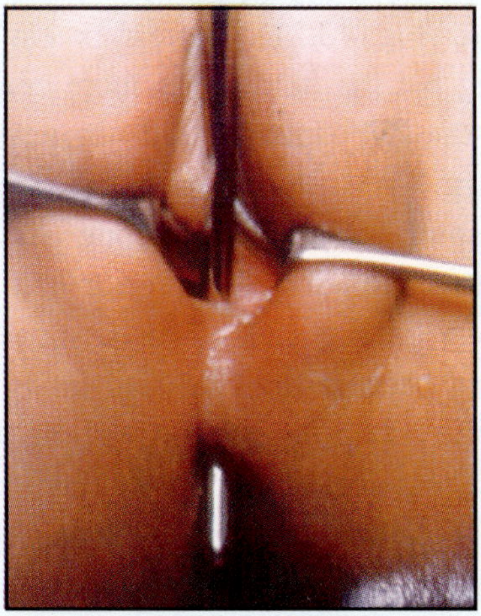

Fig. 13.18 Photograph of above.

With the patient prone and a catheter in the urethra, a sagittal incision was made between the fourchette and anal verge; anteriorly it was extended along the posterior margin of the fourchette and posteriorly, extended along the anterior half of the anal verge. The fistula was exposed and cut open. A meticulous dissection was begun to separate the anterior wall of the rectum from the posterior wall of the vagina. They shared a common muscular wall for a considerable distance above the upper limit of the fistula. After full thickness bowel wall was reached, it was freed laterally. Its caliber was reduced by anterior tapering and consequent excision of tissue surrounding the fistula. The striated muscle complex was then repaired in front of the reconstructed bowel. The lower margin of the bowel was then sutured in place to the anterior half of the anal verge. The posterior half of the bowel and the muscles behind it were left undisturbed. Then the posterior wall of the vagina was tapered after excising the tissue around the fistula, and the free inferior margin of the new vagina was sutured in place at the cut posterior margin of the vestibule. The perineal muscles were repaired behind it and the wound closed (Fig. 13.19).

Healing was uneventful. Three months later the colostomy was closed and

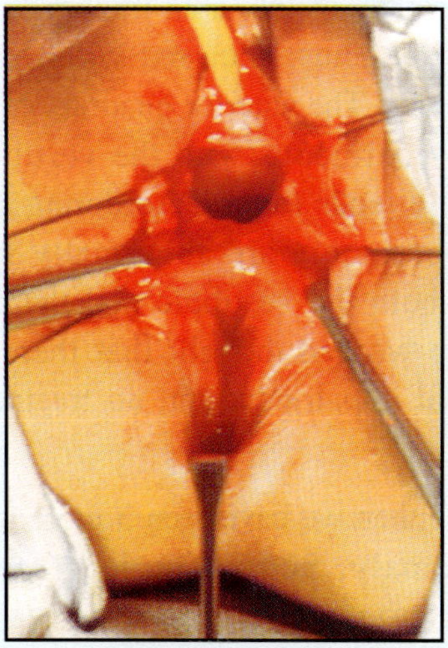

Fig. 13.19 Phtograph of operation for above.

defecation is now normal. She was brought to us recently for a premarital consultation.This fistula resembled in every way the usual form of rectovaginal fistula associated with anorectal agenesis.

IN BOTH SEXES

A visible perineal fistula

This can coexist with a normal anorectum; it has been described by Brem *et al* (1989) in a boy of Asian origin living in the US. We have a single case. A boy aged 6 years came with a normal anorectum and a subcutaneous tract leading from the anal canal up to the penoscrotal junction.The parents did not agree to surgery.

Perineal groove

We had earlier thought that PERINEAL GROOVE was a variant of perineal canal occurring only in girls; it had been described by Stephens and Smith (1971) and had been encountered by us only once. In girls, it is a wet groove between the fourchette and the anus. Prominent folds extend from the posterior ends of the labia minora to the two sides of the anus; enclosed within the folds is the sulcus. The anterior quadrant of the anal canal is continuous with the vestibule, and its mucosa tends to prolapse during straining. The labia majora are abnormally long and enclose both the vestibule and the anus. At that time we had thought that there was no functional impairment and no treatment was necessary.

Since then we have seen 3 more girls with this anomaly. Scharli in 1997 described perineal groove in a boy. We have 2 boys; one has not been treated (Fig. 13.20).

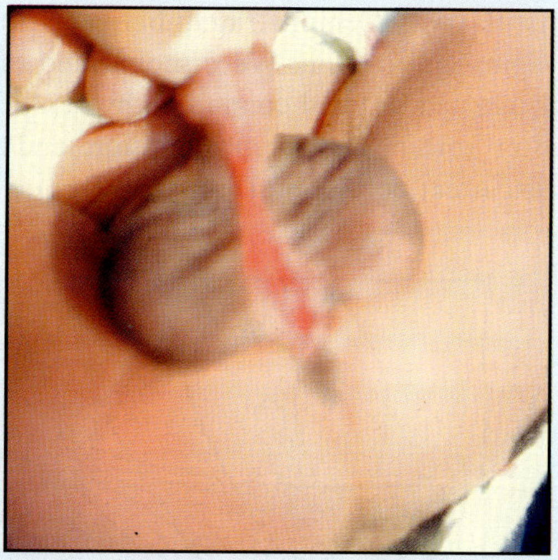

Fig. 13.20 Photographs of perineal groove.

The other has been reported (Chatterjee *et al*, 2003). He came at the age of 7 years with penoscrotal hypospadias and perineal groove (Fig. 13.21). There was some fecal soiling but the family was more concerned with the hypospadias and not with fecal soiling. We therefore corrected the hypospadias first using a long perimeatal flap that included the anterior half of the perineal groove; this could be successfully utilized because the epithelial lining of the groove was nonkeratinizing and transitional and much more vascular than the normal skin of the region. He was brought back 1½ years later because the fecal soiling had increased and there was a large mucosal prolapse in the anterior quadrant of the anus. At the second operation, the posterior half of the groove together with the prolapsed mucosa was excised, the striated muscle complex repaired and epithelial continuity restored. There was uneventful healing and continence was restored (Fig. 13.22).

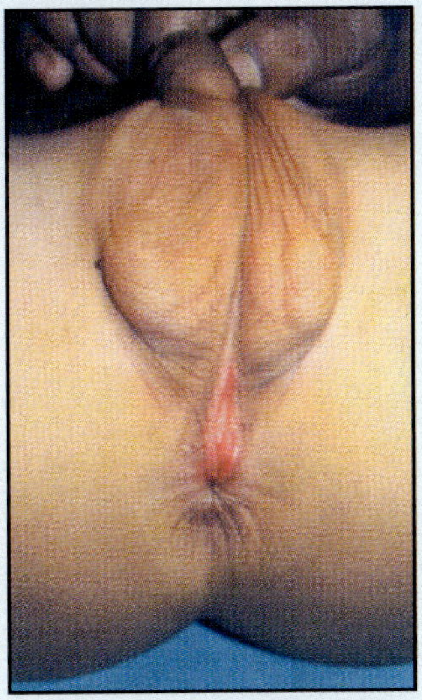

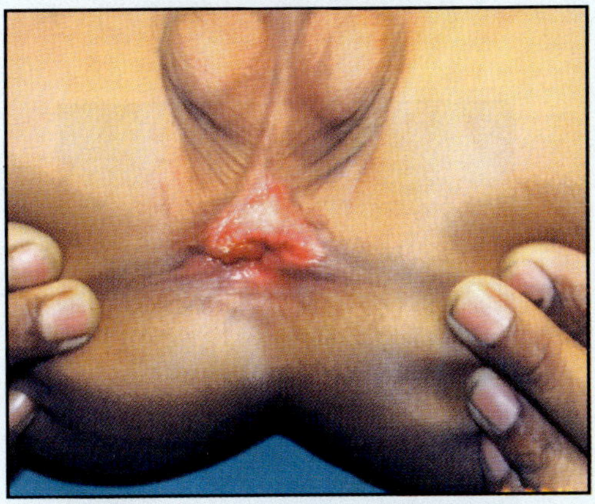

Figs. 13.21-22 Photographs of perineal groove with hypospadias.

Tubular duplication

We have two cases, a girl and a boy, the girl's case has been described earlier. She was 3 months old when first seen in 1988. She had a normal anus, in addition, the bowel opened through a second opening in the vestibule. The external appearance suggested a rectovestibular fistula with a normal anus but the internal anatomy was found to be entirely different.

Bowel washes were given through catheters introduced into both openings, but fluid introduced into one opening did not emerge from the other. Xray after instillation of contrast fluid through the vestibular opening delineated the entire colon; the entire colon was also delineated after instilling contrast fluid through the anus. However on a lateral Xray the vestibular channel was seen in front of the anal channel.

The diagnosis was confirmed at laparotomy. The terminal ileum was seen to bifurcate into two; each opened into two separate cecums and the entire large gut was duplicated. The channel opening in the vestibule was identified and transected just above the peritoneal reflection. Both ends were closed. Then a long side to side anastomosis was made between the two sigmoid colons and upper rectums (Fig. 13.23). Recovery was uneventful.

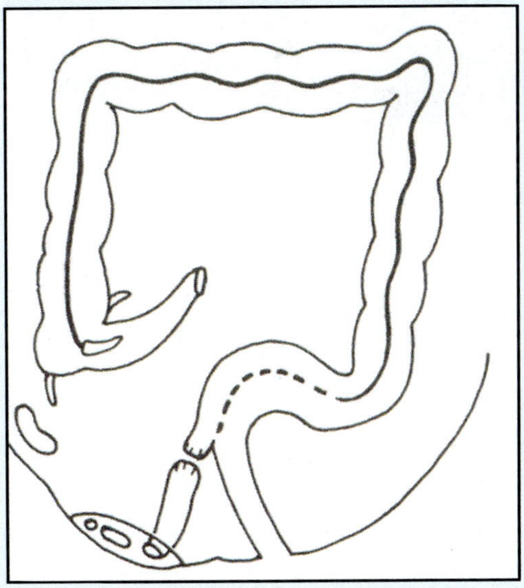

Fig. 13.23 Diagram of tubular duplication in a girl; dotted lines show planned operation.

The boy came to US Chatterjee as a newborn with multiple malformations. The most striking anomaly was duplication of the penis and urethra. The bowel opened at the normal site and also through an ectopic opening in the left buttock. (see Fig. 3.9) Total tubular duplication of the large gut was confirmed both by USG (Fig. 13.24) and by contrast Xray (Fig. 13.25). Cysto-urethgrams showed 2 urethras entering a

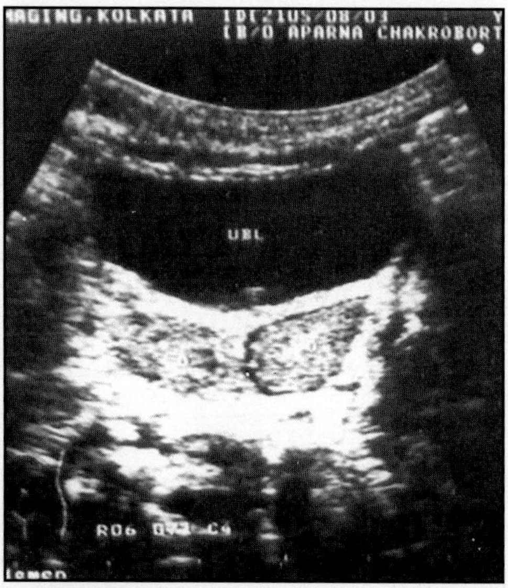

Fig. 13.24 USG of tubular duplication in a boy showing double colon & rectum.

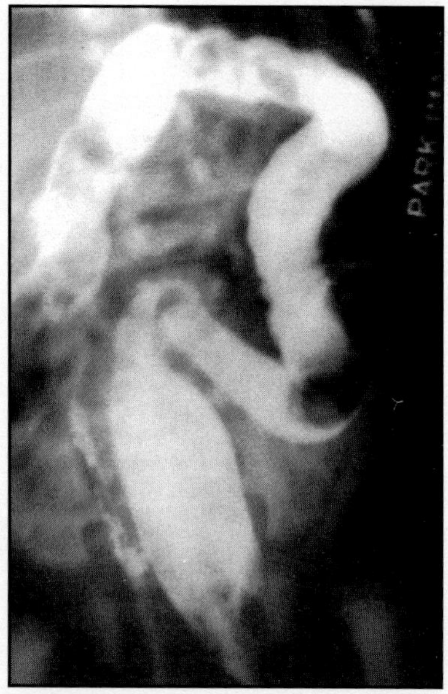

Fig. 13.25 Barium enema of tubular duplication.

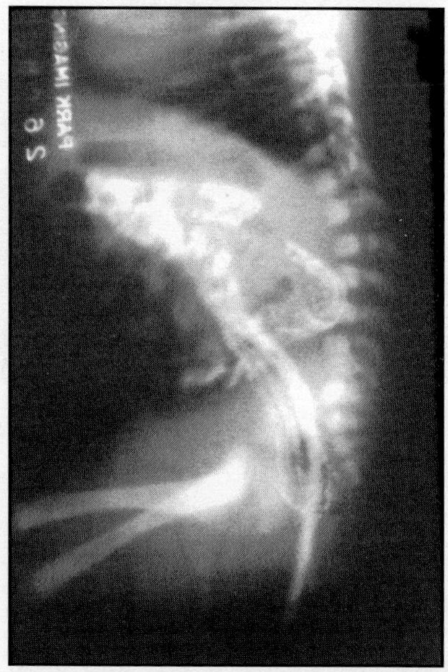

Fig. 13.26 Cysto-urethrogram of tubular duplication.

single bladder (Fig. 13.26). There were in addition cardiac, renal and skeletal anomalies. The cardiac problem was considered the most urgent and surgery for other anomalies has been postponed.

Duplications restricted to the anal canal have been described by Choi and Park in 2003. They collected 15 cases and reported 6 case of their own, all girls. They had an opening in the midline behind the normal anus and the tube ended blindly about 5 mm. above the dentate line. They were successfully excised.

CHAPTER 14

COLONIC AGENESIS, POUCH COLON, RECTAL ECTASIA AND SHARED COLON

COLONIC AGENESIS

Spriggs in 1912 appears to have been the first to describe an autopsy of a neonate with absence of the left half of the colon and the rectum. Zaidi in 1959 and Dickinson in 1967 described infants with no bowel distal to the ascending colon and Blunt and Rich in 1967 and Irving *et al* in 1983 recorded patients with complete absence of colon and rectum.

Colonic agenesis can be diagnosed during colostomy if the abdomen is widely opened. If a left lower quadrant incision is used, no colon will be seen until the wound is enlarged medially. If a right upper quadrant incision is used and the agenesis is partial, a successful colostomy will be done and the anomaly will be revealed only during a distal cologram. The cologram will mimic the cologram of a patient submitted to a sigmoid colostomy in the right upper quadrant and a proximal cologram will be necessary to differentiate between them (Fig. 14.1).

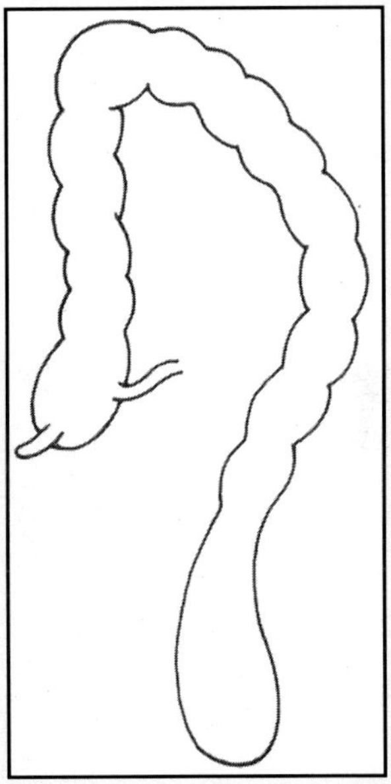

Fig. 14.1 Diagram of short colon.

We have 7 patients, all boys. The colon ended blindly in 3 and with a vesical fistula in 3. All had colostomy soon after birth and were reconstructed by APARP; in 3 the colostomy was resected and bowel proximal to this was brought down to the anus while in the other 3, the colostomy was preserved during the APARP and closed later. The seventh patient came at the age of 4 years with total fecal incontinence and massive prolapse at the neoanus. He had colostomy, APARP and discontinuance of colostomy elsewhere. We did a barium enema and then performed a revisional PSARP and a concurrent left lower quadrant colostomy. After the wound was healed, he was put up for closure of the colostomy. In the course of this operation we discovered that we had performed the left lower quadrant colostomy in the ascending colon; proximal to this was cecum with 2 appendixes and terminal ileum; distal to it was the pulled through bowel. The colos-tomy was closed without resecting bowel and uneventful recovery followed.

POUCH COLON

This is a relatively common anomaly in the northern half of the Indian subcontinent. There are only a few reports of this disorder from other parts of the world. Trusler *et al* (1959) discribed 7 cases from Canada, El Shafi (1971) 1 case from England, Chiba (1971) 2 cases from Japan, Vaezzadeh *et al* (1982) 1 case from Iran, Yuejie *et al* (1990) 8 cases from china, Lazzatto *et al* (1990) 1 case from Italy and Gopal (1978) and Kapoor (1989) 1 case each from the sourthern half of the Indian subcontinent.

The first North Indian publication on pouch colon came from Chandigarh in 1972 when Singh and Pathak described 6 cases. In 1984 Narasimharao *et al* published details of another 48 cases from the same center. Pouch colon constituted 8.3% of all their ARMs. They diagnosed pouch colon in the neonate when the diameter of the colon on an erect plain Xray was more than half the diameter of the abdomen (Figs. 14.2-4). Four types were described (Fig. 14.5).

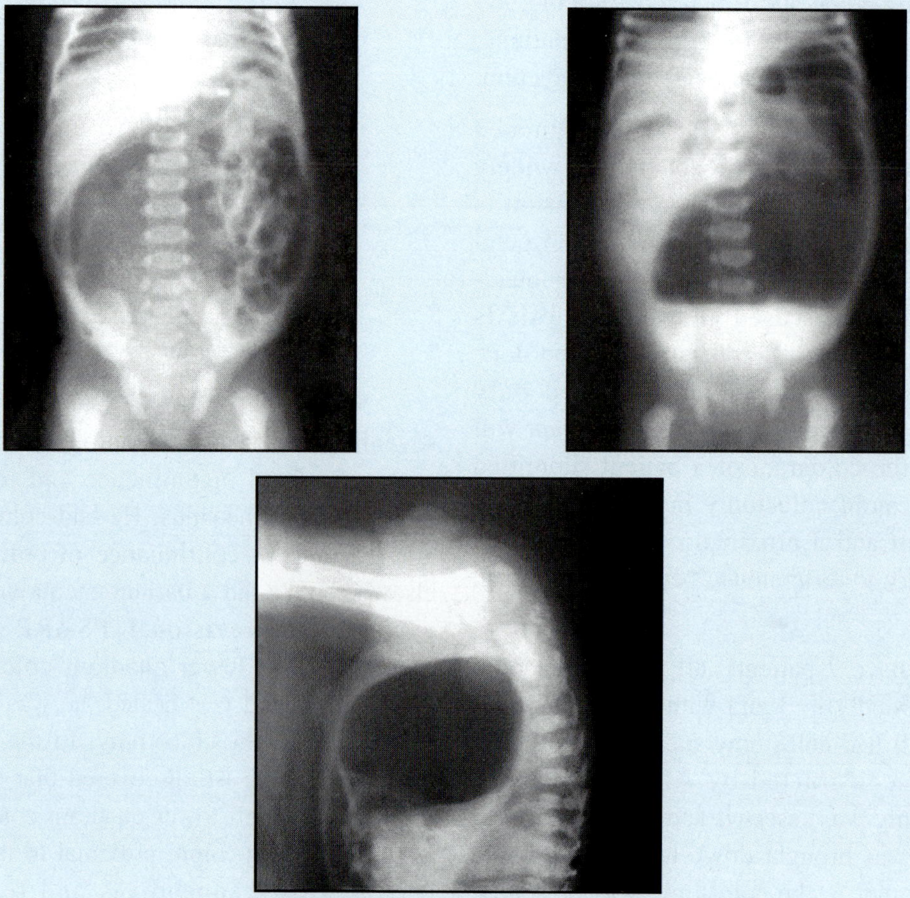

Figs. 14.2-4 Xrays of pouch colon PA erect; Lateral invertogram.

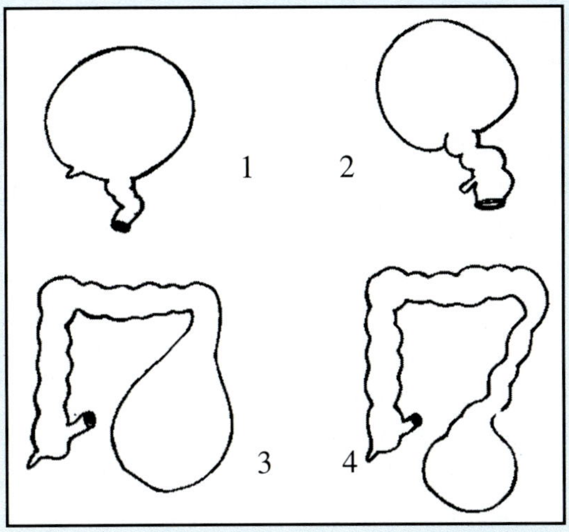

Fig. 14.5 Diagrams showing the 4 types of pouch colon.

1. Normal colon is absent and the ileum opens directly into the colonic pouch
2. The ileum opens into a short segment of cecum which then opens into the colonic pouch
3. A significant amount of normal colon intervenes between the ileum and the colonic pouch
4. Presence of near normal colon with only its terminal portion, namely rectum and sigmoid, converted into a pouch.

Over the years articles on pouch colon have appeared from Patiala (Singh *et al* 1977), Delhi (Agarwal and Patnaik, 1980, Upadhyaya, 1984, Chadha *et al*, 1994, 1998), Jaipur (Kalani and Sogani, 1984 Sharma and Harjai, 1997), Udaipur (Mathur *et al*, 2002), Lucknow (Wakhlu *et al*, 1982, 1996) and Varanasi (Wardhan *et al*, 1990). The condition has also been encountered in Pakistan (Hasan, 1985), Bangladesh (Liton 1999) and in our own center. Till 1985 we had 28 cases, subsequently we have had only 22 new cases, that is about 3% of all our cases of ARM.

On the other hand 137 cases have been encountered in Chandigarh, constituting 12.6% of all ARM cases, and 22% of high lesions. Pouch colon constituted 6% of all ARMs in the Lucknow series and nearly 20% of all high ARMs in the Varanasi series. There was a male preponderance in all the Indian series

In our series there are 37 boys, 12 girls and 1 baby of undetermined sex. This baby had neither urogenital nor anorectal openings and died after a colostomy. At autopsy, a severe dysplasia affecting the entire urogenital system was found. This, as van der Putte has explained is the predictable end result of total agenesis of the entire cloacal plate (Fig. 14.6).

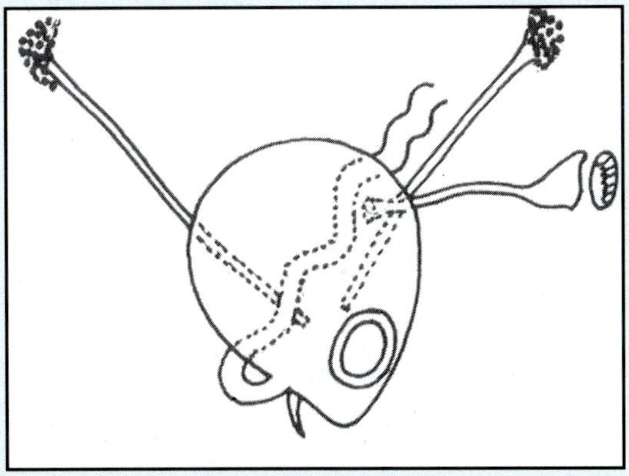

Fig. 14.6 Diagram of autopsy findings of baby with pouch and no external opening.

The breakup of our material according to the Chandigarh classification is as follows: Type 1: 8 cases; Type 2: 24 cases; Type 3: 4 cases and Type 4: 14 cases. The pouch ended blindly in 14 cases. It ended by a fistula in the others. The fistula entered into the bladder in 7 males and 1 female, into the male urethra in 10, into the vestibule in 1, into the vagina in 2 and into a common urethrovaginal canal in 7; the termination could not be determined in the others.

For all practical purposes there are only two groups of pouch colon. The larger group with a total or subtotal pouch encompasses types 1and 2 of the Chandigarh classification. Normal colon is either nonexistent or its length is less than 8 cm. and hence patients in this group are difficult to manage. The smaller group consisting of the common type 4 with a terminal pouch replacing lower sigmoid and rectum and the rare type 3 with the pouch replacing bowel from 8 cm. distal to the ileocecal valve to the lower sigmoid are relatively easy to manage.

Low birth weight and multiple associated malformations often add to the problems faced by babies with pouch colon. While major urological anomalies were found in half the babies in our series, they were found in every baby in the Chandigarh series.

Patients with pouch colon present in 3 different ways.

1. As neonates without an anus

This is the commonest presentation. The diagnosis is made on the basis of Xray as mentioned earlier. However, there is some confusion if there is perforation with pneumoperitoneum or a large collection of gas in a greatly distended vagina of a girl with a cloacal malformation.

Patients thought to have a pouch colon are submitted to laparotomy with a right upper transverse incision. The pouch is partially emptied, and the loop of bowel entering it is identified. This loop is isolated and divided as close to the pouch as possible. The distal end is closed and the proximal end is brought out as an end enterostomy through a separate incision. The location of this depends on the type of pouch. In types 1 and 2 this second incision is in the right lower quadrant; in type 1 the ileum and in type 2 the proximal colon is exteriorized and fixed in place. In type 3 the colon is exteriorized through a left upper quadrant incision. The pouch is then completely emptied and marsupialized at the main wound leaving a balloon catheter in the lumen. The wound is then closed in layers around the site of marsupialization in layers (Fig. 14.7). The balloon catheter is removed from the pouch before the patient goes home; the family can be trained to clean the mucoid discharge that emerges. The pouch is visualized by Xray after contrast is instilled into it (Fig. 14.8).

Unfortunately, some stomas tend to prolapse (Fig. 14.9).

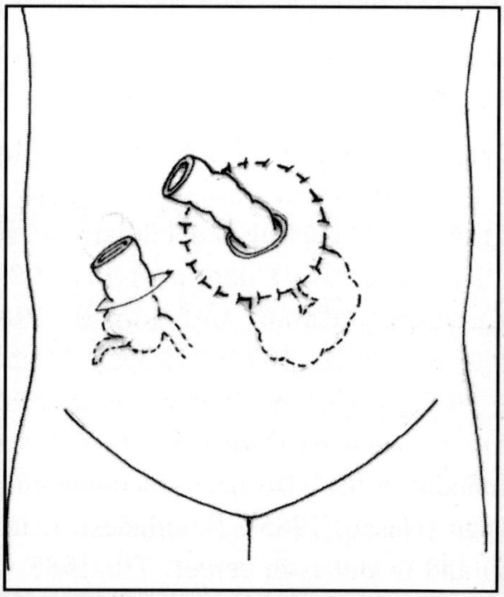

Fig. 14.7 Diagram of operation on neonate; proximal enterostomy and pouchostomy.

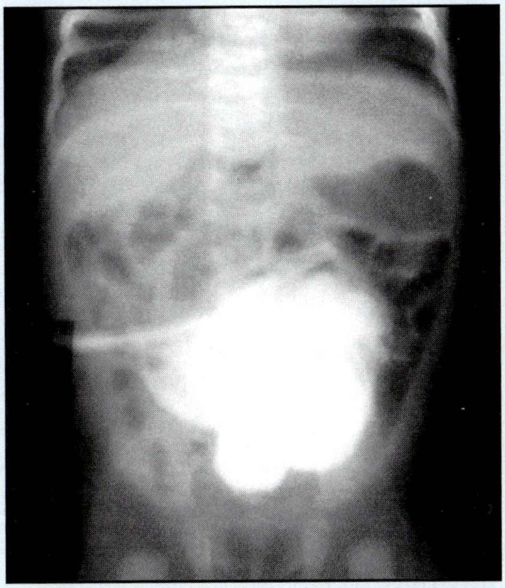

Fig. 14.8 Xray with contrast into pouch.

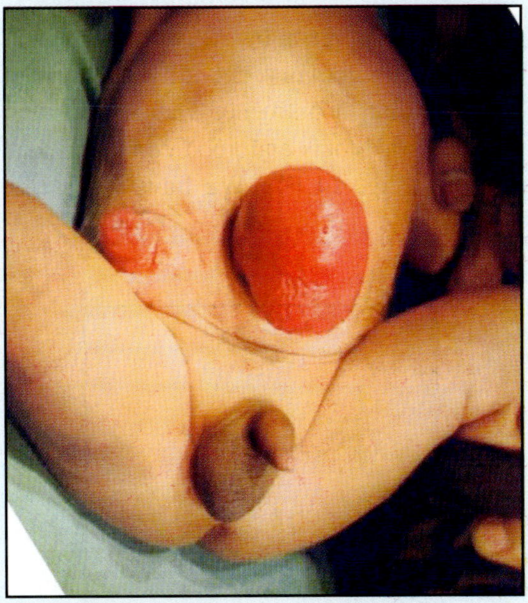

Fig. 14.9 Photograph after the above operation; minor prolapse of pouch.

This is minimal if the wall of the pouch had been accurately sutured to the muscles of the abdominal wall and if adequate nutrition is given in the postoperative period. Diarrhea is a serious problem in types one and two and the effluent from the ileum or proximal colon has to be replaced by intravenous fluids. Parenteral nutrition has to be given for varying lengths of time and oral imodium helps to solidify the stools. Type 2 patients can be managed more easily if there is a reasonable length of functioning colon distal to the ileocecal valve.

For patients with a type 4 or terminal pouch, we do a high sigmoid loop colostomy. Patients with types 3 and 4 anomalies generally have an uneventful postoperative period.

Before we embarked on this plan our results with types 1 and 2 patients were depressing and very few patients came back for reconstruction. Six cases were studied at autopsy. In the last decade, primary mortality has been eliminated, but babies, particularly girls still tend to get lost.

Reconstructive surgery is carried out when the baby is thriving and weighs about 8 kg.

Alternative strategies

A reasonable alternative is to resect a type 1, 2 or 3 pouch and close the fistula if any during the first operation which is concluded by performing an endenterostomy (Chadha). Bhaumik has recently done this on a type 3 pouch. Problems associated with pouchostomy are thus eliminated.

A neonatal onestage abdominoperineal pullthough after pouch resection appears to be an unreasonable alternative to us at the present time although Gangopaghyay's team (2003) has had successes.

2. After an operation elsewhere

The operation that has been generally

performed elsewhere is a window colostomy done by a surgeon unaware of the problems of pouch colon. The colostomy either prolapses or stenoses.

Patients who present with a massive prolapse of a window colostomy (Figs. 14.10-11) are treated by a proximal end enterostomy. Bowel distal to this and the window colostomy are then closed or the pouch is resected.

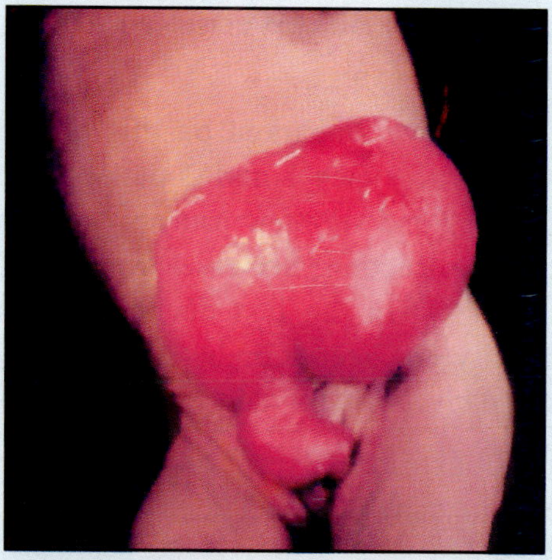

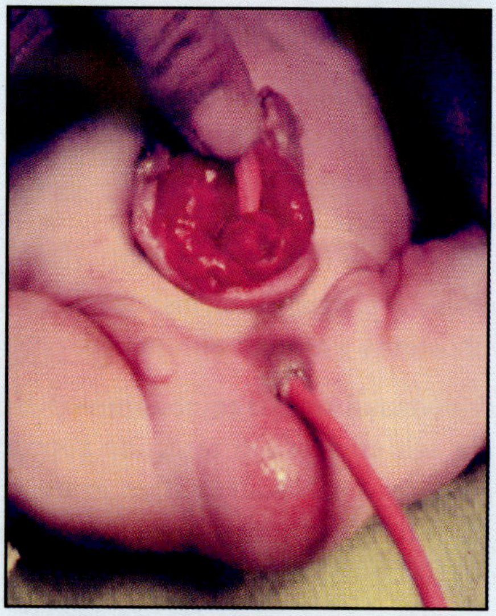

Figs. 14.10-11 Photographs of babies after window colostomy showing massive prolapse.

If the patient presents with a stenosed colostomy (Figs. 14.12-13), the diagnosis is not easy. A contrast Xray is necessary to demonstrate the presence of an underlying pouch. The opening may have to be dilated to permit the instillation of contrast, and even with contrast it may not be possible to delineate the anatomy fully. One of our earliest patients presented at 6 months of age with a stenosed right upper quadrant colostomy. Since contrast Xray was inconclusive, revision of the colostomy was planned. At operation, we found that the opening was in fact a stenosed window colostomy done on a pouch that had replaced the colon distal to the hepatic flexure. The pouch was resected and the normal right colon was pulled through to the normal anal site by APARP. There was uneventful recovery; an initial period of diarrhea and incontinence was followed by near normal stools and good continence and growth (Fig. 14.14). We have a 20 year follow up.

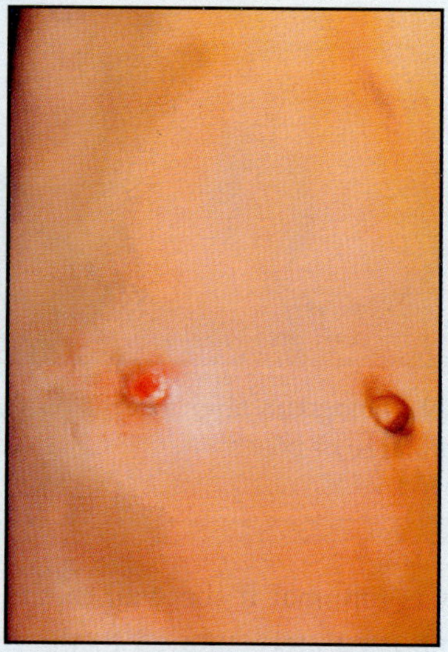

Fig. 14.12 Photograph of baby with stenosis after window colostomy in left lower quadrant.

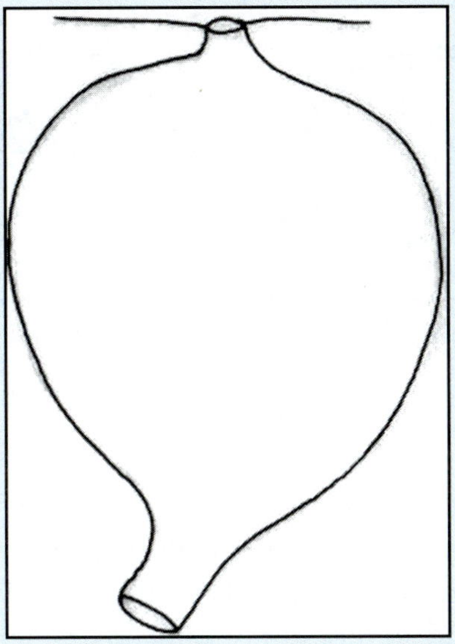

Fig. 14.13 Diagram of baby with stenosis after window colostomy in right upper quadrant.

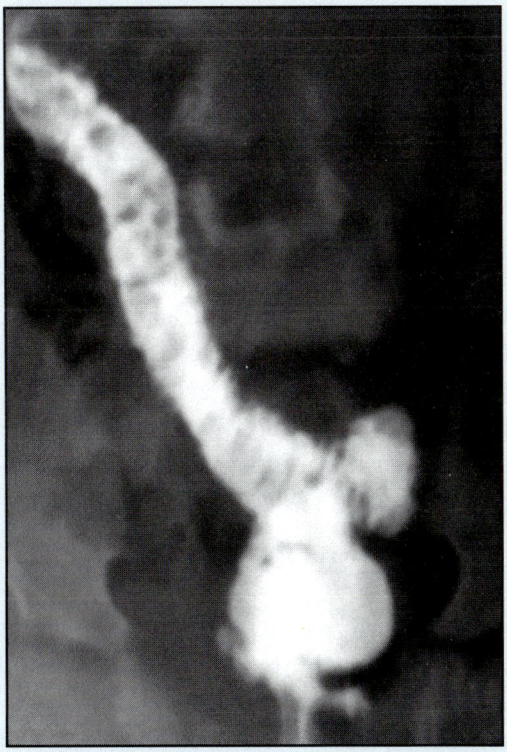

Fig. 14.14 Xray Barium enema after pullthrough of bowel proximal to type 2 pouch.

3. *With a fistula and chronic intestinal obstruction*

A girl who presents with chronic intestimal obstruction, protein-energy-malnutrition, a vestibular, vaginal or cloacal fistula and recurrent urinary infection and is kept alive by periodic dilatations and washouts may be harboring a pouch colon with a fistula. The pouch is seen on Xray after instillation of contrast fluid through the fistula. A proximal colostomy is indicated and reconstruction is carried out when the child's general condition has improved.

Reconstruction in patients with terminal pouch.

If the distal cologram shows that the terminal pouch is at or below the 3rd sacral vertebra, the bowel can be brought down with a standard PSARP after a somewhat exaggerated tapering; the colostomy is closed another day. If the bowel ends above this level an abdominoperineal procedure becomes necessary; the colostomy is resected with the pouch and normal bowel is pulled through (Figs. 14.15-16).

Reconstruction in patients with total or subtotal pouch; resection or colonorrhaphy?

This basic question can be answered correctly after studying the longterm clinical results and the pathophysiology of the pouch.

Resection of the pouch and pullthrough of the proximal bowel together with the enterostomy to the normal anal site, either by APARP or by PSARP and laparotomy was done by us in the early days. The initial problems associated with loss of large bowel gradually diminished and the quality of life improved.

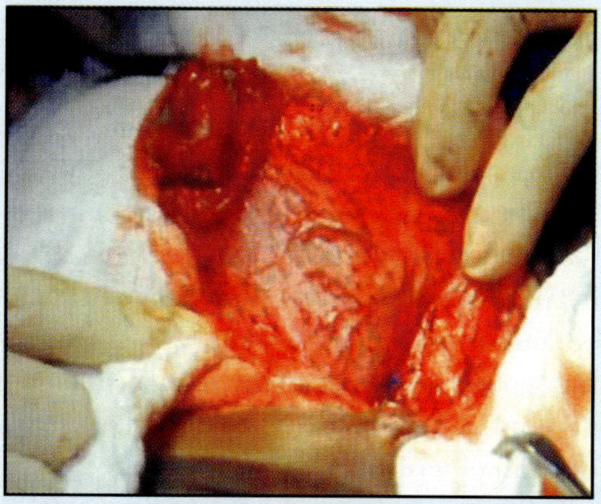

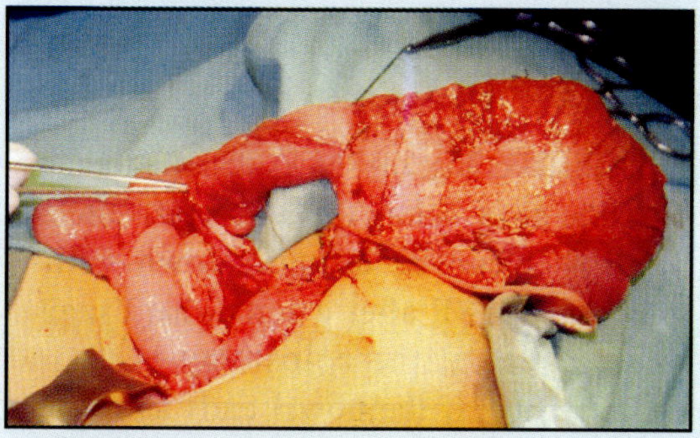

Figs. 14.15-16 Photographs of operation on type 3 pouch with colovesical fistula.

Subsequently, after studying the experience of surgeons with a much greater experience of this malformation than ours we began to perform Colonorrhaphy. This was done after carefully studying the vasculature of the pouch. In all our patients the inferior mesenteric vessels were absent; the pouch was supplied by hypertrophic terminal branches of the superior mesenteric artery and corresponding veins. We resected the antimesenteric portion of the pouch and sutured the remaining portion of the bowel longitudinally so that it resembled normal colon Fig. 14.17). In our earlier cases we had not done pouchostomy and had found the pouch difficult to handle. It was filled

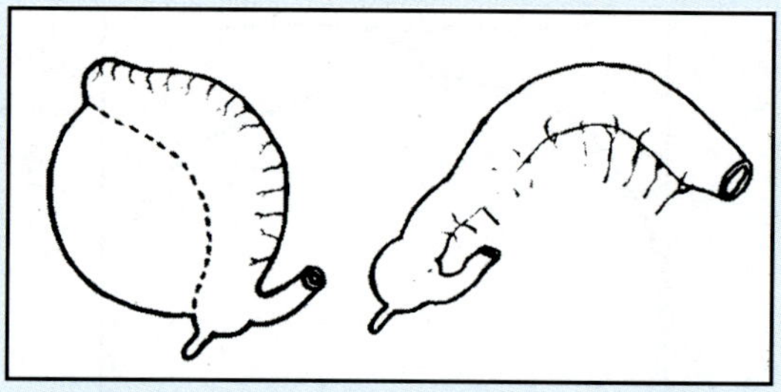

Fig. 14.17 Diagrams showing colonorrhaphy.

with stagnant intestinal contents and its epithelium was inflamed. Pouchostomy prevented this. Nevertheless, in all cases, we brought out the reconstructed colon as an end enterostomy and postponed the pullthrough for another day. Some of our colleagues in centers with more patients completed the reconstruction in one sitting.

Our results of colonorrhaphy with end colostomy were encouraging. Patients passed stool through this and gained weight. However after the pullthrough was done, they began to suffer from bouts of intractable constipation and the colon dilated to an unmanageable size (Fig. 14.18). Our results of resection and pullthrough of healthy proximal bowel were much better, and we abandoned colonorrhaphy. We find today that early enthusiasm for this operation has waned even in centers where the procedure was strongly advocated earlier and reformation of the pouch has been reported (Pathak 1999, Chadha *et al* 2002).

We have recently revised a colonorrhapy. A boy aged 4 months came in 1995 with a massive prolapse of a right upper quadrant colostomy. Cologram confirmed that there was a subtotal pouch. At laparotomy after adequate bowel preparation, it was established that the pouch ended blindly. The colostomy was mobilized and

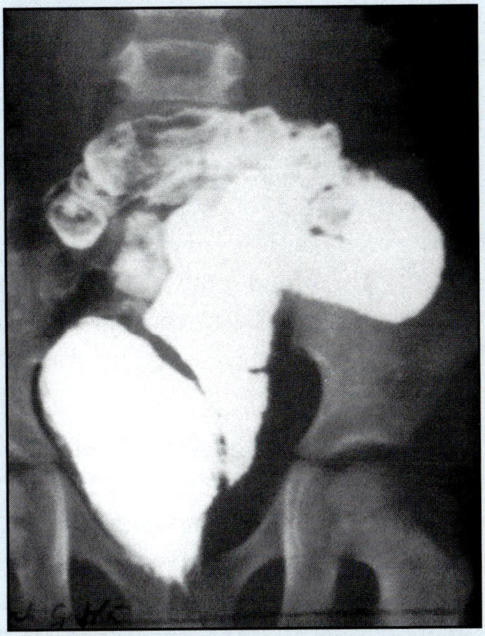

Fig. 14.18 Xray Barium enema showing reformation of pouch after colonorrhaphy and pullthrough.

colonorrhaphy was carried out. There was 8 cm. of normal colon between the ileocecal valve and the pouch. The distal end of the pouch was brought out in the left lower quadrant as an endcolostomy. It was brought down to the normal anal site by APARP 6 months later. He began to pass normal stools but follow up was poor. He continued to have intractable constipation and was brought for reexamination only when there were multiple perianal abscesses and fistulas. The caliber of the neoanus was normal but a contrast Xray showed reformation of the pouch. Readmission was advised in 1998, and in all subsequent years but the father agreed to further surgery only in 2003 when there was discharge of blood and mucus. Preoperative contrast Xray showed that the condition had worsened. This was confirmed at laparotomy. The reformed pouch was mobilized with great difficulty. The distal bowel leading down to the neoanus was left alone and the reformed pouch was excised. The stump of ascending colon was brought out as a proximal end colostomy in the left lower quadrant; the upper end of the distal colon that was retained was brought out through the right lower quadrant, also as an end colostomy. Recovery was uneventful but he again disappeared for a year. When re-examined in 2004, he had stenosis at the anus and the pouch had reformed. The anus was dilated with effect. We then tried to resect the megarectum and perform an end to end anastomosis. We failed and left him with his end colostomy.

Another boy has also been left with an endcolostomy. He had come in 1999 at the age of 7 weeks in a very ill state with a massive prolapse of a left lower quadrant window colostomy (Figs. 14.19-20). He had severe respiratory and urinary infection, sacral truncation and bilateral hydroureteronephrosis. After he was resuscitated, he was operated upon. We found that the pouch had replaced all his large bowel and was partially ischemic. It ended as a colovesical fistula. The fistula was closed, nonviable pouch was resected; colonorrhaphy was done and the terminal bowel was brought out as an endcolostomy. He subsequently had vesicostomy to control urinary retention and after this was closed we did left sided ureteroneocystostomy to control massive reflux. His urimary status improved and we thought he was fit for pullthrough by APARP. However, we failed to find space between the urethra and the levator sling and abandoned the operation. When last seen in 2004, he was doing well with an endcolostomy and had minimum urinary incontinence

A third baby was more unfortunate. He came at the age of 6 weeks with a window colostomy that had stenosed. Contrast Xray revealed a subtotal pouch. Colon proximal to the pouch was brought out as a loop colostomy and the patient was sent home. He came back with a massive prolapse of the colostomy. After adequate preparation colonorrhaphy with APARP and revision of colostomy was done. Initial recovery was uneventful but he was lost to followup for some time. He came back with an even larger prolapse, and we decided to close the colostomy. After this was done the baby deteriorated rapidly and died. Almost certainly the blood supply to the reconstructed colon had been jeopardized during the mobilization necessary to close the colostomy.

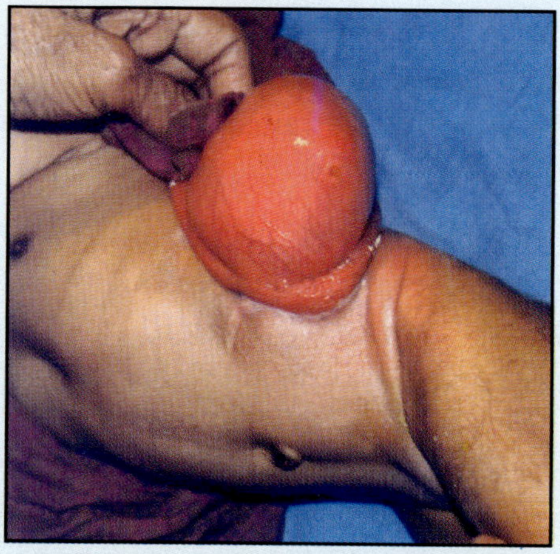

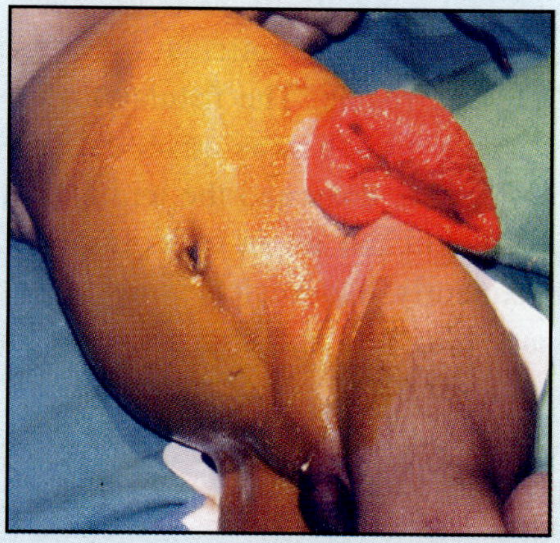

Figs. 14.19-20 Photographs of baby with massive prolapse, on crying and sleeping

The reason for poor function of the reconstructed colon seems to lie in the histology of the pouch and both its musculature and innervation have been studied. Our study of the wall of the pouch has revealed a significant difference in the structure of the total and subtotal pouches and the terminal pouches. The musculature in the latter was no different from normal colon. However, in the former, we could demonstrate focal presence of an additional muscle coat on the inner side of the normal circular muscle coat. Orientation of this additional layer was similar to the normal circular muscle from which it was clearly separated by an additional neural plexus. The muscle bundles of this additional layer were separated by broad bands of fibrous tissue (Chatterjee *et al* 2001) (Figs. 14.21-22).

Embryology

Agenesis of a part or whole of the colon or its replacement by a pouch is considered to be due to a more extensive defect in the development of the hindgut or postsplenic gut than that which causes the usual variety of ARM. The common varieties of anorectocolonic malformations indeed involve the left colon rectum and anal canal.

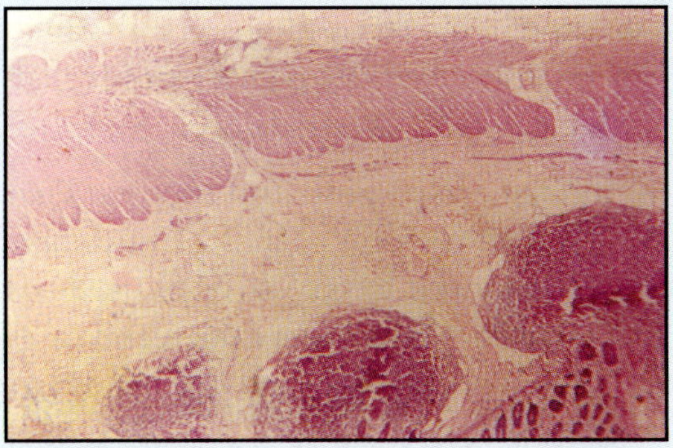

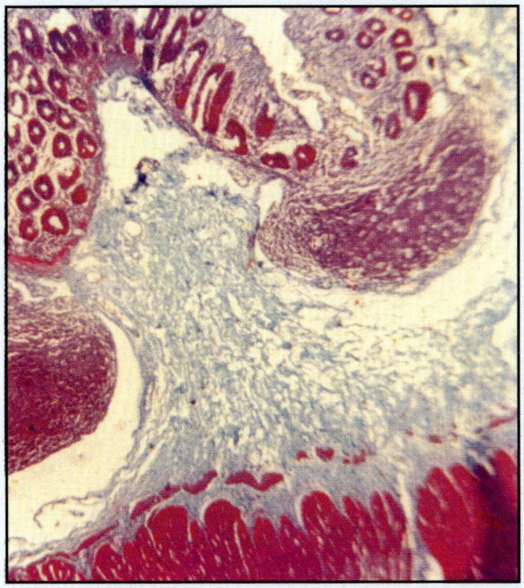

Figs. 14.21-22 Photomicrographs showing abnormal muscle layer.

However, the total or subtotal pouch can only be due to an additional defect in the right or presplenic colon. The right colon develops from the postaxial midgut. It is our hypothesis that the cecum and right colon develops normally from the postaxial midgut only when this portion of the midgut is stimulated by normally developing hindgut. Thus improper development of postaxial midgut or presplenic gut is due to a primary disorder of the proximal end of the hindgut or postsplenic gut. We had earlier proposed a similar hypothesis about the formation of the lower half of the anal canal (see Chapter 4).

RECTAL ECTASIA

Rectal ectasia is the name given by Brent and Stephens (1976) to a condition in which there is 'massive focal dilatation of the rectal terminus extending into the rectosigmoid junctional zone' accompanying some anorectal malformations. When the ectasia is present in the newborn, sigmoid colon of normal caliber empties into a dilated pouch at the pelvic brim; Brent and Stephens have shown that there is no hypertrophy of the muscle cells in this pouch, signifying a congenital or primary anomaly. According to them, secondary ectasia is due to muscular hypertrophy that follows stimulation by persisting obstruction or retained contents.

Today, we do not find any difference between a terminal or type 4 pouch colon and primary rectal ectasia. The condition may be suspected in the neonate on a straight Xray; the diagnosis is confirmed during a left lower quadrant colostomy or a fistulogram or a distal cologram (Fig. 14.23). If the patient is left with a colostomy, the pouch will enlarge with time and a distal cologram will show a huge megarectum, filling the entire pelvis (Fig. 14.24). A similar megarectum will develop if a patient with a fistula is left untreated and survives by defecating through the fistula.

Secondary megarectum may also follow an apparently satisfactory extraperitoneal reconstruction leaving a neoanus of adequate size. The patients have intractable constipation, abdominal distension and soiling, and a contrast Xray shows the megarectum. It can even show megasigmoid but in all cases the bowel proximal to the dilated segment has a normal caliber. Nine cases had been described by Powell *et al* (1982), 3 by Cloutier *et al* (1987), Cheu (1992) and Pena (1993), 1 by Chadha (1999) and 6 by Long Li (2000).

The management options are resection of the dilated segment followed by end to end anastomosis or tapering and reconstruction by PSARP. If the pouch extends high up, a laparotomy is mandatory.

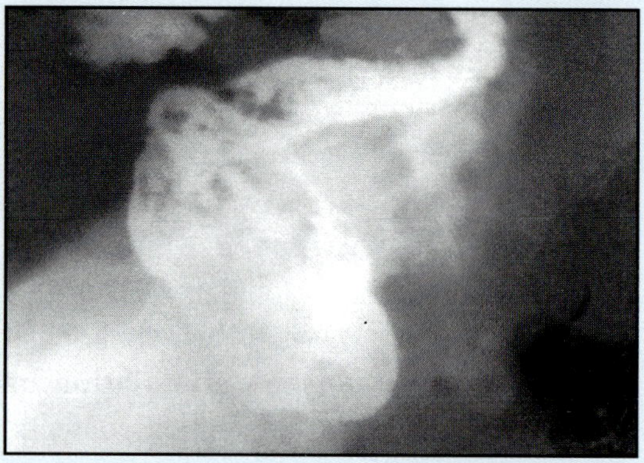

Fig. 14.23 Xray Barium enema of rectal ectasia.

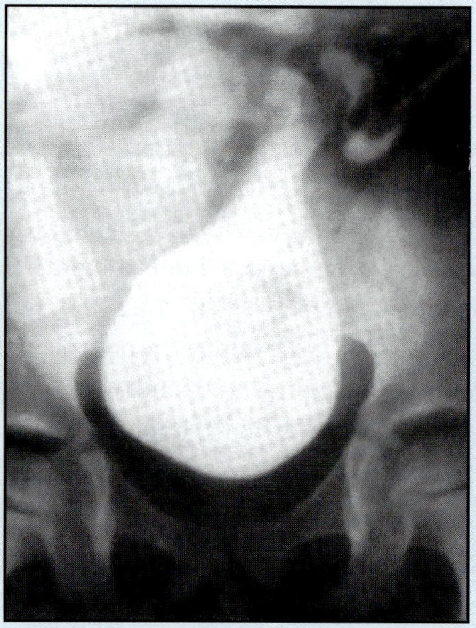

Fig. 14.24 Xray distal cologram showing ectasia.

We had earlier described 6 cases. Four of them had perineal operations elsewhere and were treated in the 1970s by methods now obsolete. Most of our more recent cases had truncated sacrums (See Chapter 15).

Patients with rectal ectasia and a normal anus and anal canal are not unknown. The patients have intractable constipation and contrast Xray shows a huge focal dilatation of the rectum with colon of normal caliber opening into it. In 1977 we treated a two year old girl with this anomaly by a Duhamel's procedure for Hirschsprung's disease. The pullthrough of normal sigmoid was easy but in the absence of a stapler it was very difficult to close the wide rectal stump. This girl is now happily married but does have some problems with fecal accumulation in the anterior pouch; she does not agree to any revisional procedure.

SHARED COLON

A PAIR OF FEMALE ISCHIOPAGUS TETRAPUS TWINS had, amongst other shared organs, a shared colon. They were brought to us in 1986 when they were 4 months old (Fig. 14.25). They had separate urethral and vaginal orifices but a single anus (Fig. 14.26). Contrast studies of the alimentary tracts revealed that these were normal up to the ileocecal region; then both ileums opened into a single shared greatly distended colon that ended in a narrow anorectum. Laxatives, bowel washes and antibiotics were given, but there was intractable enterocolitis, excoriation of the perineal skin, fecal soiling and failure to thrive. It was obvious that one stage separa-

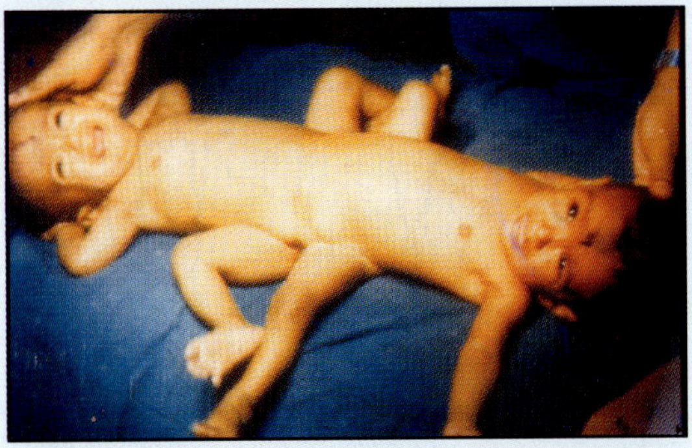

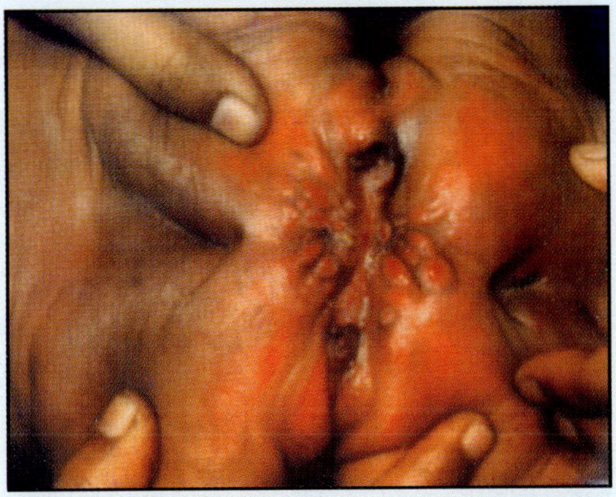

Figs. 14.25-26 Photographs of Ischiopagus conjoined twins with single opening of bowel.

tion would be hazardous; hence the separation was staged.

At laparotomy at the age of 9 months, we found that the 2 ileums opened into a single cecum and a single hugely distended large intestine ended in a narrow anorectum. The colon was transected at the level of the midtransverse colon. The proximal half in continuity with its ileum was given to Twin B and the colon was brought out as an end colostomy. The proximal end of the distal half was anastomosed to the terminal ileum of Twin A. The bowel was then transected through the lower rectum. The stump of rectum was closed and the upper rectum brought out as an end colostomy (Fig. 14.27). There was uneventful healing. The general health of both twins improved rapidly and they were fit for the final separation in 3 months time. Details of the separation have been described elsewhere (Chatterjee *et al*) and are not relevant to the present presentation. The anus was allotted to Twin A.

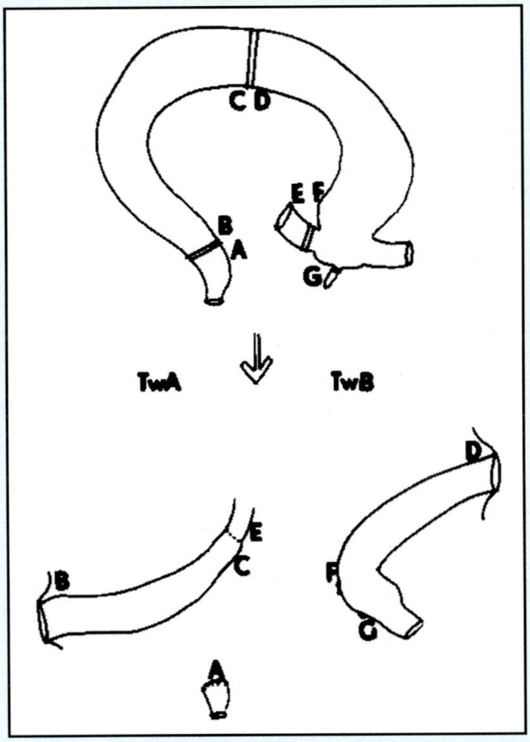

Fig. 14.27 Diagram of above showing disposition of large bowel and plan of separation.

Subsequently, the twins developed normally and led normal lives except for the colostomies. At the age of 4 years, Twin A was brought back for bowel reconstruction. The end colostomy was dismantled and the colon mobilized up to the coloileal anastomosis; this was extremely difficult. The bowel was then brought down to the normal anal site behind the anal canal as in a Duhamel procedure for Hirschsprung's disease. She passed stool through this for a few days and then became obstructed. The lumen of the pulled through bowel was found obliterated and an emergency loop colostomy had to be done. When we examined her 9 months later a septum was found between the lumen of the anal canal and the lumen of the distal colon. The situation resembled rectal atresia. We carried out the treatment suggested by Borwankar (see Chapter 12). A proctoscope was inserted into the anal canal and the septum was fulgurated with a bugbee. The lumen of the colon was entered. The opening was dilated through the colostomy from above and through the anus from below. After a few sessions of dilatation, an adequate opening was created; the bowel distal to the opening was crushed and the colostomy was closed extraperitoneally (Figs. 14.28-29). Defecation then became normal except for mild soiling when there was diarrhea. (Fig. 14.30). The unusual distribution of the blood supply of the bowel loop probably sustained it in its normal position but was inadequate when the bowel was pulled down to the anus.

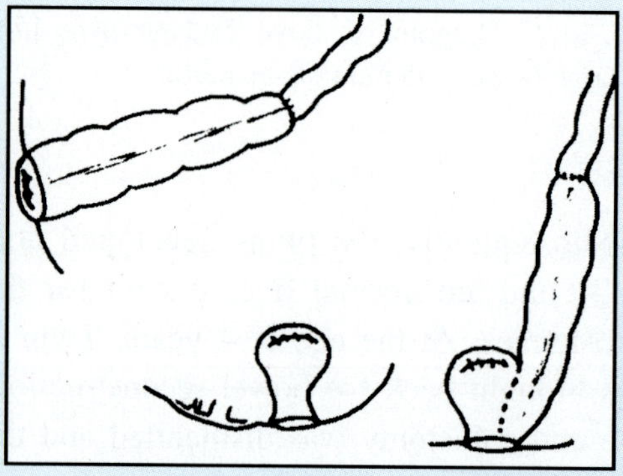

Fig. 14.28 Diagram showing plan of pullthrough of Twin A's colon.

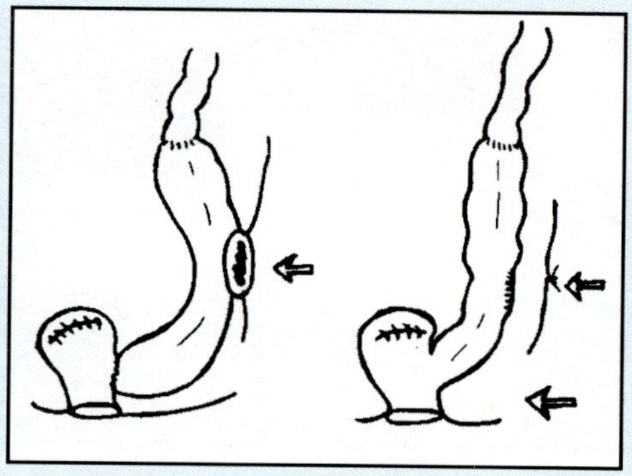

Fig. 14.29 Diagram showing plan of corrective operation of above.

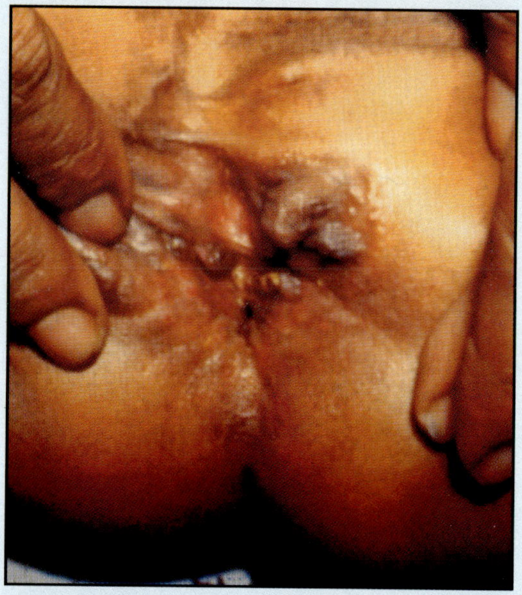

Fig. 14.30 Photograph of Twin A's perineum after surgery.

Twin B came for reconstruction when she was 5 years old. Dismantling the colostomy and mobilizing the right colon was relatively easy. Then a Mollard type of APARP was done (Fig. 14.31). There was a reasonable volume of striated muscle but it was extremely difficult to open up the space between the vagina and the levator sling, and then through the striated muscle

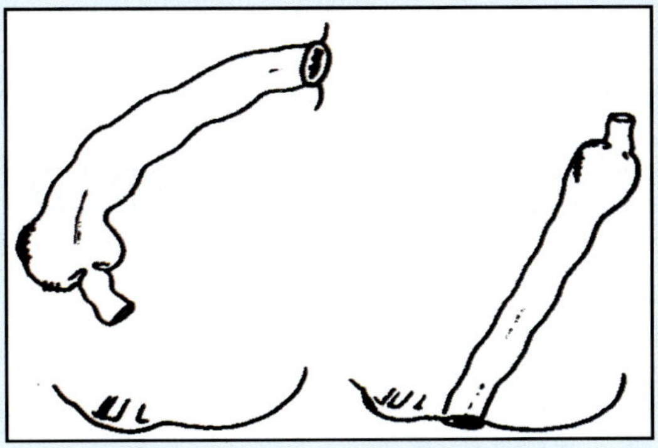

Fig. 14.31 Diagram showing plan of pullthrough of Twin B's colon.

complex. She began to pass stools well but a Y-V plasty was necessary a year later to enlarge the neoanus (Fig. 14.32).

The twins were reassessed when they were 12 years old. Twin A suffered from episodes of constipation and encopresis. We felt this was due to aganglionosis of the anorectal stump and performed anorectal myectomy. No ganglion cells were found in the excised strip, but she improved greatly and now has normal defecation. Twin B's main problem was soiling. Her pulled through bowel was just behind the vagina and there was dilated bowel above. We did a revisional anorectoplasty by the posterior sagittal route without a colostomy, Healing has been satisfactory and she also has improved greatly.

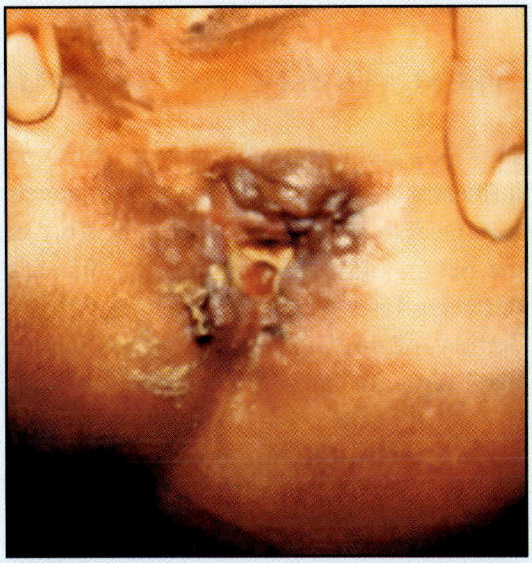

Fig. 14.32 Photograph of Twin B's perineum after surgery.

CHAPTER 15

TRUNCATION OF THE SACRUM; TETHERED CORD

TRUNCATION OF THE SACRUM

This is a condition that has a profound influence on fecal and urinary continence. It is measured by taking a straight Xray of the pelvis and by comparing the distance between line A joining the uppermost portions of the 2 iliac crests, line B joining the 2 posterior inferior iliac spines and line C parallel to the above and passing through the lowest sacral point visible radiologically. The ratio of the distances BC to AB should be 0.7 to 0.8. A ratio less than 0.4 indicates a poorly formed or truncated sacrum (Figs. 15.1-2).

The close relationship between the development of the caudal end of the vertebral column and the striated muscles of the pelvis and perineum and the pelvic viscera is well known. A normal sacrum suggests well developed levator ani muscles and normal innervation of the pelvic organs and muscles. Absence of 3 or more sacral vertebras is no doubt associated with dysplastic or absent sacral nerves and hence defective defecation and micturition. Williams and Nixon had pointed this out as early as 1957. Nevertheless, in 1971, Smith described an autopsy dissection in which the lower 3 sacral bony segments were absent but there was a full complement of nerves.

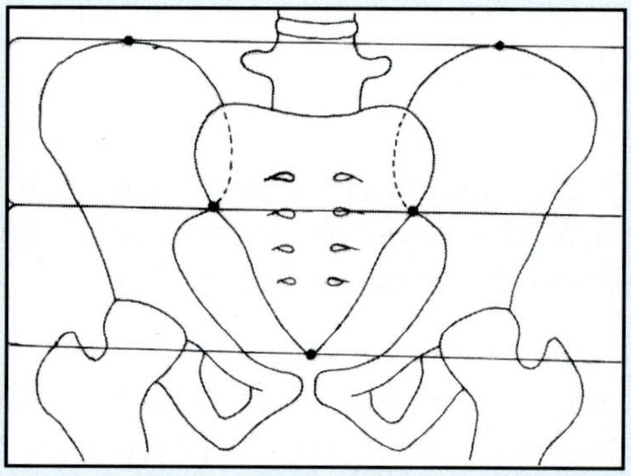

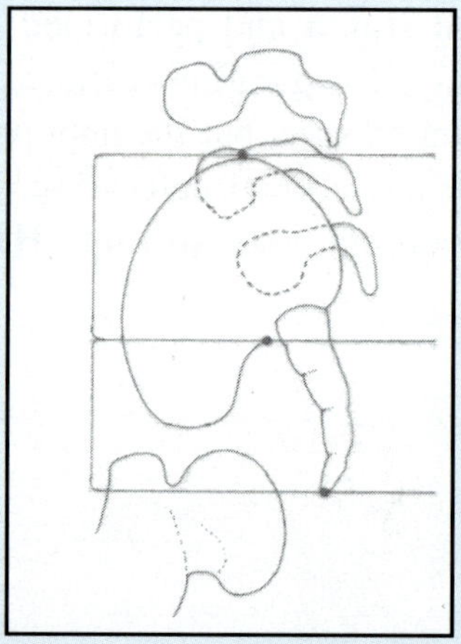

Figs. 15.1-2 Diagrams of normal sacrum AP and Lateral.

A truncated sacrum is generally present from birth, and is considered to be a congenital malformation. However, we have 2 boys born with high ARMs whom we treated by a Kiesewetter-Rehbein SAPR the

1970s. Their sacrums were complete prior to the reconstruction. However the 3 lower sacral segments did not show up on post-operative Xrays and evidences of neurological deficit were manifest during subsequent clinical examinations (Figs. 15.3-4). We believe that the excessive traction that was required to expose the presacral space to look for bowel that was not there damaged both the ossific centers as well as the emerging nerves.This operation has since been abandoned.

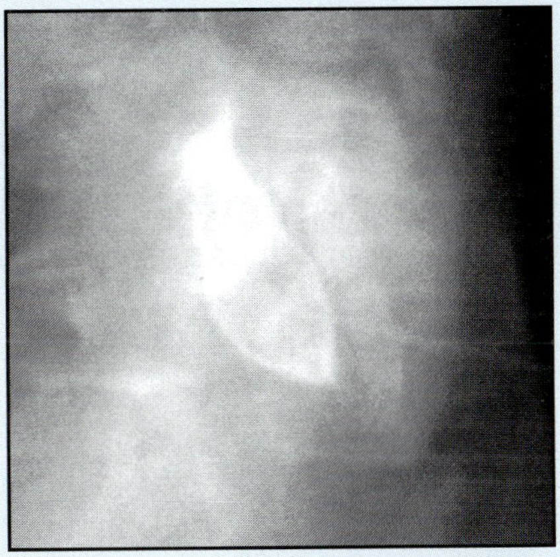

Fig. 15.3 Xray lateral showing normal sacrum of neonate.

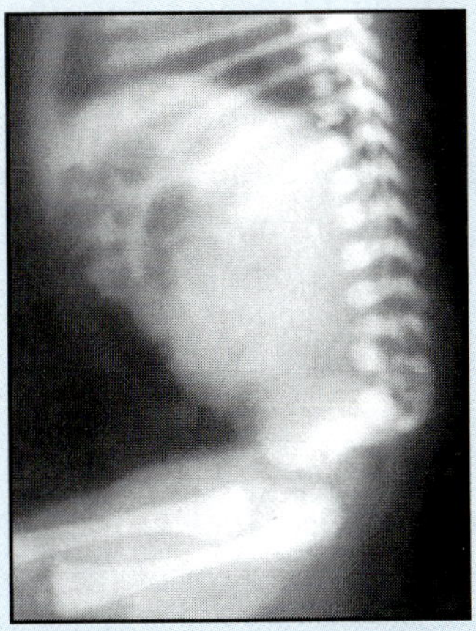

Fig. 15.4 Xray lateral showing truncation some years after SPR.

Truncation with Normal Anorectum

Truncation of the sacrum is generally thought to be a malformation associated with high or intermediate ARMs. However, we have been consulted for a number of patients with normal anorectums and truncated sacrums. They presented with constipation and fecal incontinence and urinary retention with overflow leading to chronic renal failure.

Truncation with Low Anomalies

We have 2 boys and 3 girls who had truncated sacrums and low ARMs. Both boys were aged 1 year at the time of presentation. The first came after he had a cutback elsewhere for anal stenosis; he had fecal incontinence and bilateral pes calcaneovalgus. He improved with bowel management. The second born with anoperineal fistula had been submitted to colostomy elsewhere. We have recently performed anoplasty and closed the colostomy; he is doing well but has multiple malformations. One of the girls had had Y-V plasty for vestibular fistula at 1 month, she had associated arthrogryposis and was lost to followup. The other also had Y-V plasty for a vestibular fistula at the age of 3 months. She had a lipomyelomeningocele over the sacrum and has been followed up for 12 years; she has good fecal control but suffers from some urinary incontinence and episodes of urinary infection. Her renal status is good. MRI and CIC have been advised but the parents have not agreed. The third girl had PAT for vestibular fistula at the age of 3 months; she had urinary incontinence but good fecal continence. Now at 4 years urinary continence has greatly improved.

Truncation with Intermediate Anomalies

We have 9 boys and 2 girls. One boy born in 1975 has been described in Chapter 7; he had been treated for rectovesicoperineal fistula. He has a permanent urinary diversion for urinary incontinence but has normal fecal continence.

Three other boys had been treated in the 1970s.

The first, born in 1973, had perineal operations elsewhere. He presented in 1978 with urinary and fecal incontinence and a persistent urinary fistula. We performed an intraperitoneal revision and closed the rectourethral fistula. He improved greatly and when seen in 1988, he had normal urinary continence and fecal soiling only during episodes of diarrhea. He has not reported since (Fig. 15.5).

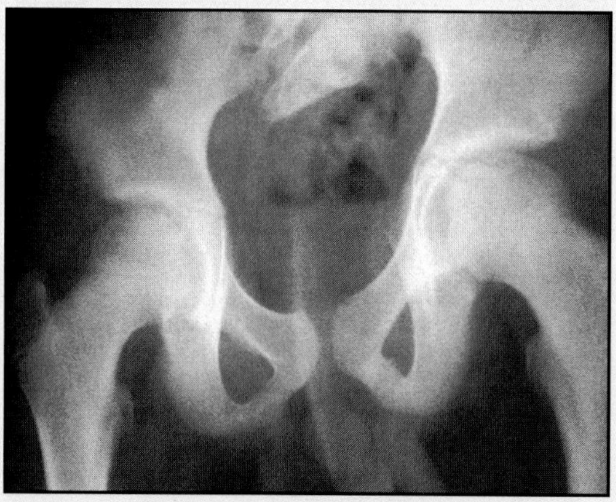

Fig. 15.5 Xray AP of patient with truncation.

The second born in 1975 also had perineal operations elsewhere and also presented in 1978 with urinary and fecal incontinence and a persisting urinary fistula; he also had prolapse at the neoanus and retained feces. We decided to do a revisional SPR (Fig. 15.6). In the process, we inadvertently opened up the subarachnoid space. We repaired the meninges and then completed the operation. His urinary

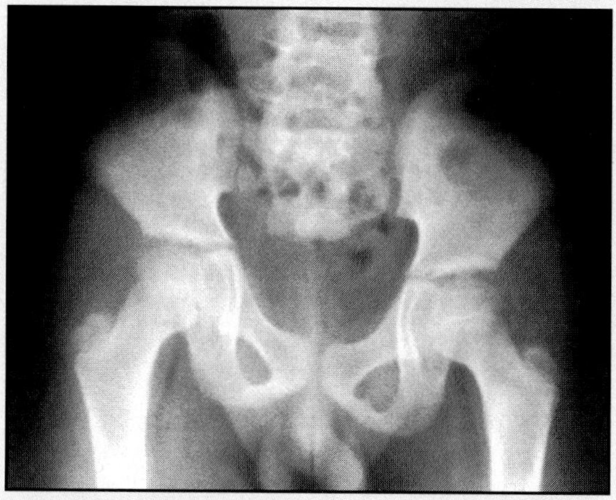

Fig. 15.6 Xray AP of patient with truncation.

continence improved but he continued to have retained feces with considerable soiling. Nothing was done for 17 years. The family finally agreed to a revisional PSARP in 1995. There was a huge megarectum that could only be tapered after opening the pelvic peritoneum. The musculature was repaired around the bowel and a concurrent colostomy was done. After colostomy closure, his continence improved remarkably. He works as a commercial artist and remains clean with a minimum of medication (Figs. 15.7-8).

This misadventure has taught us to make sure that the upper limit of the incision for PSARP should stop short of the skeleton for a patient with a truncated sacrum; separation of the levator ani should begin well below the last extant piece of sacrum.

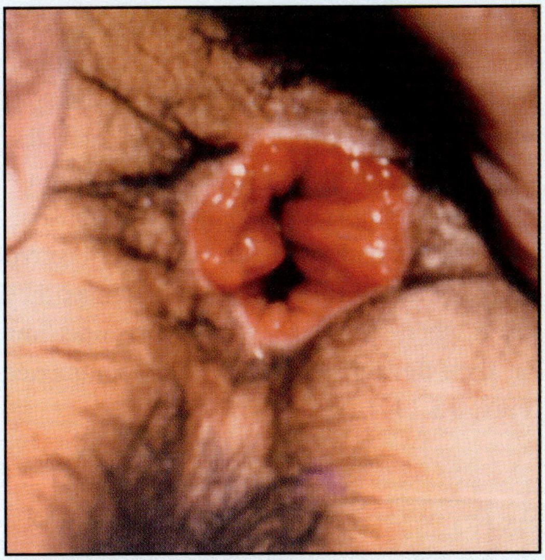

Fig. 15.7 Photograph of perineum of boy with truncated sacrum and incontinence after earlier surgery.

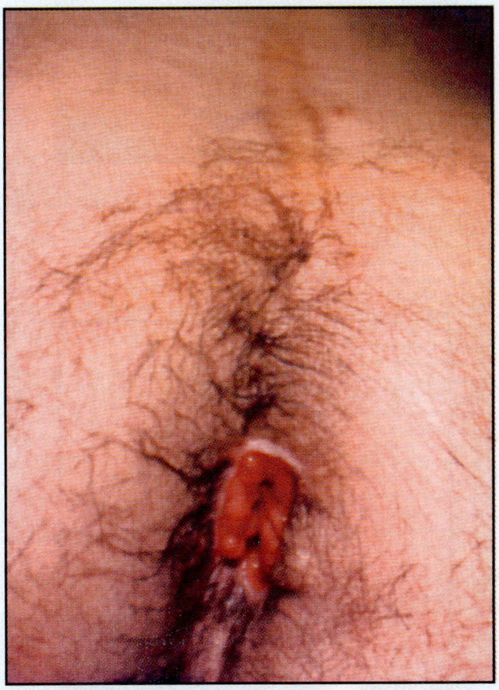

Fig. 15.8 Photograph of above after revisional PSARP showing improvement.

The third patient was born in 1977. He had a neonatal colostomy; he then had SPR with closure of the rectourethral fistula and subsequent closure of the colostomy in 1978. Since then he has had intractable constipation and fecal and urinary incntinence and reached us in 1987. He had masses of retained feces. He had a patulous anus. Sacral truncation was seen on Xray and Barium enema showed a huge rectal ectasia with colon of normal size opening into it. After routine preparation, a revisional PSARP and a concurrent colostomy was done with effect; the bowel was extensively tapered and the muscles repaired around it. Urinary function improved immediately and bowel function was restored after the colostomy was closed

We have done PSARP on 2 boys, in 1986 and in 1994. They are both improving with time. The first has normal urinary continence and requires some therapy to keep clean. The second has multiple malformations, the most disabling being agenesis of the right lung and absent right radial ray. His continence is improving with time and very little support is required. More recently, Das has done PSARP on 2 boys; one was 9 months old; he has poor urinary control and has 3-4 stools a day with soiling; the other was 21 months old, had penoscrotal transposition with chordee; he has 3-4 stools but does not soil.

Our patient with rectoperineal fistula and multiple malformations has been described in Chapter 7. He had a neonatal ASARP in 1990 and has had normal fecal continence. After surgery for perineal hypospadias with severe chordee and penoscrotal transposition, urinary continence has improved over the years and is now almost normal.

The 2 girls were pygopagus twins born in December 1982. They shared a common perineum with separate anal, vaginal and urethral orifices disposed in an L shaped fashion (Fig. 15.9).

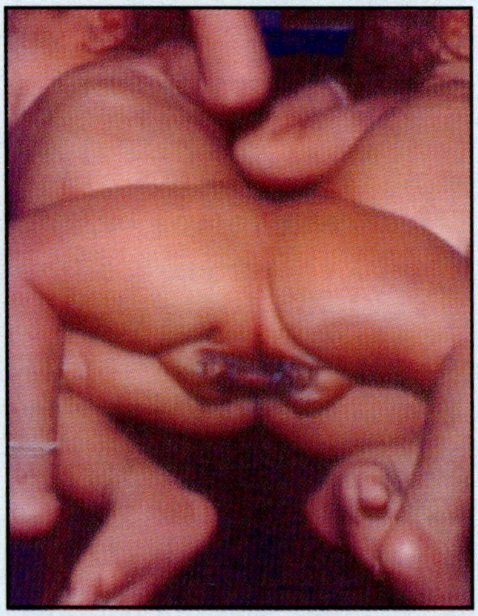

Fig. 15.9 Photograph of pygopagus conjoined twins.

They shared the striated muscle complex and muscles of the perineum and pelvic floor. They also had a common sacrum and a common subarachnoid space (Fig. 15.10).

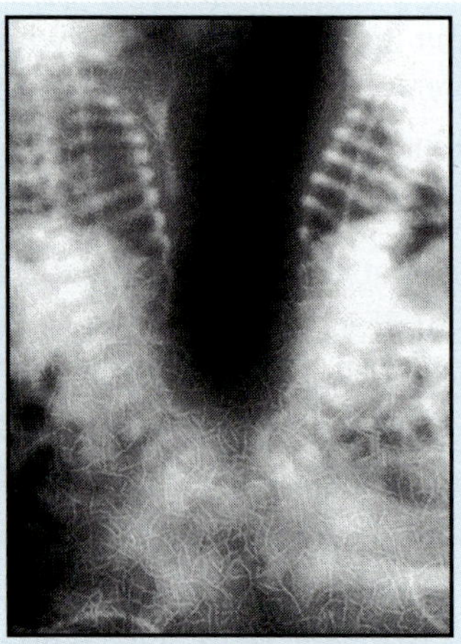

Fig. 15.10 X ray of above showing shared spine.

Defunctioning colostomies were carried out at the age of 3 months, and separation at the age of 4 months. The sacrum was split into 2 from below the level of the sacroiliac joints. The spinal cords and cauda equinas were macroscopically separate. The muscles of the pelvis and perineum could be repaired easily. After closure of the colostomies they soiled when stools were loose for some time but then developed normal fecal continence (Figs. 15.11-12).

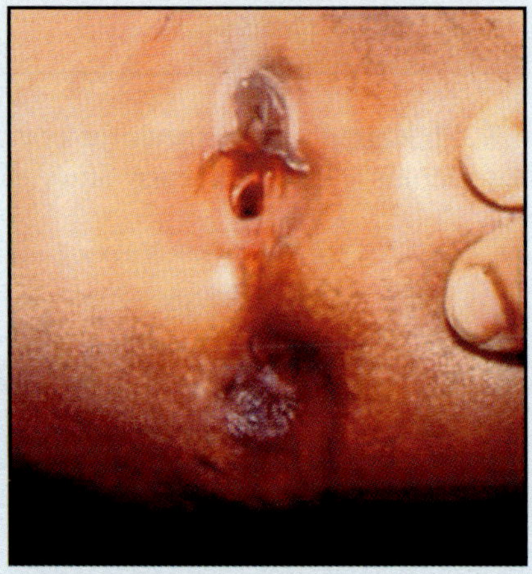

Fig. 15.11 Photograph of Twin A's perineum after surgery.

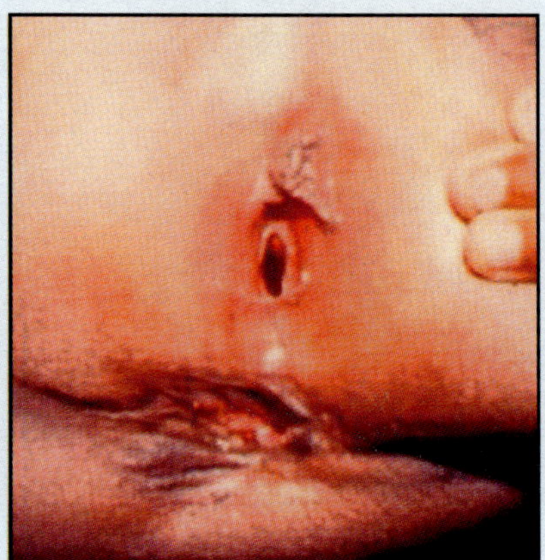

Fig. 15.12 Photograph of Twin B's perineum after surgery.

However, they had other problems connected with a shared subarachoid space and cauda equina. Each had only 2 segments of sacrum (Figs. 15.13-14). Twin B required treatment for paresis of some of the muscles of the left ankle and foot but had normal urinary continence. Twin A developed a neurogenic bladder but the foster parents would not bring her for follow-up for many years. When she ultimately turned up, she had obstructive uropathy and chronic renal failure. The magnitude of the problem was explained to the foster parents but they would not heed medical advice for its management either by CIC or by diversion. She finally died in 2002 of endstage renal disease at the age of 19 years.

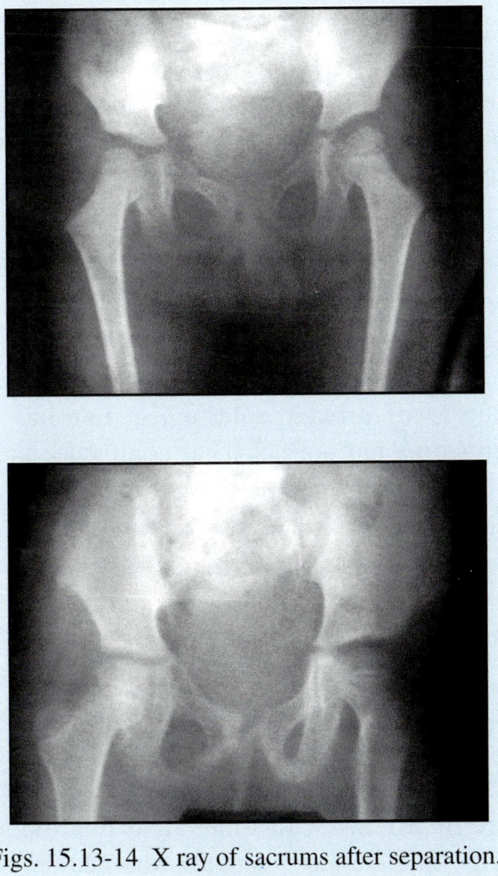

Figs. 15.13-14 X ray of sacrums after separation.

Truncation with High Anomalies

Problems of truncation in patients with high ARMs are compounded by associated malformations of the urinary tract and the fact that high anomalies are associated with poor striated muscles. Moreover whatever nerves are available are very close to the midline and hence vulnerable to injury during the course of the anorectoplasty.

We have 5 boys; 3 had been submitted to SAPR with endorectal pullthrough for a high anomaly without a fistula in the 1970s. All 3 had initially poor bowel function with accumulated feces and soiling, but one was looked after by a doting mother and the other 2 by doting grandmothers.

The first patient born in 1972 had urinary continence but suffered from urinary tract infections due to malformations that were left untreated (see Chapter 10). Fecal incontinence worsened and finally when grandmother became tired, the family agreed to revisional surgery. A revisional PSARP was done in 1993. A huge megarectum was tapered to size and the muscle complex repaired. There was considerable improvement in his bowel function. His urological problems continued and disappeared only after he agreed to a right nephroureterectomy for pyonephrosis in 2003. He leads a normal life attending to the family business but needs some therapy for constipation. His only serious complaint is erectile failure; a marriage had ended disastrously!

In the second patient born in 1974, urinary problems were worse than bowel problems, and for many years he required treatment for neurogenic bladder to control hydroureteronephrosis; this included CIC. He had a megarecrum that could be kept under control with conservative therapy and a Y-V plasty at the anus. He deteriorated when his mother died, but improved and got over both disabilities with time. He leads a normal life working in information technology but needs some support for constipation. Again his only serious complaint is erectile failure; he has fortunately not married yet!

The third patient born in 1978 has never had any urinary problem. He had unfortunately a stenosis at the site of the seromuscular cuff through which the bowel had been pulled through; this was corrected after 2 laparotomies. Intestinal obstruction was finally relieved but fecal incontinence continued and by 1990, his grandmother had also become tired. Colostomy was done. The patient however wanted to swim and he was refused entry in the club of his choice because of the colostomy. In 1994 he persuaded the family to agree to revisional surgery and closure of the colostomy. The megarectum was tapered to size and the muscle complex repaired. The colostomy was then closed and defecation became almost normal. He is an executive in the family business and requires minimum therapy. However he also is worried about erectile failure.

The fourth patient was reconstructed by APARP but died following surgery to close his colostomy (see Chapter 6). The last patient had a type 1 pouch colon and has been described in Chapter 14; he is 5 years old, has an endcolostomy and minimum urinary incontinence.

We also have 3 girls. One had a high rectovaginal fistula with a cardiac mallformation and the parents left her with a colostomy; the other 2 had cloacal malformations; one was left with a colostomy and the other has had an APARP and colostomy closure 7 years ago. She had urinary and fecal incontinence but these have improved over the years.

Das has reconstructed 2 boys by PSARP with laparotomy. One aged 2 ½ years had a short colon and bowel proximal to the colostomy had been brought down to the normal anal site. He has a reasonable amount of striated muscle complex and is improving but still has urinary incontinence and frequent stools. The other aged 3 years has almost total urinary and fecal incontinence and has been lost to followup. Both had rectovesical fistulas. His third patient has been lost to followup after colostomy.

Banerjee has also reconstructed 2 boys by PSARP with laparotomy; both had Rectovesical fistulas. The operations were done 5 and 4 years ago. Both have normal urinary continence and fecal continence is improving over the years.

Thus out of 27 patients encountered over a 30 year period, 2 have died, one after colonic surgery and the other due to renal failure. Six have been lost to followup. One has a permanent colostomy with a fair degree of urinary continence; one has a urostoma but normal fecal continence and 1 has been asymptomatic all along. Revisional PSARP has been done on 4 who had been reconstructed in the pre PSARP days and had fecal incontinence. There has been marked improvement in their quality of life. Two others treated in the pre PSARP days have improved with lesser revisions. Four patients who had PSARP and 3 who had PSARP with laparotomy in the last 2 decades are improving with time. Also improving with time are the 3 patients who had minor procedures for low anomalies.

Conclusions

1. The skeletal defect does not always permit an accurate prediction of the neurological deficit.
2. The skeletal defect and also the neurological deficit may be iatrogenic.
3. The skeletal defect may be found in patients with a normal anorectum, and also in patients with low, intermediate and high anomalies; but many more patients with high anomalies are affected.
4. The functional disability of the bowel and that of the urinary bladder do not always match; there are patients with normal urinary continence and poor bowel function, and there are patients with poor urinary function and normal fecal continence.
5. Reconstructive surgery should never be refused to a patient with a truncated sacrum. If for nothing else, the fistula with the urogenital system should be eliminated. Most patients improve if there is good parental support and an adequate cerebral function. Earlier the only support therapy available was bowel evacuation by laxatives and washouts. Today with antegrade colonic enema (ACE) life with a perineal anus is far better than with a permanent colostomy.
6. For the same reasons, revisional surgery should not be generally be refused to a patient who has been incorrectly treated in the past or who has developed a severe megarectum in spite of correct treatment. The only patient left with a colostomy had a pouch colon and severe urinary tract anomalies.
7. The results of reconstruction on patients with high ARMs are known to be worse than on those with intermediate anomalies. How much worse this can become if there is sacral truncation is a matter we need to study more fully.
8. The prime objective in the management of the urinary tract is to preserve renal function. The second objective is to ensure that the patient remains dry for a reasonable length of time. With CIC both can be reached; if required a Mitrofanoff procedure can be done.
9. All our adult male patients complain about poor erectile function. They have been referred to our colleagues in andrology to find out an acceptable solution!

We have recently been consulted for a 4 year old boy on whom Basak had performed a colostomy at birth and confirmed the presence of a high ARM with a urinary fistula and sacral truncation. An episode of epididymitis in infancy was followed by repeated episodes of urinary tract infection. Basak's advice for reconstructive surgery was not taken although the boy has normal urinary continence. The family has been led to believe that the result of reconstruction on patients with sacral truncation is poor. They have also not bothered to find out what effect the fistula is having on renal function and attempt to control the recurrent episodes of urinary infection by distal colonic washouts!

TETHERED CORD

The appearance of fecal and urinary incontinence together with lower extremity weakness, numbness and pain some time after surgery for high ARMs suggests a diagnosis of tethered cord; MRI confirms the diagnosis. The problem has been discussed by Rivosechi *et al* (1995) and Levitt et al (1997). Golonka *et al* (2002) have submitted all their ARM patients to MRI studies; this has led to their diagnosing tethered cord in one third of all patients with ARM, including those without symptoms and with low or intermediate anomalies. They have advocated early surgical release in all these patients.

In our series the association of tethered cord with ARM is relatively rare and we would advise surgical release only on the patient who has clinical evidence of neurological involvement.

CHAPTER 16

RESULTS

MORTALITY

It is tempting to write that mortality is a thing of the past as far as ARMs are concerned. Although the picture has vastly improved from the period when we first started, patients with ARM still die all over the world. The reasons are as follows

1. Associated malformations, mainly cardiac malformations, esophageal atresia, gastroschisis and vesicointestinal fissure, and gross renal dysplasia. These have been discussed in Chapter 3.
2. Complications resulting from delay in seeking treatment. Newborns still present with pneumoperitoneum, aspiration of vomit, fluid and electrolyte imbalance, and septicemia. If they survive the neonatal period without treatment or with inadequate treatment, they may present with chronic intestinal obstruction, severe urinary tract infection and protein-energy malnutrition.
3. Very low birth weight and weight well below the optimum percentile in the postneonatal period.
4. Acquired diseases, mainly infections of the gastrointestinal and respiratory tract.
5. Incorrect management. These have been discussed in earlier chapters. Faults in management begin with the inability of the persons conducting the delivery of the baby to detect the ARM immediately after birth and to advise the family about what to do. Subsequently there is delay in seeking treatment in a proper place because of failure of pediatricians and other providers of health care to appreciate the problem posed by ARMs that are not instantly lethal but potentially lifethreatening. The surgeon who sees the patient first has to decide whether he will treat on the spot or refer elsewhere. This is one of the most difficult decisions that a peripheral surgeon in the developing world has to make. We have tried to post guidelines and suggest three levels of management; one suitable for emergency management in a setup with limited facilities; another suitable for a good general surgery organization with basic arrangements for pediatric surgery and the third for a well equipped pediatric surgical service. If management is tailored to the facilities available, the chances of incorrect treatment should be much less.

In PCC, neonatal mortality over the last two decades has been restricted to five. Two died after primary reconstruction, one had long gap esophageal atresia and a cardiac malformation and had ASARP, and the other had septicemia after PSARP. There were three deaths after colostomy; one came with pneumoperitoneum and two others had necrotizing enterocolitis in the postoperative period.

In a busy public hospital like the NRS Medical College, the picture is a lot worse for the reasons mentioned earlier. Out of the 135 neonates admitted annually with ARM, 80 had colostomy with 25 deaths, 24 had surgery for low anomalies with 2 deaths and 31 were not operated upon; of these 12 died. Deaths were mostly due to delayed presentation, associated anomalies and very low birth weight. These figures can be compared with Cook's 1990 report from Liverpool in which the mortality was 15.6% in babies with high and intermediate anomalies and 5.4% in babies with low anomalies. A further problem in NRS is that a sizeable number of neonates do not report back after discharge and some undoubtedly die.

Deaths after treatment in the postneonatal period have been rare in both institutions in the last 2 decades; they have been mainly due to renal failure and to complications following laparotomy. There have been deaths after abdominoperineal reconstruction, colonorrhaphy for pouch colon and difficult colostomy.closure. In PCC there have been only 2 deaths. Both followed discontinuance of colostomy. One had a left upper quadrant colostomy elsewhere and then an APARP for a high anomaly. Resection of the colostomy and end to end anastomosis was carried out, but after 5 days, peritonitis and septicemia set in. No doubt the left branch of the middle colic artery which was the sole artery supplying the pulled through bowel had been damaged during the mobilization. The second patient had a colonorrhaphy for a type 2 pouch followed by APARP. After discontinuance of the ascending colostomy, he also developed overwhelming peritonitis and septicemia. There have been no deaths in the last 15 years and none have followed extraperitoneal reconstructions.

MORBIDITY

Three factors are responsible for morbidity.

1. **The anomaly has been left untreated**. The results of not treating the different anomalies have already been discussed.
2. **The anomaly has been incorrectly treated**. Incorrect treatment may be due to:
   i) Failure to assess the patient as a whole. Assessment includes a proper systemic study of the patient to discover and deal with the myriad of disorders that an infant in the developing world is prone to suffer from; namely anemia, malnutrition, tuberculosis, diarrhea, helminthiasis and respiratory infections. Secondly, the associated anomalies already described have to be detected and attended to; the most important anomalies that need attention are those of the urinary tract.

   ii) Failure to control wound infection. The main source of infection is of course the large bowel. The methods of containing this have greatly improved over the years. With good bowel preparation, infection of the wound or the peritoneum should not occur in the course of elective surgery. They have not occurred in our patients in the last 2 decades; earlier we have had wound disruptions after PAT, PSARP and colostomy closure.

iii) Failure to minimize tissue trauma by deft handling of the tissues and careful repair with appropriate suture material. Of the structures that are likely to be injured in the course of reconstructive surgery the most vulnerable is the small bowel. Loops of small bowel adhere to the colostomy site and the pelvic floor and need to be carefully separated; if the injury is recognized and repaired there should be no problem. Injuries to normally placed urological structures should not occur at all. The only structure that we have injured is the urethra, once during a neonatal reconstruction by SPR and once during a redo; it was repaired on the spot. We have divided a vas deferens once in the course of one of our earliest PSARPs and a seminal vesicle once in the course of a redo. We are surprised to note that there were 19 injuries in 572 patients in a leading center and that 110 patients were referred to this center with urological injuries (Hong *et al*, 2002). The reason suggested was failure to do a preoperative distal cologram. We have twice injured the vagina, once in the course of a difficult cloacal reconstruction and once during a redo for a duplex vagina; the vagina was repaired on the spot. We have pointed out in Chapter 2 that the pelvic nerves run on either side of the bowel and almost reach the midline when the bowel ends high up. They are thus extremely vulnerable if the dissection strays to one or other side, and the endresult is neurogenic bladder and loss of erectile function. Also, the diaphragm fibers of the levator ani and the striated muscle complex can be damaged in the course of a difficult abdominoperineal pull-through, and in the course of a sagittal procedure if the dissection strays away from the midline. If not recognized and repaired, some degree of fecal incontinence is inevitable. The most critical injury is the one that involves the blood supply of the bowel used for the reconstruction. A successful repair demands an adequate blood supply to the tissues used. If perfusion is insufficient, the wounds will not heal and some tissue will necrose and be lost. We have lost segments of pulled through bowel twice; once during an APARP with insufficient bowel distal to the colostomy and once during bowel reconstruction of one of the ischiopagus twins, described in Chapter 14.

iv) Failure to provide meticulous postoperative surveillance so that complications are recognized early and steps are taken in time. The role of the anesthesiologist in reducing morbidity cannot be overemphasized.

3. In the present state of our knowledge, **the problems posed by the anomaly cannot be completely resolved**. These are:

i) Sacral truncation with loss of nerve supply to the bowel and the lower urinary tract discussed in Chapter 15.
ii) Type 1 and type 2 Pouch colon discussed in Chapter 14.
iii) High cloacal anomalies with their attendant urinary and genital problems discussed in Chapter 11.
iv) Very high lesions in both boys and girls associated with poorly formed levator ani and striated muscle complex; during pullthrough a compromise has to be made between narrowing the bowel and preserving the muscular trajectory.

LONG TERM RESULTS

We have stated in Chapter 5 that the three objectives of management are

1. to prevent or relieve intestinal obstruction
2. to establish normal defecation and
3. to preserve or restore normal urogenital function.

It is convenient to start with **urogenital function** and to discuss the *2* others later.

Normal urogenital function implies in the first place **that all fistulous communications are eliminated.** This can be achieved in all patients, either at the end of the first definitive operation or by a revisional operation. In our series, all fistulas in boys and most fistulas in girls have been eliminated.

Second, **renal structure and function needs to be preserved.** Renal status deteriorates if there is vesicoureteral reflux and unrelieved obstruction in the ureter, the bladder outlet, the male urethra or the female urethra. All of these predispose to recurrent upper tract infection and all of these are curable with appropriate therapy.

Third, **bladder function needs to be preserved**. The objective of normal urinary continence with no residual urine may not be achievable if there is congenital or acquired loss of bladder innervation. If a tethered cord is the cause, this can be released. The bladder can be kept empty by simple procedures like CIC or by some form of diversion. A continuous involuntary passage of urine with a relatively empty bladder is troublesome but less harmful than retention with overflow. If the latter is left untreated as it sometimes is, chronic renal failure sets in.

Fourth, **sexual function needs to be preserved**. The problems differ in boys and girls.

The major problem in boys is erectile failure due to congenital or acquired loss of sacral nerves. Most boys with truncated sacrums regain bowel and bladder function in course of time, but none of the 6 boys in our series who are now adults have satisfactory erections. This complication has not occurred in any of the boys with normal sacrums on whom we have done anorectoplasty. Three boys had reflux into the ejaculatory ducts and consequent epididymitis; it was so serious in one that the vas had to be divided to give relief. One patient who did not have erectile problems was infertile because of an acquired fistula between the seminal vesicles and the bowel. If there is reflux into the ejaculatory ducts in childhood sperm counts are likely to be low in adult life.

The problem is different in girls. Associated malformations of the uterus and vagina give rise to urological complications in infancy and childhood, and these may lead to progressive loss of renal function. Undetected, untreated and incompletely treated malformations give rise to problems during menarche in the form of amenorrhea and dysmenorrhea, and this is the time that parents wake up and bring the girls for followup. Girls treated for cloacal anomalies occasionally require revisional surgery to enlarge the size of the vagina at this time. Two of our cloaca patients are happily married but neither have conceived so far; Both have duplex systems but they have not yet had studies to assess the state of their uterine tubes. On the other hand, girls with a capacious vagina do not have problems with intercourse even in the presence of an untreated fistula between the bowel and the urogenital tract.

Relief of intestinal obstruction is of course the prime objective of surgery for ARM. It is relatively easy to ensure an unobstructed pathway for bowel contents to pass to the exterior, but not so easy to ensure that this passage shall be under voluntary control. The elements necessary for this have been described in Chapter 2. The clinical methods of assessing function have been described in Chapter 1.

THE FINAL FUNCTIONAL RESULT

This depends on several factors

1. The basic anatomy of the malformation

Most elements for good function are present in patients with low anomalies like anal stenosis, anoperineal fistula, anovesti-bular fistula, low agenesis without fistula, funnel anus, low fistula with a normal anus and perineal groove; they are also present in patients with rectal atresia and stenosis. These are Category A patients (40% of our patients). They should indeed gain normal continence after correct treatment. However the exquisite sensation of the anal canal is absent in all of them except in those with rectal atresia and its variants.

There are major deficiencies if the bowel ends high up with or without a colonic malformation; intraperitoneal reconstruction is necessary. and the deficiencies cannot be fully compensated by present day surgery. Patients with these lesions are placed in Category C (10% of our patients). They are unlikely to gain normal continence but a reasonable quality of life can be attained

All the other patients fall in Category B (50% of our patients); results depend on type of management.

2. The quality and timing of the surgery

A great deal depends on the surgeon 'who performs the first operation on the malformed rectum' (Potts). A reckless perineal exploration or an incorrect reconstruction can be revised to a great extent by secondary surgery, but the damage cannot be totally erased. If the procedures described in this book for the different malformations are followed, most Category B patients will enjoy a normal quality of life and most Category C patients will attain a reasonable standard of social acceptability. A great deal also depends on the timing of the reconstruction. According to the members of 'imperforate anus initiative', an early reconstruction is more important than a meticulous reconstruction.

We studied the effect of timing on 50 boys with intermediate anomalies who had PSARP after a neonatal colostomy; 25 were treated in NRS and 25 in PCC. The colostomy was discontinued at the mean age of 34 months in the first group (12 to 84 months) and at the mean age of 15 months in the second (5 to 30 months). Bowel function improved much earlier in the latter.

3. Postoperative care

The development of the human brain depends on nutrition and on inputs by the family and the environment. Fecal continence depends a great deal on afferent impulses from the anorectal area; the sooner and more frequently these reach the brain, the better is function likely to be. Dilatation of the neoanus and anorectum should commence soon after reconstruction; then when the children can cooperate they are asked to squeeze on the examiner's finger in the rectum. Later they are taught to empty the bowels by coordinated contraction of the abdominal and perineal muscles and to hold the bowel contents by contraction of the sphincter complex. In order to ensure proper emptying, the stools should be kept at an optimum consistency with diet containing proper roughage; also, items that cause diarrhea should be withheld. The family has to be taught to avoid fecal retention at all costs; if necessary by the use of laxatives, suppositories and washouts. The majority of patients do well with relatively simple management. Some continue to suffer from incontinence either with constipation or with diarrhea; they require a more elaborate bowel management program; one such program has been outlined by Pena *et al* in 1998. The socioeconomic and educational status of the family and the efforts made by it for the child's development are of paramount importance. The role of the parents in managing a child with treated ARM has been described by Hassink *et al* in 1998.

4. Associated anomalies

These have beendescribed earlier. The anomalies that greatly affect quality of life are urological disorders, disorders of the brain and special senses.

ASSESSMENT OF CONTINENCE

Subjective

Our subjective assessment of continence is based on a procedure that we name 3P.

The first P stands for **Parents**. Parents are questioned about the child's performance at home, at school and with his peers; with particular emphasis on whether there is improvement or regression. They are also questioned about whether any therapy is given by way of medicine or dietary measures and the effect of discontinuance of such therapy. Finally a parent can often predict the functional result fairly early in the child's life by observing his or her efforts when the anorectum is full.

The second P stands for **Pants**. These should be counted and examined for fecal staining or worse.

The third P stands for the **Patient**. Examination includes a general survey to assess nutritional and intellectual status, an abdominal examination for evidences of fecal and urinary retention and an examination of the perineum. The position, shape and size of the anus, and the presence or absence of a fistula, prolapse or scarring is recorded. If there is no scarring, a digital examination of the anorectum is carried out to assess the caliber of the bowel, its sensory perception, the musculature of the region and the volume of accumulated feces if any. Finally the efficiency of bladder emptying is observed.

Objective

A variety of methods are available.

Imaging

Defecograms were suggested as early as 1969 by Kelly and Stephens. The child sat on a radiolucent commode after a solution of contrast was instilled into the large gut. Lateral Xrays were taken at rest, when the child evacuated and during attempted holding. The size of the bowel was seen, and also the presence or absence of the anorectal angle, the ability to empty and the ability to hold back bowel contents. The advent of CT and MRI has made this investigation obsolete.

CT scans have been particularly useful for patients who are not doing well after reconstructive surgery. It shows a megarectum, if present, it also shows whether the pullthrough had missed the sphincter complex or whether the muscles of the region were too hypoplastic to be of use (Figs. 16.1-3). The advent of spiral CT has greatly improved the accuracy of this investigation.

MRI scans, free from ionizing radiation, give more information than CT. If cost is not a factor, it is today the method of choice for showing the post reconstruction scenario It also shows in the course of a single examination, the state of the urogenital organs and the spine, spinal cord and cauda equina (Figs. 16.4-8).

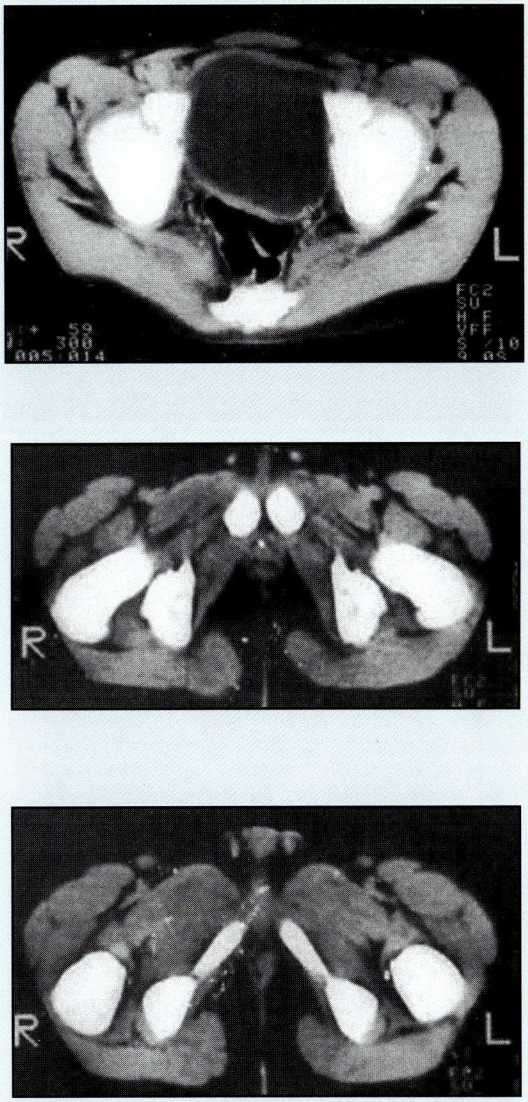

Figs. 16.1-3 CT scan of boy with truncated sacrum after SAPR showing poor striated muscles but good position of bowel; has become continent in adolescence.

The latest entry is **anal endosongraphy**. According to Emblem and his colleagues

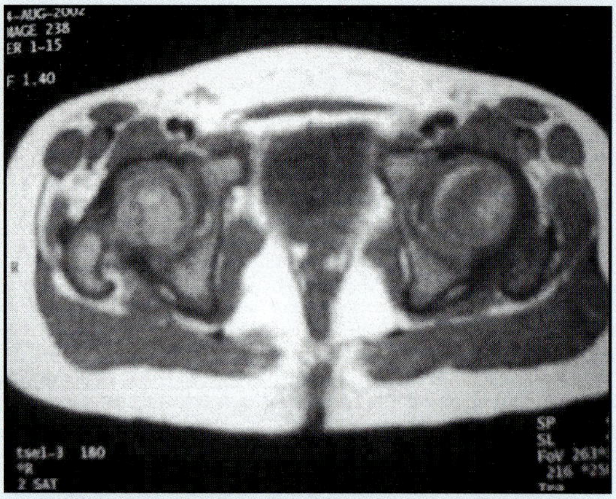

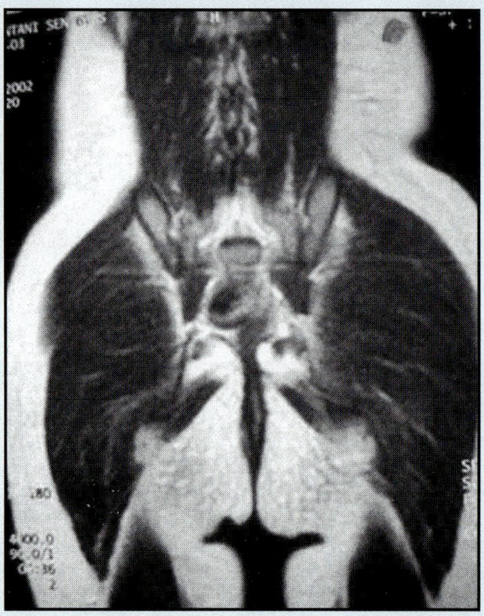

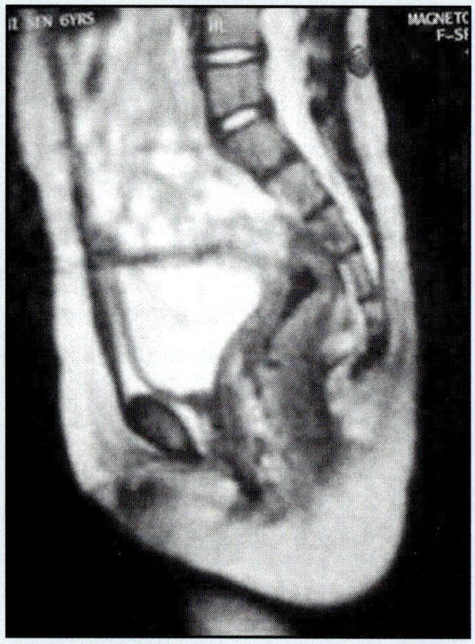

Figs. 16.4-6 MRI scan of girl after PSARVUP, showing good disposition of muscles, gut and urogenital organs; she has normal fecal and urinary continence.

(1994,1997), this is the least uncomfortable procedure of all, even less than a digital examination of the anorectum. It clearly showed internal anal sphincter (IAS) and external anal sphincter (EAS) in the 14 normal adolescents they studied. They also studied 16 adolescents operated for high and intermediate anomalies and 17 operated for low anomalies. They found that IAS was absent in all and varying degrees of scarring was seen in EAS. Moreover, the investigation revealed eccentricity of the anal canal if present. The findings corresponded with the functional state of the patient; they were normal in those who had normal continence, greatly abnormal in those who had soiling and mildly abnormal in those with only staining. We have no experience.

Electrical

By **Electromanometry** we record the pressure at different levels of the anorectum at rest, during voluntary activity and in response to artificial stimulation. Sensing catheters with balloons are placed in the lumen of the bowel at 3 different levels and connected to sensitive transducers. We can measure the mean basal pressure, the squeeze pressure and the postinflation pressure in cm. of water using a computerized instrument made by Readystock. We can also record the minimum pressure in ml. of air that produced a sensation of fulness.

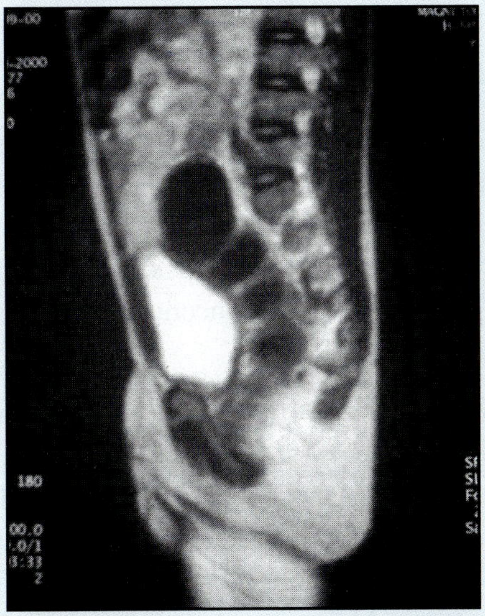

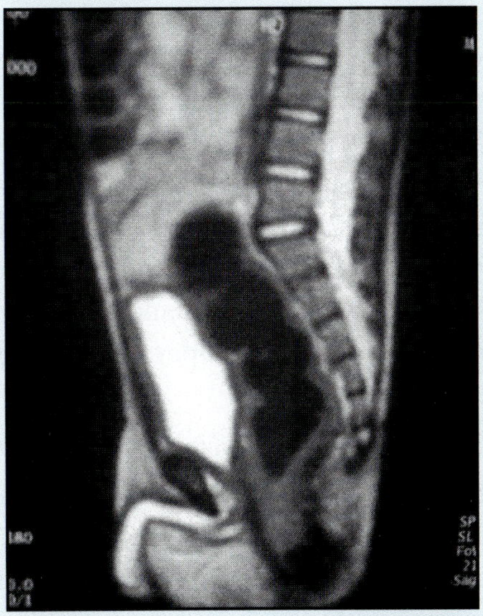

Figs. 16.7-8 MRI scan of boy after PSARP elsewhere, showing anterior placement of bowel with stenosis and proximal dilatation; had successful revisional surgery.

An extension of the above is **Biofeedback** (Engel 1974, Olness *et al* 1980, Rintala *et al* 1988). This can be used to improve the functional status of children who remain incontinent. The patient is given an opportunity to compare the manometric response to his own squeeze with that of a normal subject, and he is encouraged to try and reduce the gap.

By **Electromyography** the electrical changes in different striated muscle groups at rest and during different types of activity is recorded in millivolts.

In the course of our studies on truncated sacrums in 1995, we examined with the above mentioned devices 10 boys with repaired ARMs between the ages of 5 and 15 years. Four had normal sacrums and 6 had truncated sacrums; of the latter 4 had revisional surgery and 2 although advised redos had not had this done at the time. The patients complained about the discomfort and the inconvenience and the information by and large corroborated our clinical assessment. The investigation was subsequently abandoned but while it was in use biofeedback did motivate some children to improve on their efforts.

FINAL PLACEMENT

We believe that a simple classification based on the Wingspread chart is very necessary. We place our patients in 3 baskets, as suggested by Suruga (1998).

Those in the first basket are **HAPPY**. They have no serious uncorrected associated anomaly. Their fecal and urinary continence is almost normal, soiling is either absent or minimal, and fecal retention is also either absent or minimal They need little or no therapy to remain clean. They thus fall into Wingspread groups 1 and 2.1. Almost all our Category A patients and the majority of Category B patients become HAPPY before they reach the school going age. About half of our Category B patients require therapy up to the age of 5 years to keep them HAPPY.

In the third basket are the **GLOOMY** patients. They are shunned by their peers and cannot lead a normal life. They remain in the Wingspread groups 3.2 and 4. They become socially acceptable only if they are given a great deal of therapy by the families and by the doctors. We have several examples of such patients. They were Category C patients and the initial surgery also was not up to the standard of the 21st century; nevertheless with the support of their families they coped with their disabilities and lead a reasonably normal life as adults.

All other patients fall in the **INTERMEDIATE** basket, namely in Wingspread groups 2.2 and 3.1. Most become happy in course of time if they are properly managed. If they are not properly managed at home and do not report for follow up at proper intervals, they suffer from retention with overflow and ultimately slide into the gloomy group. This is the common story of patients in the lower socioeconomic strata of society. In spite of good reconstructive surgery, they do not become happy.

Unfortunately, a few Category A patients do not become happy in spite of good initial therapy. They have an adequate neoanus but suffer from intractable constipation with soiling because they have developed rectal ectasia (Chapter 14) with massive dilatation of the rectum and sometimes of part of the sigmoid.

We have been struck by the similarity between Suruga's baskets and the 3 groups suggested by Kiesewetter and Chang in 1977. Their groups were 'good' 'fair' and 'poor'. The 'good' category were continent most of the time, suffering occasional soiling during diarrhea or stress, the 'fair' category had soiling or staining with normal consistency of stool and the 'poor' category were frankly incontinent with only occasional control.

We believe that the status of most GLOOMY patients can be improved by revisional surgery of some kind or other. Minor revisions include enlarging a stenotic orifice or eliminating a superficial fistula or a prolapse. Major revisions require disconnection of deep fistulas, tapering or resecting dilated bowel and placing the bowel within the striated muscle complex. Pena 1983, Brain and Kiely (1989), Chadha (1993), Li *et al* (2000), Kulshrestha *et al* (2000), Tsugawa *et al* (2000) and Hrabovszky and Dewan (2002) have described their experience with revisional PSARP. Except for Brain and Kiely all the others feel that the reoperation has been worthwhile.

We have done **Revisional PSARP** on 17 boys and 5 girls; 5 had sacral truncation and 4 had rectal ectasia. In one the colostomy had not been closed; all the others were done with a concurrent colostomy. The quality of life of most patients improved greatly and they climbed to groups 2.12 or 2.22. However, a few gloomy patients with a bad family history and low intelligence did not improve even after revisional surgery.

Over the last 2 decades, numerous longterm studies have been reported. Templeton and Dietsheim's study of 1985 describing 61 patients treated by SPR, SAPR and APR is the most interesting because the second author himself was one of the subjects studied; 70% of the SPR, 38.5% of the SAPR and 50% of the APR had good results. Ong and Beasley in 1991 studied 20 patients operated by SPR and 17 by SAPR and found that 20% had poor results.

In 1988, Pena described his study of the first 322 patients treated by PSARP; 171 were available for followup and their voluntary bowel movement, soiling and constipation was recorded; patients with low anomalies did better and patients with sacral anomalies fared less well. Langemeljer and Molenaar found that of their 37 patients treated by PSARP and available for study in 1991, only 1 was fully continent and 2 were continent with soiling. Bliss *et al* reporting in 1996 on 48 patients treated by PSARP found that 20 did well, 20 were occasionally well and 8 had no awareness.

Low lesions were studied by Yeung and Kiely (1991); of 32 patients 10% had soiling and 25% had intractable constipation. Ong and Beasley's figures for low lesions (1990) were better; while 90% had acceptable continence 5 patients required prolonged therapy. In 1997, Rintala's group compared 40 children operated for low anomalies with 54 normal children and found that only half of the operated children had normal bowel function.

Earlier, in 1995, Rintala and Lindahl had compared 46 patients treated by PSARP with preservation of the internal sphincter with 70 healthy children; they found that 35% had normal continence and another 35% had good continence.

In 2 articles in 1995 and 1996, Ludman and Spitz described coping strategies adopted by children after surgery for ARM. They collected as many as 160 children between the ages of 6 and 16 with fecal incontinence. They suggested that regardless of level of continence, these children were at risk for difficulties with psychological adjustments; hence psychological evaluation and guidance to the parents should be started early.

In 1998, Kiely and Pena analysed nearly 250 patients operated for ARM. They found that 74.3% had voluntary bowel movement, 57% had soiling and 40.8% were totally continent. Patients with low anomalies and those with rectal atresia and stenosis did better than the others.

In 2001, Rintala's group reported on 22 pubertal and postpubertal patients. They found that bowel function improved with age in 19; half the patients were fully continent, 14% had occasional soiling and 22% had frequent soiling.

Varma our colleague in Calicut reported on 84 patients in 1991, 16 treated by APR, 25 by SAPR and 43 by SPR. This appears to be the only longterm Indian study apart from our own published in the same year.

We find it very difficult to compare results because while the word 'low' is relatively clear, the words 'intermediate' and 'high' appear to mean different things to different authors. Our definitions stated in Chapter 5, does not leave any scope for ambiguity and if these are followed comparisons will be much easier.

The 2 operations that we have done most commonly for patients with intermediate lesions are PAT for vestibular fistula and PSARP for a variety of anomalies. Not a single patient with an intact sacrum has true fecal incontinence. The commonest long-term problem is constipation, seen in about 50% in the first year and gradually declining to about 5% in 5 years. If constipation is not treated, there will be staining or soiling and there will be overflow incontinence if diarrhea is induced by laxatives. Constipation may be due to narrowing at the outlet or higher up or to associated aganglionosis or hypothyroidism. It may also be due to ectasia.

Patients who continue to remain incontinent either after correct treatment or after revision can now be offered **Antegrade Continent Enema (ACE)**. The operation first described by Malone in 1988 consisted of an appendicostomy through which an antegrade colonic enema could be given; this avoided the insertion of a tube through the anus for the same purpose. The initial complex operation of disconnecting the appendix and reversing it has now given place to a simpler procedure of using the tip of the appendix as a stoma. It can be done laparoscopically relatively easily. The main complication is stomal stenosis; this may require correction by a relatively easy procedure (Graf *et al* 1998, Wilcox and Kiely, 1998,Curry *et al*, 1999).

However, while we have done this operation for myelomeningocele, we have not had an opportunity to do it even once for ARM. The reasons are as follows.

i) a successful enema takes about one hour to perform and it should be done daily

ii) there must not be any distal stenosis; if there is, it should be treated first; this means an additional operation

iii) there must be an adequate length of colon; thus patients with pouch colon who really need this kind of support are debarred.

The final option is reversion to **permanent colostomy.** We have seen a number of adults operated elsewhere for ARM and living with this; they would not submit themselves to another attempt. Three patients treated by us are living with a permanent colostomy. Two had pouch colons and have been described in Chapter 14; reconstruction failed in one and could not be done in the other. The third had vesicointestinal fissure; he has had multiple operations, as a result of which he has urinary continence and a satisfactory end colostomy. He does not want any more operations. All other patients, even those with fecal retention with overflow are surviving with some kind of bowel management program and are not asking for colostomy.

There may be many reasons why our results are generally better than what has been reported from the developed world. The one striking difference in postoperative manage-ment is the mode of defecation. The vast majority of persons in the developing world **defecate in the squatting position** (Fig 16.9). The role of squatting both for parturi-tion and for defecation has recently been evaluated. Squatting realigns the pelvis to increase the opening at the bottom by up to 15 to 30%. The abdominal muscles and abdominal contents are supported by the thighs and this assists elimination of both fetus and feces. Evacuation of feces is also easier in the squatting position because the colon aligns itself naturally with the rectum and anus, which then opens completely and effortlessly. It is time that we undertake a double blind control study to find out whether or not squatting improves the longterm results of operations for ARM.

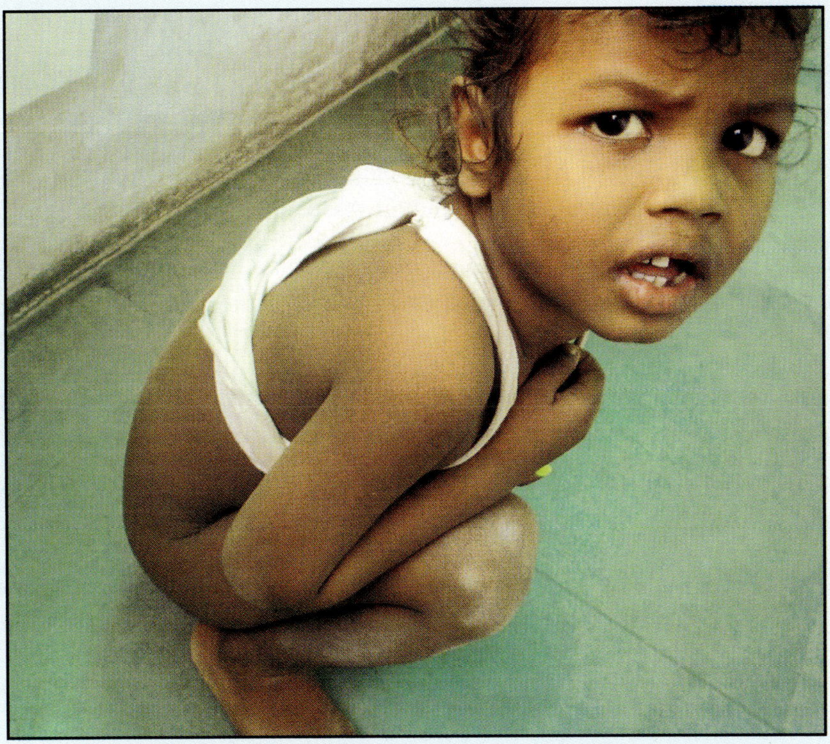

Fig. 16.9 Position adopted by our babies during defecation.

BIBLIOGRAPHY

Agarwal S, Patnaik R. Review of cases of short colon, World Congress of Pediatric Surgery, Bombay, 1980.

Agarwal S, Srinivas M, Bajpai M, *et al.* Associated anomalies in anorectal malformation . Paper read at the 29th Congress of the Indian Association of Pediatric Surgeons, 2003.

Al-Basam A, Sheikh MA, Al-Smayer A *et al.* Congenital H-type anourethral fistula with severe urethral hypoplasia : Case report and review of literature. J Pediatr Suirg 1998; 33: 1550-1553.

Aluwihare A. Primary perineal rectovaginoanoplasty for supralevator imperforate anus in female neonates. J Pediatr Surg 1990; 25: 278-281.

Aluwihare A. Imperforate anus in male children a new operation of primary perineal rectourethroanoplasty. Annals Royal Coll Surg (Eng) 1989; 71: 14-19.

Amussat JJ. Histoire d'une operation d'anus artificial practique avec success par un nouveau procede. Medical Gazette (Paris) 1935; 3: 753.

Arora M. Poster presentation at 29th Congress of Indian Association of Pediatric Surgeons, 2003.

Aslam A, Grier DJ, Duncan AW *et al.* The role of magnetic resonance imaging in the pre-operative assesment of anorectal anomalies. Pediatr Surg Int 1998; 14: 71-73.

Banerjee S. Haque J. An indigenous method of enterotomy management. J Indian Assoc Pediatr Surg 2001; 6: 77-79

Basak D, Banerjee S, Basak M *et al.* Cystic duplication of the Rectum – Our experience. J Indian Assoc Pediatr Surg 1995; Inaug No: 35-38.

Basak D. Is all cutaneous fistula with ARM a low anomaly 28th Congress of the Indian Association of Pediatric Surgeons 2002.

Basu AK, Bomayya N, Banerjee S *et al.* Pulmonary Agenesis – our experience. J Indian Assoc Pediatr Surg 2000; 5: 117-121.

Bellinger MF, Duckett JW. Accessory phallic urethra in the female patient. J Urol 1982; 127: 1159-1164.

Belman JJ. The repair of congenital H-type urethrorectal fistula using scrotal flap urethroplasty. J Urol 1977; 118: 659-661.

Bianchini MA, Fava G, Cortese MG, Vinardi S *et al.* A rare anorectal malformation: a very large H-type fistula. Pediatr Surg Int 2001; 17: 649-651

Bill AH jr, Johnson RJ. Failure of migration of the rectal opening as the cause for most cases of imperforate anus. Surg Gynec Obstet 1958; 106: 643.

Bill AH jr. Common denominators in rectal anomalies on both sides of the Atlantic. Arch Dis Child 1964; 39: 149.

Bliss DP, Tapper D, Anderson JM, *et al.* Does PSARP in patients with high imperforate anus provide superior fecal continence. J Pediatr Surg 1996; 31: 26-32.

Blunt A, Rich GE. Congenital absence of colon and rectum.Am J Dis Child 1967; 114: 405.

Bodenhammer W. Aetiology, pathology and treatment of the congenital malformations of the rectum and anus. (1860) Quoted by deVries, 1988.

Borwankar SS, Deshmukh SS. Endoscopic management of rectal atresia, 13th Conference of Indian Association of Pediatric Surgeons, Madras, 1987.

Brain AJL, Kiely EM. Posterior sagittal anorectoplasty for reoperation in children with anorectal malformation. Br J Surg 1989; 76: 57.

Brem H, Guttman FM, Laberge JM. Congenital anal fistula with normal anus. J Pediatr Surg 1989; 24: 183-185.

Brent L, Stephens FD. Primary rectal ectasia. Prog Pediatr Surg 1976; 9: 41.

Browne D. Some congenital deformities of rectum, anus, vagina and urethra. Ann Roy Coll Surg Eng 1951; 8: 173.

Browne D. Congenital deformities of the anus and rectum. Arch Dis Child 1955; 30 : 42.

Bryndorf F, Matsen CM. Ectopic anus in the female. Acta Chir Scand 1959; 118: 466.

Canil K, Fitzgerald P, Lau G *et al.* Button-pexy fixation for repair of ileostomy and colostomy prolapse. J Pediatr Surg 1995; 30: 1148-1149.

Carson JA, Barnes PD, Tunell WP *et al.* Imperforate anus : The neurological implication of sacral abnormalities. J Pediatr Surg 1984; 19: 838.

Chadha R, Bagga D, Malhotra CJ *et al.* The embryology and management of congenital pouch colon associated with anorectal agenesis. J Pediatr Surg 1994; 29: 439-446.

Chadha R, Bagga D, Mahajan JK *et al.* Congenital pouch colon revisited. J Pediatr Surg 1998; 33: 1510-1515.

Chadha R, Gupta S, Mahajan JK, *et al.* Congenital pouch colon in females. Pediatr Surg Int 1999; 15: 336-342.

Chadha R Megasigmoid associated with anorectal malformation J Indian Assoc Pediatr Surg 1999; 4: 151-155

Chadha R, Gupta S, Tanwar US *et al.* Congenital pouch colon associated with segmental dilatation of the colon. J Pediatr Surg 2001; 36: 1593-1595.

Chadha R, Bagga D, Gupta S *et al.* Congenital Pouch Colon – massive redilatation of the colon pouch after pullthrough surgery, J Pediatr Surg 2002; 37: 1376-1379

Chatterjee H. Perineal canal. 9th Congress of Asian Association of Pediatric Surgeons, Singapore, 1988.

Chatterjee SK. Rectourethral fistula. Calcutta Med J 1957; 54: 134.

Chatterjee SK, Talukder BC. Double termination of the alimentary tract in female infants. J Pediatr Surg 1969; 4: 237.

Chatterjee SK, Das S. The spreadeagled position. 34th Conference of the Association of Surgeons of India, Cuttack, 1974.

Chatterjee SK. The relation between the levator ani and the bowel in patients with anorectal malformations. Hari Om Award Lecture : Conference number – Association of Surgeons of India, 1976, p.211.

Chatterjee SK. The value of inversion radiography (invertography) in the assessment of anorectal malformations. J Indian Med Assoc 1976; 67: 165.

Chatterjee SK. Double termination of alimentary tract: A second look. J Pediatr Surg 1980; 15: 623.

Chatterjee SK, Debmaulik T, Talukder BC *et al.* Separation of pygopagus twins. Pediatr Surg Int 1986; 1: 74-78.

Chatterjee SK, Chakravarti AK, Debmaulik T *et al.* Staging the separation of ischiopagus twins. J Pediatr Surg 1988; 23: 73-75.

Chatterjee SK. Anorectal Malformations. Oxford University Press, New Delhi, India 1991; Oxford University Press, Oxford, UK, 1993.

Chatterjee SK, Banerjee S. Perineal anal transplant for vestibular fistula. Asian J Surg 1999; 22: 142-145.

Chatterjee SK, Chakravarti AK, Haque J. Conjoined Twins – Life after separation. Asian J Surg 1999; 22(3): 321-326.

Chatterjee SK. Revisional posterior sagittal anorectoplasty. J Indian Assoc Pediatr Surg 2000; 5: 43-50.

Chatterjee SK, Banerjee S, Basu AK *et al.* Rectourinary fistula with a narrow urethera. Pediatr Surg Int 2001; 17: 410-413.

Chatterjee U, Mitra J, Chatterjee SK. Pouch Colon with enteric smooth muscle abnormality. Poster at 49th Conference of the Indian Association of Pathologists and Microbiologists, 2001.

Chatterjee SK, Chatterjee US, Chatterjee U. Perineal groove with penoscrotal hypospedias. Pediatr Surg Int 2003; 19: 554-556.

Cheu HW, l Grossfeld JL. The atonic baggy rectum : A cause of intractable obstipation after imperforate anus repair. J Pediatr Surg 1992; 27: 1071-1073.

Chiba T, Kasai M, Asakura Y. Two cases of coloplasty for congenital short colon. Arch Jap Chair 1976; 45: 40.

Choi SO, Park WH. Anal canal duplication in infants. J Pediatr Surg 2003; 38: 758-762.

Cloutier R, Archambandt H, D 'Amours C *et al.* Focal ectasia of the terminal bowel accompanying low anal deformities. J Pediatr Surg 1987; 22: 758-760.

Cook RCM. Anorectal malformations, in Neonatal Surgery, Eds. Lister 3rd *et al*, 2nd Edn, Butterworths, 1990, p.556.

Cripps H. Quoted by Moore TC. Challenges in pediatric surgery. Med Intelligence Unit, R G Landes Co., Austin 1994.

Cruz E. Management of imperforate anus. 7th Congress of Asian Association of Pediatric Surgeons, 1984.

Currarino G, Coln D, Votteler T. Triad of anorectal, sacral and presacral anomalies. Am J Radiol 1981; 137: 395-396.

Curry JL, Osborne A, Malone PS. How to achieve a successful Malone ante grade continence enema. J Pediatr Surg 1998; 33: 138-141.

Curry JL, Osbome A, Malone PS. The MACE procedure. Experience in the United Kingdom. J Pediatr Surg 1999; 34: 338-40.

Demirbilek S, Atayurt HF. Anal transposition without colostomy: functional results and complications. Pediatr Surg Int 1999; 15: 221-223.

Deshpande AV, Sanghani HH, Sanghavi BV *et al.* Delayed presentation of vaginal agenesis with anorectal malformation – A unique problem. J Indian Assoc Pediatr Surg 2003; 8: 242-244.

De Vries PA, Friedland GW. Congenital H type anourethral fistula. Radiology 1974; 113: 397.

DeVries PA, Friedland GW. The staged sequential development of the anus and rectum in human embryos and fetuses. J Pediatr Surg 1974; 9: 755.

DeVries PA, Pena A. Posterior sagittal anorectoplasty. J Pediatr Surg 1982; 17: 638-643.

DeVries PA, Cox KL. Surgery of anorectal anomalies. Surg Clin North Am 1985; 65: 1139.

DeVries PA. Results of treatment and their assessment. Anorectal malformations in children, update. Eds. Stephens FD, Smith ED. Liss, 1988, p.481.

Dickinson SJ. Agenesis of the descending colon with imperforate anus. Am J Surg 1967; 113: 279.

Donaldson JS, Black CT, Reynold M *et al.* Ultrasound of the distal pouch in infants with imperforate anus. J Pediatr Surg 1989; 24: 465-468.

Dinnick T. Origins and evolution of colostomy. Br J Surg 1934; 22: 142.

Dobbing J, Sands J. Quantitative growth and development of the human brain. Arch Dis Child 1973;48: 757.

Dorairajan T. Anorectal atresia, Anorectal malformation in children, update, Eds. Stephens FD, Smith Ed, Liss, 1988, p.105.

Dorairajan T 1989 personal communication.

Dorairajan T. Colostomy in infancy. 16th Conference of Indian Association of Pediatric Surgeons, 1990.

Dougherty CM, Spencer R. Quoted by Bellinger MF and Duckett JW, 1982.

Dubowitz V, Pearce A. Reciprocal relationship of phosphorylase and oxidative enzymes in skeletal muscles. Nature 1960;185: 701.

Duhamel B. From the mermaid to anal imperforation : The syndrome of caudal regression. Arch Dis Child 1961; 36: 152.

Duthie HL, Watts JM. Contribution of the external anal sphincter to the pressure zone in the anal canal. Gut 1965; 6: 64.

Duthie HL, Dynamics of the Rectum and Anus Clin. Gastroenterol 1975; 4: 467.

Ein SH. Stephens CA. Vaginal construction in children with vaginal agenesis and imperforate anus. J Pediatr Surg 1971; 6: 435-439.

Ein SH. Imperforate anus (anal agenesis) with rectal and sigmoid atresias in a newborn. Pediatr Surg Int 1997; 12: 449-451.

Elshafie M. Congenital short intestine and cystic dilatation of the colon associated with ectopic anus. J Pediatr Surg 1971; 6: 76.

Emblem R , Diseth T Morkrid L *et al.* Anal endosonography and physiology in adolescents with corrected low anorectal anomalies. J Pediatr Surg 1994; 29: 447-51.

Emblem R, Diseth T, Morkrid. Anorectal anomalies : Anorectal manometric function and anal endo-sonography in relation to functional outcome. Pediatr Surg Int 1997; 12: 516-519.

Engel BT, Nikoomanesh P, Schuster MM. Operant conditioning of rectosphincteric responses in the treatment of fecal incontinence. N Eng J Med 1974; 290: 646.

Fitzgerald RJ, Watters K, Bissett WH *et al.* Translevator anal anomalies with cutaneous fistulae deep to the scrotum. J Pediatr Surg 2002; 37: 1326-1329.

Fowler R Jr. Landmarks and legends of the anal canal. Austr NZJ Surg 1957; 27: 1.

Freeman NV, Burge DM, Soar JS *et al.* Anal evoked potentials. Z Kinderchair 1980; 31: 22.

Freeman NV, Bulut M. High anomalies treated by early neonatal operation. J Pediatr Surg 1986; 21: 218-220.

Gangopadhyay AN, Gopal CS, Gupta DK *et al.* Management of pouch colon with anorectal malformation. J Indian Assoc Pediatr Surg 1996; 1: 55-59.

Gangopadhyay AN, Sinha CK, Sahoo SP. Combined rectal atresia and rectal stenosis. Pediatr Surg Int 1997; 12: 605-606.

Gangopadhyay AN, Gopal SC, Mohan V *et al.* Single stage management of all variants of pouch colon in new born. 29th Congress of the Indian Association of Pediatric Surgeons, 2003.

Gans SL, Friedman NB, David JS. Congenital anorectal anomalies : Changing concept in management. Clin Pediatr 1963; 2: 605.

Gans SL. Classification of anorectal anomalies : A critical analysis. J Pediatr Surg 1970; 5: 511-513.

Gans SL, Berci G Advances in endoscopy of infants and children. J Pediatr Surg 1971; 6: 199-234.

Georgeson KE, Inge TH, Albanese CT. Laparoscopically assisted anorectal pull through for high imperforate anus – a new technique. J Pediatr Surg 2000; 35: 927-931.

Goligher JC. Surgery of the anus rectum and colon. 5th Edn, Bailliere Tindall, 1984, p.1, `285.

Golonka NR, Haga LJ, Keating RP *et al.* Routine MRI evaluation of low imperforate anus reveals unexpected high incidence of tethered spinal cord. J Pediatr Surg 2002; 37: 966-969.

Goon HK. Repair of anorectal malformations in the neonatal period. Pediatr Surg Int 1990; 5: 246-249

Gopal CS.Single stage anerectoplasty in newborns. Workshop on Anorectal Malformations in Varanasi, 2001.

Gopal G. Congenital rectovesical fistula with colonic reservoir. Indian J Surg 1978; 40: 447.

Gough MH.Anorectal agenesis with persistence of cloaca. Proc Royal Soc Med 1959; 52: 886.

Graf JL, Strear C, Bratton B *et al.* The antegrade continence enema procedure : A review of the literature. J Pediatr Surg 1998; 33: 1294-1296.

Gross RE. The surgery of infancy and childhood. WB Saunders, 1953, p.348.

Gupta DK, Dave S. Complications following PSARP. Workshop on Anorectal Malformations in Varanasi, 2001.

Gupta DK, Dave S. Management of associated anomalies with anorectal malformations. Workshop on Anorectal Malformations, Varanasi, 2001.

Halimul EM, Adang QM, Kartono D. Rectal atresia treated by modified Duhamel's procedure. Ann Acad Med Surg 1981; 10: 476.

Hamada Y, Sato M, Hioki K. Anal canal duplication in childhood. Pediatr Surg Int 1996; 11: 577-579.

Hamza AF, Soliman HA, Abdel Hay SA *et al.* Total urogenital sinus mobilization in the repair of cloacal anomalies and congenital adrenal hyperplasia. J Pediatr Surg 2001; 36: 1656-1658.

Hasan NU. Personal communication. 1988.

Hassink EAM, Brugman-Boezeman ATM, Robbroeckx LMH *et al.* Parenting children with anorectal malformations : implications and experience. Pediatr Surg Int 1998; 13: 337-383.

Hendren WH. Surgical management of urogenital sinus abnormalities. J Pediatr Surg 1977; 12: 339-357.

Hendren WH. Constipation caused by anterior location of the anus and its surgical correction. J Pediatr Surg 1978; 13: 505.

Hendren WH. Construction of female urethra from vaginal wall and a perineal flap. J Urol 1980; 123: 657.

Hendren WH.Urogenital sinus and anorectal malformations. J Pediatr Surg 1980; 15: 628-641.

Hendren WH. Further experiences in reconstructive surgery for cloacal anomalies. J Pediatr Surg 1982; 17: 695-717.

Hendren WH. Repair of cloacal anomalies – current techniques. J Pediatr Surg 1986; 21: 1159-1176.

Hendren WH. Cloacal malformations: experience with 105 cases. J Pediatr Surg 1992; 27: 890-901.

Hendren WH. Construction of a female urethra using the vaginal wall and a buttock flap : experience with 40 cases. J Pediatr Surg 1998; 33: 180-187

Hiatt RB, Santulli TV. Important factors influencing the treatment of imperforate anus. Dis Colon Rectum 1962; 5: 110.

Holschneider AM. The problem of anorectal continence. Prog Pediatr Surg 1976; 9: 85.

Holschneider AM. Function of the sphincters in anorectal malformations and postoperative evaluation. Anorectal malformations in children, update. Eds. Stephens FD, Smith ED Liss, 1988, p.425.

Hong AR, Croitoru DP, Nguyen LT *et al.* Congenital urethral fistula with normal anus : A report of two cases. J Pediatr Surg 1992; 27: 1278-1280

Hong AR, Acuna MF, Pena A *et al.* Urologic injuries associated with repair of anorectal malformations in male patients. J Pediatr Surg 2002; 37: 339-344.

Hrabovszky Z, Dewan PA. Revision anorectoplasty in the management of anorectal anomalies. Pediatr Surg Int 2002; 18: 4: 269-272.

Husburg B, Lindahl HG, Rintala R *et al.* High and intermediate imperforate anus : results after surgical correction with special respect to internal sphincter function. J Pediatr Surg 1992; 27: 185-189.

Ikawa H, Yokoyama J, Sanbonmatsu T *et al.* The use of computerized tomography to evaluate anorectal anomalies. J Pediatr Surg 1985; 20: 640-644.

Ismail A. Perineal canal: a simple method of repair. Pediatr Surg Int 1994; 9: 603-604.

Ito H, Sano H, Ando S *et al.* Congenital rectovestibular fistula without imperforate anus. Geka (surgery) 1976; 38: 525.

Iwai N, Yanagihoma J, Tokiwa K *et al.* Voluntary anal continence after surgery for anorectal malformations. J Pediatr Surg 1988; 23: 393-397.

Johnson RJ, Palken M, Derick W *et al.* The embryology of high anorectal malformations in the female. Surg Gynec Obst 1972; 135: 759.

Jit I. Prenatal and postnatal structure of the anal canal and development of its sphincters. J Anat Soc India 1974; 23: 37.

Jit I. Creeping epithelium of the human anal canal. Indian J Med Res 1975; 63: 411.

Japan Study Group of anorectal anomalies. J Pediatr Surg 1982; 17: 302-308.

Jones NM. Smilgin-Humphreys, M.Sulivan PB *et al.* Pediatric anal endosonography. Pediatr Surg Int 2003; 19: 703-706.

Kalani BP, Sogani KC. Short colon associated with anorectal agenesis: Treatment by colonorrhaphy. Ann Pediatr Surg 1984; 1: 83.

Kapoor V. Congenital short colon, International conference on incontinence. Munster, 1989.

Karrer FM, Flannery AM, Nelson MD *et al.* Anorectal malformations : Evaluation of associated spinal dysraphic syndromes. J Pediatr Surg 1988; 23: 45-48.

Keibel F, Mall FP. A manual of human embryology. Vol. 2, J B Lippincott Co, London, 1912, p.322.

Keith A. Three demonstration on malformations of the hindend of the body-I : Specimens illustrating malformations of the rectum and anus. Br Med J 1908; 2: 1736.

Keith A. Human embryology and morphology, 1948, 6th Ed., Arnold Co. London, p. 536.

Kelly JH. Cine radiography in anorectal malformations. J Pediatr Surg 1969; 4: 538-546.

Kelly JH. The radiographic anatomy of the normal and abnormal neonatal pelvis. J Pediatr Surg 1969; 4: 432.

Kiely EM, Pena A. Anorectal malformations. Pediatric Surgery. 5th Ed. Vol. 2, Eds. O'Neill JA, Rowe MI, Grosfeld JL *et al.* Mosby – Year Book Inc., 2000, pp.1425-1448.

Kiely EM 2004. Personal communication

Kluth D, Hillen M, Lambrecht W. The principles of normal and abnormal hindgut development. J Pediatr Surg 1995; 30: 1143-1147.

Krasna IH. A simple pursestring suture technique for treatment of colostomy prolapse and intussusception. J Pediatr Surg 1979; 14: 801-802.

Krstic ZD, Lukac M, Lukac R *et al.* Surgical treatment of cloacal anomalies. Pediatr Surg Int 2001; 17: 329-333.

Kubota Y, Shimotake T, Yanagihara J *et al.* Development of anorectal malformations using Etretinate. J Pediatr Surg 1998; 33: 127-129.

Kulshrestha S, Kulshrestha M, Yadav A *et al.* Posterior sagittal approach for repair of rectourethral fistula occurring after perineal surgery for imperforate anus at birth. Pediatr Surg 2000; 35: 1155-1160.

Kulshrestha S, Gangopadhyay AN, Sahoo SP. An unusual variant of rectal atresia with rectovestibular fistula. J Pediatr Surg 1997; 32: 921-2.

Kulshrestha S, Kulshrestha M, Prakash G *et al.* Management of congenital and acquired H type of Anorectal fistulae in girls by anorectal vaginoplasty. J Pediatr Surg 1998; 33: 1224-1228.

Kulshrestha S, Kulshrestha M, Yadav A *et al.* Posterior sagittal approach for repair of rectourethral fistula occurring after perineal surgery for imperforated anus at birth. J Pediatr Surg 2000; 35: 1155-1160.

Kuwashima S, Limura F, Kono T *et al.* Fetal MRI : value and limitations – a review of 55 lesions. Nippon Igaku Hoshasen Gakkai Zasshi 2001; 61: 9: 491-495.

Laberge JM, Bose O, Yazbeck S *et al.* The anterior perineal approach for pullthrough operation in high imperforate anus. J Pediatr Surg 1983; 18: 774-778.

Ladd WE, Gross RE. Congenital malformations of anus and rectum. Am J Surg 1934; 23: 167.

Lal P, Gupta A, Krishna K *et al.* Congenital H-type urethroanal fistula. Pediatr Surg Int 1998; 13: 193-194.

Lambrecht W, Lierse W. The internal sphincter in anorectal malformations : Morphological investigations in neonatal pigs. J Pediatr Surg 1987; 22: 1160-1168.

Langemeijer RATM, Molenaar JC. Continence after posterior sagittal anorectoplasty. J Pediatr Surg 1991; 26: 587-590.

Lawson J. The functional anatomy of the pelvic floor muscles and associated sphincters. Recent advances in Pediatric Surgery. Ed. Wilkinson AW, Churchill, 1969.

Leape LL, Ramenofsky M. Anterior anus: A common cause of constipation in children. J Pediatr Surg 1978; 13: 627-630.

Leditschke JF, Pena A: An unusual cloacal anomaly – late recognition and operative correction. Pediatr Surg Int. 1991; 6: 52-55.

Levitt MA, Patel M, Rodriguez G *et al.* The tethered spinal cord in patients with anorectal malformations. J Pediatr Surg 1997; 32: 462-68.

Levitt MA, Stein DM, Pena A. Rectovestibular fistula with absent vagina a unique anorectal malformation. J Pediatr Surg 1998; 33: 986-990.

Li L, Yan-Xia W, Xia-Na W *et al.* Posterior sagittal approach: Megasigmoid resection and anal reconstruction for severe constipation and fecal incontinence after anoplasty. J Pediatr Surg; 2000; 35: 1058-62.

Louw JH. Congenital abnormalities of the rectum and anus. Current problems in surgery, Year Book Medical, 1965.

Ludman L, Spitz L. Coping strategies of children with faecal incontinence. J Pediatr Surg 1996; 31: 563-567.

Luzzatto C, Zanardo V, Guglielmi M. Imperforate anus with congenital short colon : combined abdominal and posterior sagittal approach. Pediatr Surg Int 1990; 5: 375-376.

Magnus RV. Congenital rectovesical fistula and its associated anomalies. Aust NZJ Surg 1972; 42: 192.

Magnus RV. Urinary abnormalities in children with congenital rectovesical fistula. Aust Pediatr J 1974; 10: 82.

Mahmoud MIS. New transanal approach for surgical correction of perineal canal. Br J Surg 1995; 82: 182-183.

Martins JL, Martins ECS. Anorectal anomaly associated with caudal regression: late evaluation after posterior sagittal anorectoplasty. Pediatr Surg Int 2003; 19: 1-1: 106-108.

Matas R. The surgical treatment of congenital anorectal imperforation. Transactions of the American Surgical Association 1897; 15: 87.

Mathur P, Prabhu K, Jindal D Unusual presentation of pouch colon. J Pediatr Surg 2002; 37: 1351-1353.

McHugh K, Dudley NE, Tam P. Pre-operative MRI of anorectal anomalies in the newborn period. Pediatr Radiol 1995; 25: S33-S36.

Mirza I, Zia-ul-Miraj M. Management of perineal canal anomaly. Pediatr Surg Int 1997; 12: 611-612.

Mishra BN, Narasimhan KL, Chowdhary SK *et al.* Neonatal PSARP versus staged PSARP – A comparative analysis. J Indian Assoc Pediatr Surg 2000; 5: 10-13.

Mitchell ME, Hensle TW, Crooks KK. Urethral reconstruction in the young female. J Pediatr Surg 1982; 17: 687-694.

Mollard P, Marechal JM, Debeaujin M. Surgical treatment of high imperforate anus with definition of the puborectalis sling by an anterior perineal approach. J Pediatr Surg 1978; 13: 499-504.

Mollard P, Souey P, Louis D *et al.* Preservation of infralevator structures in imperforate anus. J Pediatr Surg 1989; 21: 1023-1026.

Moore TC. Advantages of performing the sagittal anoplasty operation for imperforate anus at birth. J Pediatr Surg 1990; 25: 276-277.

Moore TC. Challenges in pediatric surgery. Med Intelligence Unit, pp.1-25, R G Landes Co., Austin, 1994.

Nainan KM, Mitra SK, Pathak IC. Perineal anal transplant in anorectal malformations in female patients. Surg 1975; 77: 697.

Nakayama DK, Templeton JM, Ziegler MM *et al.* Complications of posterior sagittal anorectoplasty. J Pediatr Surg 1986; 21, 488.

Narasimarao KL, Prasad GR, Katariya S *et al.* Prone cross-table lateral view : An alternative to the invertogram in imperforate anus. Am J Radiol 1983; 140: 277.

Narasimarao KL, Yadav K, Mitra SK *et al.* Congenital short colon with imperforate anus (pouch colon-syndrome). Ann Pediatr Surg 1984; 1 : 159.

Narasimarao KL, Chaudhury SR, Samuj R *et al.* Perineal canal – repair by a new surgical technique. Pediatr Surg Int 1993; 8: 449-450

Nievelstein RAJ, Vos A, Valk J *et al.* Magnetic resonance imaging in children with anorectal malformations: Embryologic implications. J Pediatr Surg 2002; 37: 1138-1145.

Ninh TN, Bohn GL. Rectovestibular fistula in South Vietnam. Proceedings of the Pediatric Surgical Congress, Melbourne, 1970.

Nixon HH. Colostomy, a simple technique and observations on indications. Z Kinderchir 1966; 3: 98.

Nixon HH. Congenital deformities of the anorectal region in Surgery of the anus, rectum and colon. 5th Ed., Eds. Goligher JC, Bailliere Tindall. 1984.

Norris WJ, Brophy TW, Brayton D. Imperforate anus : A case series and preliminary report of the one stage abdominoperineal operation. Surg Gynec Obstet 1949; 88: 623.

Oguzkurt P, Tanyel FC, Buyukpamukeu N. Acute scrotum due to epididymo-orchitis associated with vasal anomalies in children with anorectal malformations. J Pediatr Surg 1998; 33: 1834-1836.

Okada A, Kamata S, Imura K, *et al.* Anterior sagittal anorectoplasty for recto and anovestibular fistula. J Pediatr Surg 1992; 27: 85-88.

Olness K, Mcparland FA, Piper J. Biofeedback, a new modality in the management of children with faecal soiling. J Pediatr Surg 1980; 96: 505-508.

Ong NT, Beasley SW. Comparison of clinical methods of assessment of continence after repair of high anorectal anomalies. Pediatr Surg Int 1990; 5: 233-237.

Ong NT, Beasley SW. Long term functional results after perineal surgery for low anorectal anomalies. Pediatr Surg Int 1990; 5: 238-240.

Ong NT, Decampo M, Fowler R Jr. CT in the management of imperforate anus patients following rectoplasty. Pediatr Surg Int 1990; 5: 241-245.

Ong NT, Beasley SW. Long term continence in patients with high and intermediate anorectal anomalies treated by sacroperineal (Stephens) rectoplasty. J Pediatr Surg 1991; 26: 44-48.

Palken M, Johnson RJ, Derrick W *et al.* Clinical aspects of female patients with high anorectal agenesis. Surg Gynec Obstet 1972; 135: 411.

Paidas CN, Morreale RF, Holoski KM *et al.* Septation and differentiation of the embryonic human cloaca. J Pediatr Surg 2000; 34: 877-884.

Partridge J, Gough MH. Congenital abnormalities of the anus and rectum. Br J Surg 1961; 49: 37.

Pathak IC. Evolution of concepts of sphincteric anatomy and surgical procedures in anorectal malformations. J Indian Assoc Pediatr Surg 1997; 2: 1-13.

Pathak IC. Pouch colon syndrome: A changing scenario. Ann Nat Acad Med Sci (India) 1999; 35, 69-81.

Patwardhan N, Kiely EM, Drake DP *et al.* Colostomy for anorectal anomalies : High incidence of complications. J Pediatr Surg 2001; 36: 795-798.

Pellerin D, Fekete C, Yandza T *et al.* Traitement chirurgical definitive en periode neonatale sans derivatione prealable des malformations anorectales hautes – Resultats. Chirurg Pediatr 1986; 27: 274.

Pena A. Posterior sagittal anorectoplasty : International Symposium of Pediatric Surgery in Acapulco, 1980.

Pena A, De Vries PA. Posterior sagittal anorectoplasty – important technical considerations and new applications. J Pediatr Surg 1982; 17: 796-811.

Pena A. Posterior sagittal anorectoplasty as a secondary operation for the treatment of fecal incontinence. J Pediatr Surg 1983; 18: 762-773.

Pena A. Surgical treatment of high imperforate anus. World J Surg 1985; 9: 236.

Pena A. Surgical management of anorectal malformations : A unified concept. Pediatr Surg Int 1988; 3: 82-93.

Pena A, Filmer B, Bonilla E *et al.* Transanorectal approach for the treatment of urogenital sinus : Preliminary report. J Pediatr Surg 1992; 27: 681-685.

Pena A, Behery ME. Megasigmoid : A source of pseudoincontinence in children with repaired anorectal malformations. J Pediatr Surg 1993; 28: 199-203.

Pena A. Total urogenital mobilization – an easier way to repair cloaca. J Pediatr Surg 1997; 32: 263-268.

Pena A, Guardino K, Tovila JM, *et al.* Bowel management for fecal incontinence in patients with anorectal malformations. J Pediatr Surg 1998; 33: 133-137.

Pena A, Kessler O. Posterior Cloaca : A unique defect. J Pediatr Surg 1998; 33: 407-412.

Pena A. Posterior sagittal anorectoplasty : Results in management of 332 cases of anorectal malformations. Pediatr Surg Int 1998; 3: 94-104.

Penington EC, Hutson JM. The absence of lateral fusion in cloacal partition. J Pediatr Surg 2003; 38: 9: 1287-1295.

Potts WJ, Riker WL, Deboer A. Imperforate anus with rectovesical, rectourethral, rectovaginal and rectoperineal fistula. Ann Surg 1954; 140: 381.

Potts WJ. The Surgeon and the child. WB Saunders, 1959.

Powell RW, Sherman JO, Raffensperger JG. Megarectum : A rare complication of imperforate anus repair and its surgical correction by anorectal pullthrough. J Pediatr Surg 1982; 7: 786-795.

Pringle KC, Sato Y, Soper RT. Magnetic resonance imaging as an adjunct to planning an anorectal pullthrough. J Pediatr Surg 1987; 22: 571-574.

Rafensperger JG, Ramenofsky M. The management of a cloaca. J Pediatr Surg 1973; 8: 647-657.

Raghupati RK, Moorthy PK, Rajamani G,et.al Laparoscopically assisted anorectoplasty for high ARM J Indian Assoc Pediatr Surg 2003; 4: 202-207.

Rehbein F.Imperforate anus: Experiences with abdominoperineal and abdomino-sacroperineal pullthrough procedures. J Pediatr Surg 1967; 2: 99.

Rhoads JE, Pipes RL, Randall SP. Simultaneous abdominal and perineal approach in operation for imperforate anus with atresia of the rectum and rectosigmoid. Ann Surg 1948; 127 : 552.

Rintala RJ, Lindahl HG, Louhimo I. Biofeedback conditioning for fecal incontinence in anorectal malformations. Pediatr Surg Int 1988; 3: 418-421.

Rintala RJ. Postoperative internal sphincter function in anorectal malformations. Pediatr Surg Int 1990; 5: 127-130.

Rintala RJ, Lindahl HG, Marttinen E *et al.* Constipation is a major functional complication after internal sphincter-saving posterior sagittal anorectoplasty for high and intermediate anorectal malformations. J Pediatr Surg 1993; 28: 1054-1058.

Rintala RJ, Lindahl HG. Internal sphincter saving PSARP for high and intermediate anorectal malformations : technical considerations. Pediatr Surg Int 1995; 10: 345-9.

Rintala RJ, Lindahl HG. Is normal bowel function possible after repair of intermediate and high anorectal malformations? J Pediatr Surg 1995; 30: 491-9.

Rintala RJ, Mildh L, Lindhal H. H-type anorectal malformations : Incidence and clinical characteristics. J Pediatr Surg 1996; 31: 559-562.

Rintala RJ, Lindahl HG, Rasanen M. Do children with repaired low anorectal malformations have normal bowel function? J Pediatr Surg 1997; 32: 823-6.

Rintala RJ, Lindahl HG. Posterior sagittal anorectoplasty is superior to sacroperineal sacroabdominoperineal pull-through A long term follow-up study in boys with high anorectal anomalies. J Pediatr Surg 1999; 34: 334-337.

Rintala RJ, Lindahl HG. Fecal continence in patients having undergone posterior sagittal anorectoplasty procedure for a high anorectal malformation improves at adolescence, as constipation disappears. J Pediatr Surg 2001; 36: 1218-1221.

Rivosechi M, Lucchetti MC, Zaccana A *et al.* Spinal dysraphic defect by MRI in patients with ARM. J Pediatr Surg 1995; 30: 488-490.

Rizalar R, Demirbilek S, Bernary F *et al.* H-type urethrorectal communication and complete urethral stenosis with unilateral renal agenesis. Eur J Pediatr Surg 1992; 4: 49-50.

Romualdi P. A new technique for surgical treatment of some rectal malformations. Arch Klin Chir 1960; 296 : 371.

Rosen NG, Hong AR, Soffer SZ *et al*. Rectovaginal fistula : A common diagnostic error with significant consequences in girls with anorectal malformations. J Pediatr Surg 2002; 37: 961-965.

Sadler TW Langman's Medical Embryology, 8th Ed., Lippincott Williams & Wilkins Philadelphia 2000

Sai K, Uchino J, Kasai Y. Congenital rectovestibular fistula with a normal anus. J Jap Soc Pediatr Surg 1975; 11: 521.

Santulli TV. Imperforate anus, in Pediatric Surgery. 1st Ed., Benson *et al*, Year Book Publishers, 1962, p.821.

Santulli TV, Schullinger JN, Amoury RA *et al*. Malformations of the anus and rectum. Surg Clin N Am 1965; 45: 1253.

Santulli TV, Schullinger JN, Kiesewetter WB *et al*. Imperforate anus: A survey from the members of the surgical section of the American Academy of Pediatrics. J Pediatr Surg 1971; 5: 484-487.

Sarin YK. Two orifices in the perineum of the girl with imperforate anus, possibility of uterovaginal agenesis associated with rectovestibular fistula. J Pediatr Surg 2002; 37: 1217-1219.

Sarin YK, Sinha A, Gupta A. High anorectal malformation in boys : Need for clarity of definition and management. J Pediatr Surg 2002; 37: 1637-1639.

Saxena N, Bhattacharya N, Katariya S *et al*. Perineal anal transplant in low anorectal anomalies. Surgery 1981; 90: 464.

Scharli AF, Kiesewetter WB. Defecation and continence : Some new concepts. Dis Colon Rectum 1970; 13: 89.

Scharli AF. Anorectal incontinence : Diagnosis and treatment. J Pediatr Surg 1987; 22: 693-701.

Scharli AF Perineal groove 7th Colorectal Club meeting, Rome, 2000.

Schuster SR, Tiele RL. An analysis of ultrasound scanning as a guide in determination of high or low imperforate anus. J Pediatr Surg 1979; 14: 798-800.

Scott JES, Swenson O, Fisher JH. Some comments on the surgical treatment of imperforate anus. Am J Surg 1960; 99: 137.

SenGupta PC Personal communication, 1990.

Sengupta PC. Atypical female intersex. Br J Obstet Gynecol 1992; 99: 689-696.

Senocak ME, Buyukpamuken N. One-stage correction of congenital urethral atresia with urethrorectal communication. Pediatr Surg Int 1990; 5: 221-223.

Shafik A. New concept of the anatomy of the anal sphincter mechanisms and physiology of defecation. Invest Urol 1975; 12: 412.

Shah AA, Kothari MR, Bhattacharjee N, *et al.* Magnetic resonance imaging in anorectal malformations. J Indian Assoc Pediatr Surg; 2001; 6: 4-13.

Shambhogue LKR, Langemeijer RATM, Madern GC, Molenaar JC. Rectoperineal fistula in newborn boys. J Pediatr Surg 1994; 29: 536-537.

Sharma AK, Chaturvedi V, Wakhlu A. Anal agenesis associated with rectal atresia. J Pediatr Surg 1995; 30: 113-114.

Sharma AK, Kothari SK, Menon P, *et al.* Congenital H-type rectourethral fistula. Pediatr Surg Int 2002; 18: 2-3: 193-194.

Singh A, Singh R, Singh A. Short colon malformation with imperforate anus. Acta Ped Scand 1972; 71: 781.

Singh A. Pouch colon, workshop on anorectal malformations. Chandigarh, 1988.

Smith ED. Congenital anomalies of the sacrum. Aust NZJ Surg 1959; 29: 165.

Smith ED. An overview of anorectal anomalies. J Pediatr Surg 1987; 22: 335.

Smith ED, Saeki K. Associated anomalies in Anorectal malformations in children, update, Eds., Stephens FD, Smith ED, Liss, 1988, p.501.

Smith ED, Stephens FD, Holschneider AM *et al.* Operations to improve continence after previous surgery. Anorectal malformations in children, update, Ed., Stephens FD, Smith ED Liss, 1988, p.447.

Spriggs WJ.Congenital occlusion of the gastrointestinal tract.1912. Quoted by Narasimharao *et al*, 1983.

Sripathi V, Anand Kumar D, Lakshmi Devi G. Perineal canal in a male. International Workshop on Anorectal Malformations, Lucknow, 2003.

Stephens FD, Smith ED. Malformations of the anus. Aust NZJ Surg 1953; 23: 9.

Stephens FD. Imperforate rectum: A new surgical technique. Med J Aust 1953; 2: 202.

Stephens FD. Congenital imperforate rectum, rectourethral and rectovaginal fistulas. Aust NZJ Surg 1953; 22 : 161.

Stephens FD. Congenital malformations of the rectum and anus in female children. Aust NZJ Surg 1961; 31: 90.

Stephens FD. The female anus, perineum and vestibule, embryogenesis and deformities. Aust NZJ Obstet Gynaecol 1968; 8: 55.

Stephens FD, Smith ED. Anorectal malformations in children. Year Book Medical Publishers, 1971.

Stephens FD, Donnellan WL. H type urethra-anal fistula. J Pediatr Surg 1977; 12: 95-102.

Stephens FD. Normal and abnormal embryology of the cloaca. Congenital malformations of the urinary tract. Praeger, New York, 1983, p.3.

Stephens FD, Smith ED. Classification, identification and assessment of surgical treatment of anorectal anomalies : A report of a workshop. Ped Surg Int 1986; 1: 200-205.

Stephens FD, Smith ED. Anorectal malformations in children, update, Liss. 1988.

Stone HH, Wilkinson AW. Experimental production of rectal stenosis and atresia in the rabbit. J Pediatr Surg 1983; 18: 89-90.

Suruga K. Postoperative disorder of anorectal function are quality of life. 15th Congress of Asian Association of Pediatric Surgeons, 1998

Swenson O, Donnellan WL. Preservation of the puborectalis slihg in imperforate anus repair. Surg Clin N Am 1967; 47; 173.

Swenson O, Donellan WL. In : Pediatric Surgery, 3rd Ed., Meredith & Co., 1969, pp.948-962.

Tam PK, Chan FL, Saing H. Direct sagittal CT scan : A new diagnostic approach for surgical neonates. J Pediatr Surg 1987; 22 : 397-400.

Templeton JM, Ditescheim JA. High imperforate anus : Quantitative results of longterm fecfal continence. J Pediatr Surg 1985; 20 : 645-652.

Thomas GG, Molenaar JC. Management of a fistula between the rectum and the lower urinary tract. J Pediatr Surg 1979; 14: 65-73.

Trusler GA, Mastel AL, Stephens CA. Colon malformation with imperforate anus. Surgery 1959; 45: 320.

Tsuchida Y, Saito S, Honna T *et al*. Double termination of the alimentary tract in females : A report of 12 cases and a literature review. J Pediatr Surg 1984; 19: 292.

Tsugawa C, Nishijima E, Muraji T *et al*. Surgical repair of rectovestibular fistula with normal anus. J Pediatr Surg 1999; 34: 1703-5.

Tsugawa C, Hisano K, Nishijima E *et al.* Posterior sagittal anorectoplasty for failed imperforate anus surgery. J Pediatr Surg 2000; 35: 1625-1629.

Upadhyaya P. Midanal sphincteric malformation : Cause of constipation in anterior perineal anus. J Pediatr Surg 1984; 19: 183.

Upadhyaya P. Pouch colon syndrome : A high anorectal anomaly. Ann Pediatr Surg 1984; 1: 155.

Vaezzadeh K, Gerami K, Kalani P *et al.* Congenital short colon with imperforate anus : A definitive surgical care. J Pediatr Surg 1982; 17: 198-200.

Vaidya A, Adyanthaya K, Patil V. Total urogenital mobilisation for the correction of an unusual anorectal malformation. 29th Congress of the Indian Association of Pediatric Surgeons, 2003.

Van Der Putte SCJ, Neeteson FA. The normal development of the anorectum in the pig. Acta Morphol Neerl Scand 1983; 21: 107.

Van Der Putte SCJ, Neeteson FA. The pathogenesis of the hereditary congenital malformations of the anorectum in the pig. Acta Morphol Neerl Scand 1984; 33: 17.

Van Der Putte SCJ. Normal and abnormal development of the anorectum. J Pediatr Surg 1986; 21: 434.

Varma KK. Long term continence after surgery for anorectal malformations. Pediatr Surg Int 1991; 6: 32-35.

Wakhlu A, Tandon RK, Kalra R. Short colon associated with anorectal malformations. Indian J Surg 1982; 44: 621.

Wakhlu A, Pandey A, Tamdon RK *et al.* Coloplasty for congenital short colon. J Pediatr Surg 1996; 31: 344-48

Wakhlu A, Pandey A, Prasad A *et al.* Anterior sagittal anorectoplasty for anorectal malformations and perineal trauma in the female children. J Pediatr Surg 1996; 31: 1236-1240.

Wakhlu A, Pandey A, Prasad A, Kureel SN *et al.* Perineal canal. Pediatr Surg Int 1997; 12: 283-285.

Wakhlu A, Wakhlu AK. Anterior sagittal anorectoplasty. J Indian Assoc Pediatr Surg 2004; 9: 74-79.

Wangensteen OH, Rice CO. Imperforate anus. Ann Surg 1930; 92: 77.

Wardhan H, Gangopadhyay AN, Singhal GD *et al.* Imperforate anus with congenital short colon (pouch colon syndrome). Pediatr Surg Int 1990; 5: 124-126.

Webster R. Historical review, In : Anorectal malformations in Children. Eds. Stephens FD, Smith ED, Year Book Medical, 1971, p.1

White JJ, Haller JA, Scott Jr *et al.* N type anorectal malformations. J Pediatr Surg 1978; 13: 631-637.

Wilcox DT, Kiely EM. The Malone (Ante grade colonic enema) procedure; early experience. J Pediatr Surg 1998; 33: 204-206.

Wilkins S, Pena A. The role of colostomy in the management of anorectal malformations. Pediatr Surg Int 1988; 3: 105-109.

Wilkinson AW. Congenital anomalies of the anus and rectum. Arch Dis Child 1972; 47: 960.

Williams DI, Nixon HH. Agenesis of the sacrum. Surg Gynec Obst 1957; 105: 84.

Williams PL Gray's Anatomy 38th Ed., Churchill-Livingdtone, 1996.

Willital GR. Advances in the diagnosis of anal and rectal atresia by ultrasonic echo examination. J Pediatr Surg 1971; 6: 454.

Wilson PM. Anchoring mechanisms of the anorectal region. S Afr Med J 1967; 41: 1127.

Yamataka A, Segawa O, Yoshida R *et al.* Laparoscopic muscle electrostimulation during laparoscopy assisted anorectal pull-through for high imperforate anus. J Pediatr Surg 2001; 36: 1659-61

Yeung CK, Kiely EM. Low anorectal anomalies: a critical appraisal. Pediatr Surg Int 1991; 6: 333-335.

Yeung personal communication 2001.

Yntema CC, Hammond WS. Origin of intrinsic ganglia of trunk viscera from vagal neural crest in chick embryo. J Comp Neurol 1954; 101: 515.

Yuejie WU, Rong DU, Guie Z *et al.* Association of imperforate anus with short colon. J Pediatr Surg 1990; 25: 282-284.

Zaidi ZH. Colostomy without survival in infant with no colon or rectum beyond the ascending colon. Am J Dis Child 1959; 98: 385.

Zhang J. Acquired rectovestibular fistula. Chinese J Pediatr Surg 1984; 5: 35.

INDEX